The Science of the Brain

Function, Dysfunction and Disease

The Science of the Brain

Function, Dysfunction and Disease

Ari Rappoport
The Hebrew University of Jerusalem
Jerusalem, Israel

ELSEVIER

ACADEMIC PRESS
An imprint of Elsevier

Academic Press is an imprint of Elsevier
125 London Wall, London EC2Y 5AS, United Kingdom
525 B Street, Suite 1650, San Diego, CA 92101, United States
50 Hampshire Street, 5th Floor, Cambridge, MA 02139, United States

ISBN: 978-0-443-45008-2

For information on all Academic Press publications
visit our website at https://www.elsevier.com/books-and-journals

Publisher: Megan Ball
Acquisitions Editor: Joslyn Chaiprasert-Paguio
Editorial Project Manager: Pat Gonzalez
Production Project Manager: Punithavathy Govindaradjane
Cover Designer: Mark Rogers

Typeset by VTeX

Contents

Foreword

Ari Rappoport has produced an extraordinary work of scholarship, likely unique in the modern era. He immersed himself for nearly two decades in the vast literature on the brain, studying hundreds of thousands of papers, and winnowing tens of thousands of particular significance. He discovered logical threads through the mass of information, pertinent to basic brain function and to many brain disorders and diseases. He recorded his discoveries in meticulously expounded and referenced essays, which were never published. Now for the first time, his entire oeuvre is available to the scientific and general public.

Rappoport presents his discoveries in the form of theories, theories of causes and theories for treatments of disorders and diseases. Like all theories, they represent targets for testing through research and clinical investigation. Like all theories, their value lies in the testing they stimulate, as well as in their validation. And like all theories, they face the ultimate test, the test of time.

Regardless of the outcome of testing, the essays will be of value to readers for their comprehensive nature and their inherent interest. The essays are authoritative reviews, organized around thematic ideas. It may be off-putting to authorities in the relevant fields that the author is not himself a recognized authority. As a computer scientist with no formal medical or related training, he nevertheless became an expert through years of intensive study, and through great analytical ability and critical acumen.

Reviews of important topics are common. There are many on all the subjects in this book. What is uncommon is the grounding in an overarching theory, Rappoport's general theory of brain plasticity, and going beyond theory to proposals for treatment of disease. The book is an invitation to clinicians to address extraordinary challenges in very specific ways. Regardless of the validity of the theories, any success in alleviating debilitating conditions will make it all worthwhile.

Roger Kornberg
Winzer Professor in Medicine
Stanford University School of Medicine
Nobel Laureate (2006)

The science of the brain

1 Contribution of this book

This book presents novel complete theories for almost all important brain disorders. It covers autism spectrum disorder (ASD), schizophrenia (SZ), attention-deficit hyperactivity disorder (ADHD), obsessive-compulsive disorder (OCD), anorexia and bulimia, major depressive disorder (depression (MDD)) and bipolar disorder, multiple sclerosis, parkinson's disease (PD), alzheimer's disease (AD), migraine and cluster headache, amyotrophic lateral sclerosis (ALS), and frontotemporal dementia (FTD). These are the top mysteries of psychiatry and neurology.

At present, practically nothing is known about what causes these disorders. The chance discovery of drugs (mainly serotonergic) that are effective at reducing some MDD and SZ symptoms has led to serotonin (SER)-based theories of these disorders. However, nobody has managed to show a convincing SER problem in MDD and SZ patients [1]. Likewise, amyloid beta is blamed for AD, but its causal role is highly controversial [2]. The degeneration of dopamine neurons is known to induce the movement symptoms of PD, but it is not known what causes this degeneration.

Thus, psychiatry and a large part of neurology do not have a solid scientific basis at present. This book provides such a basis, and is the first to do so.

Nature of theories. The chapters of this book are not "reviews". They present theories, i.e., a new synthesis. My theories are all 'complete', in the sense that they describe the etiology (core cause) of the disease (often accompanied by the identity of the 'bad' protein), symptoms (a mechanistic description), pathophysiology (e.g., abeta aggregation), risk factors, and protective factors. In many cases, they imply improved ways of treating the disease.

The fact that a theory is complete does not mean that it is correct. Being complete is one of the minimal strong requirements from a theory. However, in the present case, each theory is supported by a variety of previously published empirical research results (see the Methodology section). In most cases, this support is already overwhelming (e.g. SZ). In some cases (e.g., in OCD), additional support should be sought.

Naturally, science cannot prove theories, only refute them. But when the bulk of the theory is based on significant empirical findings, the burden of refutation passes to the other side. So my theories are complete, and I firmly believe that most are correct and ready to pass the refutation challenges ahead.

2 History

I am an Associate Professor at the Hebrew University of Jerusalem, having joined the Computer Science faculty in 1992. The first 8 years of my research were done in the area of geometric modeling and computer graphics. From 2002, I switched to natural language processing (NLP) and machine learning.

My NLP interest has always been from a cognitive perspective. In 2010, I started reading about the brain, hoping to find insights as to how it implements language. I haven't found any. In fact, I found that although a lot is known about the small components (neurons, connections, ion channels, receptors, etc), and a lot is known about the phenotypic behavior that the brain drives, extremely little is known about the level that joins them, the systems levels.

In 2017, I wrote a very long paper presenting a complete theory of how the brain works. Almost nobody has understood it (they were right, it was not so accessible). After writing a few more small papers (on basal ganglia paths and sleep), I focused on brain disorders and diseases.

Between 2017-2024 I completed developing and writing papers presenting complete theories of most of the important brain disorders/diseases and for brain function.

3 Methodology

To tackle the important brain disorders, I prepared a list of the important disorders/diseases, based on textbooks. When addressing a disorder/disease, I first passed over all of the salient literature describing them. I listed what is truly known about the disease, where by "truly known" I mean that it is backed up by hundreds of papers written over decades by dozens of research groups.

Once I had this data, I formulated an initial hypothesis as to the core cause of the disorder. In most cases, this was easy. For example, anorexia nervosa is characterized by patients not eating even though their body needs additional food. A natural account for this is the activation of receptors whose role is to suppress food intake, such as 5-HT2c (SER2c) and CRH2. This type of biological explanation sidesteps the "mental" issues of the phenomenon, viewing it as a biological phenomenon instead. In the case of anorexia, CRH2 recruitment of gut SER also explains nausea and purging behaviors.

The next step was to find supportive evidence. This was also not difficult, since people have published millions of papers on many different aspects of disorders, and it is natural to expect that these papers would cover a lot already. Invariably, in over 98% of the cases, it took from one minute to one hour to find substantial evidence supporting a hypothesis.

Thus, a major difference from the mode of work of conventional researchers is that they would have devised new experiments to refute the hypothesized direction. I worked differently. I based my hypotheses only on validated data, and kept tweaking and refining it according to established facts. I would form a hypothesis, look in Google Scholar, and find experiments that people have already done years ago that validate my hypothesis. Overall, I browsed hundreds of thousands of papers, thorough reading about 45,000.

In other words, I used the available literature to arrange the theory as a forest rather than a huge number of independent trees.

During the course of this work, it was common to discover that one or some of the agents (molecules) I found were thought to be the cause for the disease. However, the logic was always of the kind "this agent accumulates, and this accumulation is what causes the disease" (amyloid beta in Alzheimer's, alpha-synuclein in Parkinson's, TDP43 in ALS, etc). This is an erroneous approach, because an agent accumulates (aggregates) whenever the brain recruits it to combat something. Blaming the agent is like blaming the firefighters.

To refine my understanding, I had to develop, in almost every case, a theory for the physiological role of the agent. Once I knew what it is supposed to be doing at health, I could phrase a hypothesis about what goes wrong in the disease. So for example, I developed a theory in which amyloid beta's normal role (in health) is to stabilize synapses after the initial 15 minutes of short-term memory. This is a crucial role, and without it, there would be no short term memory. Abeta needs cholesterol in order to initiate this role, so the problem in Alzheimer's should be lack of plasma membrane cholesterol, not direct accumulation of abeta. Lack of membrane cholesterol is consistent with the increased danger associated with the ApoE4 allele, which combines another established body of evidence for AD.

Summary. My methodology consisted of gathering the salient fact of a disease, formulating the physiological roles of the agents involved (their role in health), analyzing what could go wrong to yield the symptoms, coming up with hypotheses as to the core cause of the disease, and finding existing supporting evidence.

4 Overview of results

Here I highlight some of the key breakthroughs that have allowed me to come up with novel solutions to these major problems.

Autism. My theory states that ASD is caused by CRH-mediated stress in the months after birth. Normally, at this time, there is a process called "minipuberty" in which gonadal steroids are released in very large quantities (especially in males), to ensure the maturation of the brain and various paths. In ASD, due to CRH, what is excessively released are adrenal, not gonadal steroids. Adrenal steroids are triggered by ACTH, and their main effect is via membrane receptors. This impairs the organizational function of gonadal steroids. In addition, CRH, instead of acting on the CRH2 receptor to support glucose uptake and maturation (e.g., of vision), acts as a prolonged duration stress ligand, and opposes oxytocin signaling, which is essential for the learning of sociality. These insights allowed me to explain both the symptoms and pathology of ASD, and to propose biomarkers and treatment.

Schizophrenia (SZ). My theory states that SZ is caused by hyperactivity of calcium-independent phospholipase A2 (iPLA2), which recruits endocannabinoids (mainly anandamide (AEA)). AEA disconnects neurons from the neural network, and increases their intrinsic excitability. This yields a state in which neurons are active without being controlled by others. The theory then shows that psychosis (positive symptoms) and negative, mood, and cognitive symptoms all result from this state. Moreover, reducing the activity of iPLA2 should improve patient's state.

ADHD. My theory states that in the prototypical case, ADHD results from the brain trying to maintain somewhat higher glucose levels than normal. It does this by opening KATP channels sooner than normal, which increases cellular excitability and results in cells firing continuously without control, manifesting in the ADHD symptoms. The perfect drug treatment for ADHD already exists: sulfonylureas close KATP channels and have been used for treating people with diabetes safely for dozens of years.

OCD. My theory states that OCD involves two phenomena. First, hyperactive CRH provides the "stress" component. Second, in prefrontal cortex, CRH increases cAMP to activate HCN channels, which trigger repeated activation of pyramidal neurons. Patients cannot stop this hyperactivation, explaining unstoppable obsessions. Thus, the disorder has a biological explanation, and does not require a psyhchiatric one. Fortunately, there is an approved drug (guanfacine), an adrenergic receptor 2a2 agonist, used for treating ADHD, which is known to reduce the activation of prefrontal HCN channels.

Anorexia and Bulimia. My theory states that anorexia nervosa is caused by hyperactivity of the CRH2 receptor, whose normal role is to suppress eating. Bulimia is caused by hyperactivity of the CRH1 receptor, whose role is to promote eating. CRH2 is present in the gut and promotes serotonin to induce a feeling of nausea. Patient behavior does not stem from "mental" reasons, but from physiological biological signals.

Depression and Bipolar Disorder. My theory states that depression occurs when the person faces a problem they cannot resolve in a timely manner. In this case, my view is that one of the basic survival responses are made (charge/fight, flight, freeze). A specific contribution of the chapter is the insight that survival responses are promoted by opioids (e.g., beta-endorphin promotes charge of prey). The response that causes depression is "disengage" (give up, withdraw), which is triggered by the opioid dynorphin. DYN binds its receptor KOR, enters the cell, and continues signaling. As long as it promotes signaling, the response viewed from the outside as "depression" continues. Bipolar disorder occurs when KOR is desensitized due to overuse, and does not restrain the activity of norepinephrine and dopamine neurons, which cause the bipolar symptoms. Some substance abuse symptoms have the same account.

Parkinson's Disease. My theory states that the core cause of PD is an overabundance of mucin-degrading bacteria (mainly akkermansia muciniphila) in the gut. This pushes relatively too much galactose into the circulation, coupled with too little glucose. Galactose yields higher oxidative stress and less glycolysis than glucose, with reduced cellular protection by glutathione, and this eventually "burns" the susceptible cells. Dopamine and norepinephrine cells are the most vulnerable, as attested by the fact that they are the only ones that express neuromelanin, whose role is to protect cells from iron toxicity (ferroptosis).

Alzheimer's Disease. My theory states that AD is cause by reduced presence of lipid rafts on the cells membrane. LRs need cholesterol, so the main technical problem is reduced transfer of cholesterol from astrocytes into neurons, and reduced intracellular trafficking of cholesterol. To develop the AD theory, I developed a complete and novel theory of brain plasticity. The healthy role of amyloid precursor protein is to support cholesterol signaling during plasticity. Its alpha cleavage occurs during the first phase of plasticity, when candidates for new synapses are generated. Its beta cleavage, which produces amyloid beta (abeta), occurs during the second phase, when winners are enhanced and losers are removed. Since cholesterol terminates abeta's action, and since cholesterol is deficient, abeta accumulates outside cells, and tau, which maintains lipid rafts at the membrane as part of its cytoskeleton role, accumulates intracellularly.

Multiple Sclerosis. My theory states (like other modern theories) that MS is caused by Epstein-Barr Virus (EBV), which modifies the behavior of B cells. What my theory adds is a mechanistic account of how this yields the disease pathology. Activated B cells release TNF, which acts on ceramide to break down existing myelin sheets.

ALS/Frontotemporal Dementia. My theory states that ALS and a major form of FTD are caused by hyperactive calcium channels, where the culprit protein is most likely the a2d subunit. This yields calcium toxicity in many types of cells, including at the neuromuscular junction and pancreatic beta cells whose role is to release insulin. At some point, beta cells are damaged to the extent that they cannot respond to glucose by releasing sufficient insulin, which causes all insulin targets, mainly motor-related neurons, to collapse. Luckily, insulin treatment should normalize this situation and improve patient state.

Migraine and Cluster Headache. My theory states that migraine is caused by desensitization of the sympathetic nervous system (SNS), mainly its norepinephrine branch that acts upon baroreceptors (BRRs). This induces a state where BRRs cannot respond to increased blood pressure, which triggers the release of pain-conveying agents such a CGRP. Cluster headache is similar, this time with CO2 sensors.

The Brain's Adaptive Response Process. This chapter is different from the other chapters, which describe disorders. This chapter presents an account of how the healthy brain works to produce its responses. There are two stages: response selection (its content), and allowing the selected response to execute.

Response selection uses a four-stage process that includes (i) sensory inputs, (ii) generation of response candidates, (iii) competition, and (iv) final selection. What is beautiful here is that each stage uses different neural networks (L4, L2/3, inhibitory interneurons, L5).

Regarding post-selection execution, virtually all subcortical circuits are arranged in an "Allow, Restrain, Amplify, Respond (ARAR)" architecture that is used to allow the execution of the winning response. For example, the main such circuits for goal-directed responses are in the basal ganglia, where D1 (D2)-expressing medium spiny neurons activate during Allow, GPi (GPe) neurons are tonically active to restrain responses as long as they are not allowed, the thalamus and subthalamic nucleus Amplify the selected response, and motor circuits in cortex and subcortex execute the response. (Note that in this analysis, the role of the D2 path is not to suppress movement, as is commonly thought, but to allow learned movements.) There are also ARAR circuits rooted at the amygdala, habenula, hippocampus, superior colliculus, and cerebellum.

The roles of L5b and L5a are to support learned and novel execution, respectively. When activated, they innervate the representations of the sensory goals of the action taking place, and when these goals are met, the action is stopped and the next action in the sequence is selected (mainly according to higher level needs and sensory inputs) and starts. During action observation, this process generates what is known as predictions. Thus, goals and predictions are two terms describing the same phenomenon (as well as efference copy).

These processes can almost trivially explain how language works in the brain, and various other important phenomena (e.g., the difference between execution and imagery, emotion, consciousness, etc).

Sleep. In the theory presented here, the main driver for sleep is the need to restore normal homeostasis, with an emphasis on extruding cytosolic and mitochondria calcium into the endoplasmic reticulum (ER) and the extracellular environment. Calcium ER deficiency leads to the unfolded protein response, which has two arms, one of which leads to apoptosis. Sleep prevents the triggering of this arm, and allows the first arm to complete protein synthesis (translation). Since translation occurs after the cell has produced new synapses following execution, sleep is essential for both preventing cell (or organelle) death and for completing plasticity processes (i.e., memory).

While this explanation of the pressure for sleep has some overlap with existing accounts, my account of two other major imoprtant questions of sleep, NREMS vs. REMS, and the nature of dreams, is completely novel. The coordinated neural firing during non-REM sleep normalizes ions concentrations for most of the brain's neurons at the same time. REM sleep is needed in order to restore acetylcholine neurons, whose role is to promote focused execution paths during wake, hence they cannot be restored with other neurons (they would oppose their simultaneous firing).

Dreams occur when the neurons participating in wake focused execution paths are active during sleep. They involve a sense of reality because they use precisely the same neurons that are involved in reality perception. The content of dreams is determined by the neurons that show large calcium deficiency, which is why we dream of things that have some similarity to wake events. However, the order of the "story" is not the same as in wake, which is why dreams are in most cases unrealistic. The chapter also explains how anesthesia works by using various mechanisms used during sleep.

5 Conclusion

This book is the first to provide a scientific foundation for psychiatry and for much of neurology. It would have been easier to do this without having been diagnosed with an aggressive form of cancer (small cell lung cancer) before finishing, but I think that I have managed to complete the text satisfactorily. Hopefully, future generations will take interest, and medications based on my theories will be developed to help patients.

References

[1] J. Moncrieff, R.E. Cooper, T. Stockmann, S. Amendola, M.P. Hengartner, M.A. Horowitz, The serotonin theory of depression: a systematic umbrella review of the evidence, Molecular Psychiatry 28 (8) (2023) 3243–3256.

[2] G.P. Morris, I.A. Clark, B. Vissel, Questions concerning the role of amyloid-β in the definition, aetiology and diagnosis of Alzheimer's disease, Acta Neuropathologica 136 (5) (2018) 663–689.

Acknowledgements

I am deeply grateful to Yoav Lorch and Prof. Roger Kornberg, whose support and belief in my work have made all the difference. Their open-mindedness and readiness to take action are not only impressive but also truly heartwarming. I would also like to extend my gratitude to Yair Safrai for his invaluable help along the way.

Special thanks to Nimrod Rappoport (PhD) and Naama Rappoport (MD), who generously took the time to review some of the chapters and engage in deep, thought-provoking discussions on various biological matters. Their insights have considerably enriched this work.

I am also grateful to Profs. Omri Abend and Roi Reichart, as well as Effi Levi, for their technical support, but even more so for their friendship, which has been a source of encouragement throughout this journey.

To the incredible oncology staff at Shaare Zedek Hospital in Jerusalem, and Prof. Iris Barshack from Sheba Hospital – thank you for fighting for my life with unwavering dedication, empathy, and professionalism. I owe you more than words can express.

And finally, to my wife, Lana, my children, Naama, Nimrod, Nitay, Noga, and Noi, and my sister Galit – you have been my greatest source of strength. Your love, patience, and constant encouragement have lifted me up even in the hardest moments. You have kept my motivation high and reminded me why I do what I do. This journey would not have been possible without you.

Chapter 1

A CRH2-ACTH theory of autism spectrum disorder

1.1 Introduction

Autism spectrum disorder (ASD) is a developmental disorder defined by impaired social communication and restricted, repetitive behaviors [1,2]. The average global prevalence of ASD is around 1%, higher in high-income countries [1]. Prevalence in 8 year olds in the US in 2020 was reported to be much higher, approximately 4% of boys and 1% of girls [3].

Despite the high public profile of ASD, the extreme burden it puts on patients and caregivers, and extensive research efforts (over 77K/2.2M papers in pubmed/Google Scholar), there is currently no theory of ASD, no early biomarkers, and no preventive treatment. Post-diagnosis treatment is only behavioral (no pharmaceutical treatment), and its efficacy is limited.

Here I present a **CRH theory of ASD (T*ASD)**. T*ASD is the first complete theory of ASD, explaining its etiology, symptoms, pathophysiology, and treatment. The theory is supported by substantial evidence, and points to novel very early screening and treatment procedures.

Theory overview. According to T*ASD, the core cause of ASD is pre-, peri- or postnatal stress that induces excessive postnatal corticotropin-releasing hormone (CRH) release. The main trigger is a stress-inducing state, but the tendency for excessive stress-induced CRH can be heritable. Excessive release can start prenatally, but the ASD symptoms are mainly due to its postnatal effects. The damage is done during the first year of life, mainly at 0-9 months.

Excessive postnatal CRH impairs normal brain development. This happens via two arms, urocortins and steroids (STRDs). The common aspect of the two arms is prolonged stress-associated signaling at the expense of long-term plasticity signaling.

Urocortins (UCNs) are members of the CRH peptide family, which bind CRH receptor 2 (CRH2). UCNs are released in high glucose states, and are crucial for the utilization of glucose for growth (protein synthesis). In ASD, the excessive CRH yields prolonged binding of CRH2 by CRH instead of UCNs, which impairs the long-term growth effects of CRH2 signaling.

In the second damage arm, excessive CRH induces excessive ACTH, which (in addition to inducing cortisol) is the main inducer of adrenal dehydroepiandrosterone (DHEA), a precursor of testosterone and estrogen. STRDs

The Science of the Brain. https://doi.org/10.1016/B978-0-44-345008-2.00007-2

act via nuclear receptors to support long-term plasticity (differentiation, protein synthesis). However, they also support the initial stages of plasticity via membrane receptors. These two paths are in mutual opposition. DHEA supports rapid signaling, and its excess in ASD impairs the long-term plasticity aspects of gonadal STRDs.

The UCN and STRD arms can explain all of the major ASD symptoms and properties. Impaired social interaction, increased sensory sensitivity (including aversion to touch), impaired eye gaze, and early motor impairment are a consequence of the high CRH2/UCN expression in social, low-level sensory, eye control, and motor brain areas. Impaired social interaction and touch aversion are also explained by the suppression of oxytocin (OXT), an agent essential for social development and pleasant touch, by testosterone and CRH. Repetitive stereotypies and self-injurious behavior such as scratching are directly stimulated by CRH and ACTH.

Limited interests and aversion to novelty are present in ASD because novelty induces CRH release, which people with ASD seek to minimize. These behaviors are a form of self-treatment.

Males are more vulnerable to ASD for at least three partially overlapping reasons. First, estrogen directly supports glucose metabolism and protein synthesis. Second, males need postnatal STRD-mediated plasticity more than females do, as attested by higher release during minipuberty. Third, estrogen stimulates the release of OXT, while testosterone opposes it.

Evidence supporting T*ASD includes direct evidence for increased CRH and ACTH and their effects (e.g., on the sympathetic nervous system and mast cells), and data related to anatomical growth, growth pathways, STRDs, OXT, food intake patterns, comorbidities, and sexual characteristics.

Blood and urine tests for the agents involved in the impaired paths (CRH, ACTH, DHEA etc) during the first postnatal months, and adrenal imaging, can serve for very early identification. There are various possible preventive treatments, probably the most promising being transdermal DHT patches, which reduce CRH and ACTH release.

The paper details the theory, its supporting evidence, and possible treatments.

1.2 Theory

The core cause of ASD is pre-, peri- or postnatal stress that induces excessive postnatal CRH release. The stress event itself can be minor and/or chronic, with the response enhanced by a tendency for increased release. A large part of the genome supports stress sensing and responses, so such a tendency can involve a large number of small genetic and epigenetic changes. The excessive response can start prenatally, but the ASD symptoms are mainly due to damage done during the first postnatal year (say, 0 to 9 months). The excessive stress responses usually subside after the first year to normal or only slightly increased levels, but their effects persist. Thus, fundamentally, ASD is an 'injury' type disorder.

Excessive postnatal CRH impairs normal brain development via two arms, UCNs and STRDs. The two arms share a common aspect, prolonged stress-associated signaling of an agent at the expense of its long-term plasticity signaling.

1.2.1 Urocortins (UCNs)

The first damage arm involves **urocortins (UCNs)**, members of the CRH peptide family [4,5]. CRH acts on two receptors, CRH1 and CRH2, with higher affinity for CRH1. UCN1 binds these two receptors as well, while UCN2 and UCN3 bind only CRH2. The two receptors are G protein-coupled receptors that mainly bind Gs to induce cAMP, but also bind Gi/o and Gq.

The role of CRH1 is to trigger responses to metabolic deficiency (hypo) stress states, including hypoglycemia (hypog), cold, and hypoxia. It triggers the hypothalamus (hthal)-pituitary-adrenal (HPA) stress axis to yield ACTH and cortisol release, stimulates the counter-regulatory responses (CRRs) to hypog via the sympathetic nervous system (SNS), acts in the hthal to increase food intake, and promotes general neural excitability.

Regarding CRH2, at present there is no coherent view of its action, besides a general opposition to some of the effects of CRH1 [4,5]. T*ASD provides a novel coherent account, distinguishing between CRH2 binding by UCNs (**U-CRH2**) and by CRH (**C-CRH2**).

T*ASD presents a new theory of U-CRH2, whereby its role is to **trigger responses to metabolic excess (hyper) states**, mainly hyperglycemia (**hyperg**), and also heat. In support of this theory, we note that UCNs are released in unstressful situations in response to high meal-induced glucose [6–8], and that U-CRH2 supports glucose uptake by tissues, insulin release, and glucose utilization for growth (protein synthesis, differentiation) [9–18]. U-CRH2 opposes CRRs [19], and suppresses appetite and food intake [4].

Due to the low CRH affinity to CRH2, **C-CRH2 is activated in prolonged and/or high stress situations**. While U-CRH2 induces quick CRH2 endocytosis and recycling back to the plasma membrane [20], C-CRH2 delays endocytosis [20], opposes glucose uptake and insulin signaling [20], and promotes prolonged cAMP production [10]. As a result, **C-CRH2 opposes the growth effects of UCN signaling**.

In ASD, chronic CRH release yields chronic postnatal C-CRH2. This reduces both U-CRH2 binding (because CRH competes with UCNs for CRH2 binding) and U-CRH2 signaling, impairing the learning of all that should be learned during these crucial months. Chronic CRH may also involve chronic activation and desensitization of CRH1.

UCNs are crucial for the development of areas showing CRH2 expression and UCN release. These include the amygdala, BNST, lateral septum, visual cortex, the Edinger-Westphal (EW) nucleus, hypothalamus, auditory cortex, olfactory and touch circuits, motor circuits, and prefrontal cortex (PFC). These areas are those that support low-level sensory inputs (olfaction, vision, audition, touch), sexual and social development, executive function, and regulation of metabolism.

UCNs are also expressed in non-brain tissue, and there are indeed widespread general health problems in ASD [21]. However, the brain is more sensitive to UCN impairment, because in non-brain tissue glucose-induced growth is strongly supported by insulin. In the brain, insulin mainly acts on motor pathways.

1.2.2 Steroids (STRDs)

The second damage arm in ASD involves **sex steroids (STRDs)**. Excessive CRH induces excessive ACTH, which is known as the inducer of adrenal glucocorticoid (GC, cortisol in humans) release. However, **ACTH is also the main inducer of adrenal dehydroepiandrosterone (DHEA)** [22], the precursor of testosterone and estrogen. At the same time, high CRH reduces GSTRDs via CRH2 [23].

All steroids, including gonadal STRDs and GC, are known to act via nuclear receptors to support long-term plasticity. However, they also support the initial stages of plasticity via membrane receptors that induce rapid intracellular signaling [24]. These two paths oppose each other, because the Ca^{2+}, cAMP and MAPK signaling activated during rapid initial responses interfere with the safe DNA access needed for long-term plasticity. DHEA generally supports rapid signaling, as shown by its direct effects on Ca^{2+} [25] and by its mutual opposition with GC [25–27]. Thus, DHEA and adrenal steroids (ASTRDs) generally oppose the long-term plasticity aspects of gonadal steroids (GSTRDs).

During the first 1-6 months after birth, human babies undergo **minipuberty**, very high GSTRD release, indicating that GSTRD-mediated plasticity is crucial for early postnatal development. In parallel, the adrenal gland undergoes involution and loses about half of its volume [28,29]. In ASD, these processes are impaired, and **the excessive postnatal ASTRDs impair GSTRD-mediated development**.

1.2.3 Explaining ASD symptoms and properties

The UCN and STRD arms of ASD can explain all of the major ASD symptoms and properties, as follows.

Impaired social interaction is a defining characteristic of ASD, explained in two ways. First, there is high CRH2 expression in the areas that support social development, including the BNST, amygdala, lateral septum, and hypothalamus. This indicates that these areas need U-CRH2 signaling, which is impaired.

The second account is related to **oxytocin (OXT)**. The OXT system is one of the most important systems in early postnatal development, when human babies learn that the company of other humans is a positive thing via its association with food and pleasant touch. The role of OXT as an agent essential for the development of sociality is well accepted [30]. UCN3 greatly enhances OXT-induced accessory olfactory bulb plasticity [31]. During the first few years after birth, three is an almost complete overlap between UCN and OXT expression in the hypothalamus PVH and supraoptic nuclei [32]. OXT is directly inhibited by both testosterone [33] and C-CRH2 [34–36]. These OXT-UCN data further explain the social impairment in ASD.

Repetitive stereotypies (arm flapping, hand twirling, clapping, rocking, head banging) are a defining characteristic of ASD. CRH [37–41] and ACTH [42,43] directly induce these types of movements in animal models, including non-human primates, probably because they dramatically increase neural excitability. (See also itch below.)

Limited interests, extreme aversion to novelty, and a desire for order are defining characteristics of ASD. CRH release, which is already basally excessive in ASD, is acutely stimulated by unpredicted inputs [44,45], and makes male goats show more distress following novelty [46]. Conversely, medial amygdala UCN3 increases preference for novel conspecifics [47]. People with ASD reduce the unpleasant feeling associated with additional CRH release by restricting novel inputs. In addition, brain learning is impaired in ASD, so people with ASD naturally tend to engage in actions and thoughts that they have already learned.

Increased sensory sensitivity is a known property of people with ASD. This happens both because CRH1 promotes sensory hyperexcitability, and because CRH2 is highly expressed in low-level sensory paths. Since early postnatal development mainly involves pruning of excitatory synapses and maturation of inhibition [48,49], its impairment leads to sustained sensory overload.

Self-injurious behavior is very common in ASD [50] (some stereotypies involve self-injury as well). ACTH, aMSH, and beta-endorphin (other products of the ACTH gene POMC) induce itch and scratching [42,51], and both ACTH [52,53] and DHEA stimulate aggression [54,55].

Aversion to touch is an early sign of ASD. This can be explained by sensory hypersensitivity, ACTH-mediated itch, and reduced OXT, which mediates pleasant touch [56]. The excessive stimulation of the itch path induces an allodynia-like state in which neutral inputs evoke aversive itch signaling.

Impaired eye gaze is a known marker of ASD. The EW nucleus controls learned eye gaze [57] and contains a population of centrally-projecting neurons with very high UCN1 expression [57]. EW UCN1 is not expressed at birth and gradually increases, showing the importance of UCN signaling to EW development [58].

Early motor impairment is clearly present in ASD [59]. CRH2 is abundantly expressed in skeletal muscle neurons [60], and UCNs act via CRH2 to improve muscle metabolism and growth [61–63]. STRDs are known to be important for motor development.

Males are more vulnerable to ASD for at least three reasons. First, estrogen, which is higher in females, directly supports brain glucose metabolism and protein synthesis [64]. Thus, the relative female advantage in estrogen covers up for some of the damage done in ASD. Second, minipuberty occurs in both sexes but is much stronger in males [65]. This shows that males need postnatal GSTRD-mediated plasticity more than females do. Relatedly, EW UCN1 expression is 10-1.6 higher in males than in females [66], making male eye gaze learning more sensitive to excessive CRH. Third, estrogen stimulates the release of the social agent OXT [67,68], while testosterone opposes it [33].

The **spectrum nature** of ASD stems from the wide expression pattern of CRH, UCNs, CRH receptors, and STRD receptors, and the fact that the core cause is stress, which can be highly variable, spatially and temporally. Hence, there is large variability in the ways in which the damage can be manifested.

It is common for babies with ASD to show **excessive passivity** during their first year of life, followed by **hyperactivity** during their second year (and throughout life) [69]. This datum supports high CRH during the 1st year, which activates CRH2 to suppress hunger, cortical norepinephrine, and the SNS. CRH release gradually diminishes, until at some point it can chronically activate CRH1, promoting hypermovement, hunger, food intake, gut issues, etc. Indeed, early life stress has been shown to induce permanent CRH hyperexcitability [70].

Although the public image of **the autistic savant** is clearly unfounded, a small number of papers reported that many people with ASD excel in specific limited areas (e.g., mathematics, visual perception) [71,72]. In addition, ASD risk is higher with parents with higher IQ and technical capabilities [73]. These data can be explained by a larger number of synapses (especially excitatory ones) due to decreased pruning during postnatal development, and by chronic CRH stimulation of the release of norepinephrine, which promotes memory [74]. Conversely, **intellectual impairment** is highly comorbid with ASD, and is explained by reduced brain (specifically PFC) development.

Cortisol exerts negative feedback on CRH and ACTH secretion. Since STRDs (mainly ASTRDs) oppose GC [75], T*ASD predicts that any situation in which both CRH and ASTRDs (and GSTRDs) are high during development should increase ASD risk. People are especially vulnerable in periods with normally high GSTRDs, because they need their long-term plasticity effects in these periods. This is indeed the case (see PCOS and stress during pregnancy below).

1.3 Evidence

T*ASD is supported by extensive evidence. The main lines are related to stress, CRH, ACTH, growth (anatomy and pathways), STRDs, OXT, comorbidities, and food intake.

1.3.1 Stress, CRH, ACTH

There is strong evidence for increased CRH and ACTH, relating to the prenatal, perinatal, and post-damage periods.

Perinatal and prenatal stress. Perinatal stress, which involves high CRH release, increases ASD risk [76]. This includes complications during delivery [76,77], usage of delivery drugs such as pitocin [77], epidural analgesia [78], neonatal hypog [79], and C-section due to prolonged labor, membrane rupture, or infection (not the C-section itself) [80].

Preterm birth increases ASD risk [1,81]. This indicates high CRH, because it is a major trigger of preterm birth [82],

Direct CRH and ACTH evidence. Only one paper reported on serum CRH in ASD, and found it higher (4-10yo, n=40) [83]. With respect to ACTH, the following reports showing increased levels were made. Increased serum ACTH and cortisol, with a positive correlation between ACTH and cortisol (6-18yo boys, n=32) [84]. Higher plasma ACTH and beta-endorphin, due to more severely affected ASDs (10 ± 7yo, n=48) [85]. Higher ACTH and lower cortisol (15 ± 9.5yo, n=36) [86]. Symptoms correlated with ACTH, 16% with high ACTH, 10% low basal cortisol, 10% with decreased cortisol response to ACTH (7.35 ± 2.6yo, 3-12yo, n=50) [87]. Higher plasma ACTH in Asperger adults, n=20 [88].

Autonomic nervous system. SNS activity is chronically higher in ASD, as shown by higher basal heart rate, decreased heart rate variability, and blunted skin conductance response [89–91]. Parasympathetic activity is lower, and respiratory sinus arrhythmia data can predict the severity of repetitive behaviors in 5-10yo [92]. Since CRH triggers SNS activation, these data support chronic CRH release. As noted above, the T*ASD view is that at the time when ASD is diagnosed, CRH release is diminished to chronically activate CRH1 rather than CRH2.

Mast cells, allergies, gut. There is high activation of immune mast cells in ASD [93], and higher prevalence of allergy-related disorders in patients and their siblings [94,95]. CRH directly activated mast cells, which are involved in allergic responses.

Gut problems are common in ASD patients [94,96] and their parents [97]. CRH activation of mast cells increases gut permeability [98].

There is general pro-inflammation immune activation in ASD [94], which can be due to CRH but may simply stem from the excessive release of stress-related agents.

Eye gaze. CRH overexpression decreases UCN expression in the EW nucleus, which mediates learned eye gaze [99].

Other. There is high ASD comorbidity with anxiety [100], and maternal post-traumatic stress disorder increases ASD risk [101]. Both point to high CRH.

The cortisol response to ACTH stimulation is slower in ASD [102] and its levels are higher [103], supporting chronic activity.

ASD is associated with skin hyperpigmentation phenomena [104], which are also associated with high ACTH [105]. Recall that melanocortins, which affect skin pigmentation, are a product of the ACTH gene POMC, stimulated by CRH.

People with ASD have non-brain health problems in most organs, which are the main cause of premature death [106]. This indirectly supports the UCN path, because UCNs are expressed in these organs and are important for their healthy development.

1.3.2 Anatomical growth

Prenatal. Intrauterine growth restriction (IUGR) is associated with dramatically increased ASD risk [107,108]. This supports a growth problem in ASD, and specifically supports high CRH, since high late pregnancy maternal plasma CRH is significantly associated with preterm small for gestational age births [109]. UCNs are expressed in the placenta and fetal membranes, and are needed for prenatal glucose uptake [8,110].

Early postnatal. ASD involves increased excitation-inhibition ratio during early development [111], and decreased lateral inhibition in cortical mini-columns (mean age 12yo) [112]. This shows impaired postnatal synaptic pruning and/or impaired postnatal brain development, which is normally dominated by maturation of inhibition.

Accelerated postnatal head circumference growth is consistently reported in ASD [113–117] (but see [118]). Baby length was reported to be higher in 4-5 month old boys, with babies at the top 10% of physical size having greater symptom severity later [116]. Babies with ASD show extremely rapid weight gain in infancy [107]. These data support high postnatal ACTH, since ACTH and other POMC products directly promote bone growth [119].

ASD brains show strong local connectivity and low long-distance one [120], with hyperconnectivity at young ages [121], supporting reduced postnatal pruning and development.

Related to sensory hypersensitivity in ASD, there is auditory brainstem pathology, with delayed maturation of low- to high-level pathways [122].

Epileptic seizures are common in ASD. This can be explained by increased brain excitation by CRH (e.g., in the hippocampus), and by reduced development of brain inhibitory interneurons.

1.3.3 Growth agents & pathways

Glucose. ASD is significantly associated with a family history of hypothyroidism [94], especially with maternal hypothyroidism during pregnancy [123]. Hypothyroidism is associated with hypog, further supporting the association of reduced glucose with increased ASD risk.

Gestational diabetes increases ASD risk [1,124]. ASD risk is increased with type 1 diabetes and increased blood glucose levels [125,126]. Using the HOMA-IR model, people with ASD were shown to have insulin resistance and decreased brain glucose metabolism (4-18yo, n=60) [127]. These data show the importance of cellular glucose for opposing ASD.

Neonatal hypog is independently associated with developmental problems and ASD traits [108]. Since UCN secretion is stimulated by glucose, it is decreased in hypog states.

Protein synthesis. The Akt/mTOR growth axis is dysregulated (mainly reported decreased) in ASD [128–132]. UCNs and GSTRDs are needed for the proper activation of this axis during development.

Glautathione (GSH), which is a major agent promoting protein synthesis in the pentose phosphate pathway (PPP), is decreased in ASD [133].

ASD is associated with neonatal jaundice [79,134] (although not consistently [135]). The enzyme G6PD is essential for the PPP and protein synthesis, and neonatal jaundice indicates G6PD deficiency [136] and neonatal hypog [108]. Thus, neonatal jaundice supports reduced cellular glucose in ASD.

1.3.4 Sex steroids

Androgens. DHEA is increased in ASD, in both prepuberty males and females [137–141], showing excessive ASTRDs. Note that female androgens are mainly produced in the adrenal gland, where their production is stimulated by ACTH.

Testosterone, estrogen. Although testosterone is mainly reported to be increased in ASD (prepubertal, pubertal and in adults) [138,139,142–148], it is also reported to be decreased [149–151] or unchanged [152]. The increased DHEA in ASD explains the increased testosterone results. The conflicting results can be explained by reduced GSTRD production due to high ASTRDs.

Both an association with higher amniotic fluid estrogens [153] and no association with umbilical cord testosterone [154] were reported. No relationship between amniotic fluid testosterone and autistic traits was found in girls [155]. There are contradictory reports on the association between prenatal or early postnatal testosterone and autistic traits [156–158]. Thus, the evidence for a prenatal problem is weak.

Follicle-stimulating hormone and estrogen were reported to be decreased in both male and female ASD serum [159], supporting reduced GSTRDs.

Polycystic ovary syndrome, prenatal androgens. PCOS is a condition involving high ASTRDs, mainly DHEA. Large population studies have shown that children of mothers with PCOS have a higher risk of ASD [160,161]. Regardless of a PCOS diagnosis, mothers of children with ASD had higher testosterone [162].

As mentioned above, the T*ASD view is that high androgens during sensitive developmental periods increase risk via an association with increased CRH.

Prenatal testosterone is released during weeks 8-20 of pregnancy, so this should be a sensitive period to stress-induced ASD. Indeed, the association of ASD with maternal stress during pregnancy [163,164] may be specific to this period. An all-Denmark birth cohort showed that maternal hospitalization due to 1st/2nd trimester viral or bacterial infection increases risk about 3x [165], and increased 1st trimester maternal stress during the Quebec ice storm was associated with increased ASD risk [166].

Supporting the effect of stress on sex STRDs, prenatal stress increases anogenital distance (a masculinization index) in human females, with a trend for a decrease in males [167].

Congenital adrenal hyperplasia (CAH) involves high ACTH and androgens, and is not linked to ASD, at least in girls [155]. These PCOS and CAH data imply that CRH and ACTH are involved in PCOS but not in CAH pathogenesis.

Masculine/feminine features. ASD involves higher gender dysphoria [168], with males and females more likely to be bisexual and homosexual, respectively [169]. In the general adult population, people with autistic traits are more likely to be bisexual or with an uncertain orientation [170]. In addition, women with ASD have more masculine facial features than women without ASD [171–173], and men with ASD are more feminine in some ways [171,172] (although hyper-masculine faces were also reported in prepubertal boys with ASD [173]). These data imply lower androgens in males and higher androgens in females during sensitive developmental periods. This accords with T*ASD, because higher CRH-ACTH-DHEA increases androgens in females, and these ASTRDs opposes GSTRDs so decrease some organizational effects of GSTRD androgens in males.

There is also some evidence that CRH decreases ovary aromatase, which converts testosterone to estrogen [174]. This could be another route through which women with ASD have less estrogen and more testosterone than other women.

Endocrine disrupting chemicals (EDCs). Pre- or perinatal exposure to EDCs (e.g., some pesticides, plastics) increases risk [175,176]. Many EDCs mimic estrogen, amplifying its recruitment of CRH towards the end of pregnancy. (Note that higher postnatal estrogen is relatively protective due to protein synthesis, see above.)

Sexual behavior. CRH1 basally stimulates gonadotropin hormone-releasing hormone (and thus GSTRDs) [177], which might explain the higher sexual drive and frequent inappropriate sexual behavior shown by adolescents and adults with ASD [178].

Summary. ASTRDs are definitely increased in ASD, in both males and females. Testosterone is usually increased in males, and this is most likely due to the increase in ASTRDs. Conversely, GSTRDs are lower in males. Males are more vulnerable in developmental periods in which they need GSTRDs. These data support increased CRH-ATCH and decreased long-term GSTRD plasticity in ASD. Prenatal estrogens increase risk, probably by stimulating CRH.

1.3.5 Oxytocin

OXT is dysregulated in ASD, with most papers reporting decreased OXT [179,180], but several reporting an increase [181]. This accords with the T*ASD prediction. The decrease is due to high testosterone [33] and decreased UCN-mediated plasticity [35]. The increase happens because plasticity, including at the hypothalamus, involves maturation of inhibitory interneurons, and possibly because estrogen (which stimulates OXT [67]) is increased due to DHEA. There is also the possibility of inherently decreased OXT capacity in ASD due to epigenetics.

Pitocin usage during labor indicates delivery problems (see above), but may also increase risk by inducing a long-term desensitization of OXT receptors [182]. Usage of the OXT antagonist tractocile during labor is associated with later social communication problems [183].

Several wide cohort studies showed a strong association of ASD with **reduced breastfeeding** [184–190]. This can be because human milk contains OXT [30], and because breastfeeding is accompanied by longer human touch, which reduces CRH [191] (even beyond puberty [192]) and increases OXT.

There is one report of decreased fMRI activity in the insula following affective touch in ASD, coupled with increased activity in the primary somatosensory cortex following neutral touch [193].

1.3.6 Food intake

Babies and toddlers later diagnosed with ASD show decreased satiety and increased desire for food intake (non-stop suckling, decreased nursing strike) [194–197]. In the general population, autistic traits at age 6 years are associated with being hungry/not satisfied, or no breastfeeding, or small drinking quantities at age 2 months [198]. These data can be explained by the fact that part of the role of OXT is to signal satiety and decrease food intake (mainly sugars) [199], so reduced OXT prolongs the time to satiety. Another account is that the deficiency of glucose for growth in ASD is sensed (via an unknown mechanism, although see CRRs below), and this stimulates continued food intake.

Children with ASD show restricted food preference and an unwillingness to try novel food [200]. This may be due to their general avoidance of novelty to prevent higher CRH release.

At later ages, there is high obesity in ASD [21], which could be due to chronically high activation of CRH1, which stimulates the counter-regulatory responses (CRRs) to hypog and food intake [19]. In addition, in ASD, less ingested glucose is channelled to protein synthesis, which leaves excessive blood glucose. In this situation, serotonin promotes the storage of glucose in adipose tissue as fat [201]. Supporting this account, blood serotonin is elevated in patients [202] and correlates with symptom severity [203].

1.4 Treatment

1.4.1 Detection

Postnatal levels of blood, urine, saliva, hair and/or CSF CRH, ACTH, cortisol, UCNs, testosterone, estrogen, DHEA/cortisol ratio, and OXT, can be used for early screening. The most promising biomarker may be **ACTH**, because it is directly related to both CRH and ASTRDs. Levels at birth would probably be less informative than levels at the age of 3 months, since at this age adrenal involution, coupled with a dramatic decrease in DHEA, should already have happened. However, as indicated above, there are reports in which adrenal involution occurs much earlier. Normal timelines for CRH and ACTH decrease and adrenal involution should be investigated more in order to devise the optimal detection schedule for ASD. Prenatal (maternal plasma and amniotic fluid) levels, mainly of CRH and ACTH, would be useful too.

Direct demonstration of higher adrenal volume using imaging would also point to a problem, because reduced ACTH is a major factor in adrenal involution [204], with both CRH and ACTH increasing adrenal volume [205].

1.4.2 Preventive treatment

Is it justified? When discussing preventive treatment, we must keep in mind that so-called 'autistic traits' are part of the vast repertoire of human properties, and are not necessarily a bad thing to have. Nonetheless, it is clear that many people with ASD are simply unable to conduct an independent fulfilling life, which justifies treatment.

Definition. By 'preventive treatment', I mean treatment made during the damage period, since it is generally not possible to reduce high pre- and perinatal CRH. Nonetheless, it may be a good idea not to take certain medications during pregnancy. For example, selective serotonin reuptake inhibitors, which are a very common treatment for depression, are associated with increased 2nd trimester CRH (although causality has not been shown) [206].

Behavioral. A general principle is that drug treatment should be accompanied by behavioral treatment. The problem is impaired brain plasticity (learning), but the brain still has learning capacity, and the impairment can be greatly alleviated by repeated training [207].

Pleasant postnatal human **touch**, and **breastfeeding**, should reduce risk by increasing OXT and reducing CRH in the brain.

CRH, DHT. The best treatment would be to **reduce CRH levels**. Antibodies to CRH have been isolated in mice [208]. However, the main damage is done in the brain. RNA interference methods can be used to reduce CRH production, but the drug needs to penetrate the brain.

There is a promising way to reduce CRH. DHT mediates many of the organizational effects of GSTRD androgens [209]. Probably as part of this role, it suppresses ASTRDs, decreasing HPA axis activity and the release of its driving agents, including CRH and ACTH [210,211]. DHT synthesis during male minipuberty takes place only in the testis, with adrenal production being extremely high at birth but dropping to very low levels at 10 weeks [29]. Conversely, ACTH inhibits 5a-reductase, the rate limiting enzyme in DHT production [212].

Thus, **exogenous DHT, which is readily available, could ameliorate or even prevent the ASD phenotype** if used at the right time. DHT is available in transdermal patch form, making its administration to babies very easy.

Obviously, this treatment may be suitable only for males, but males comprise 80% of the ASD population. DHT mediates some or all of its anti-CRH effects via its conversion to 3b-diol (by 3beta-hydroxysteroid dehydrogenase) [210], which binds estrogen receptor beta but not the androgen receptor. Like estrogen, 3b-diol phasically increases OXT [67]. Thus, 3b-diol treatment may be suitable for females (and possibly males as well).

This DHT proposal may seem paradoxical in light of the increased levels of androgens reported in ASD. However, recall that according to T*ASD, these increased levels are mainly due to ASTRDs, not GSTRDs, which are the normal source of DHT during minipuberty.

Other. There are additional possible treatments. Cortisol reduces CRH release, so postnatal **exogenous glucocorticoids (GCs)** might help. GC doses should be lower than those that desensitize the GC receptor (GR).

ACTH suppression (e.g., with somatostatin analogues such as pasireotide) could be helpful, mainly to reduce damage done in the ASTRD. This treatment may need to be supplemented by exogenous GCs.

Exogenous OXT during the first postnatal months might be beneficial. Some intranasal OXT crosses the blood-brain barrier (BBB) [213], but there is no evidence that it reaches the hypothalamus. Blood OXT needs assistance in order to cross the BBB in meaningful amounts and to remain active for more than a short time.

Exogenous UCNs diffuse across the blood-brain barrier [214], and may be beneficial by competing with CRH for receptor binding.

1.4.3 Symptomatic treatment

ACTH suppression (e.g., with DHT) may be a good treatment for aggression symptoms exhibited after the initial damage period (recall that ACTH and DHEA promote such aggression). Reducing CRH should also counter aversion to novelty and repetitive movements and habits.

1.5 Discussion

ASD is one of the major brain disorders, and one of the largest mysteries of modern science, medicine and human society. Here I presented the first complete theory of ASD, complete in the sense that it explains the etiology, symptoms, and pathology of ASD, and relies on substantial empirical evidence.

Other theories. At present, there is no theory of ASD that mechanistically explains even its symptoms, let alone its etiology and pathology [215]. Several hypotheses have been articulated regarding the nature of ASD. The 'extreme male brain' hypothesis [216] posits a difference between systematizing, which is supposedly a male way of behavior, and empathizing, supposedly female. These notions are very hard to define, and in any case do not provide any mechanistic account. T*ASD agrees that females with ASD are more masculine in some ways, but as the evidence brought above shows, males with ASD can be argued to be more feminine than males without ASD.

The idea that OXT is central in ASD has been raised [217], which is natural in light of the role of OXT is social development. However, mechanisms have not been detailed, and although OXT dysregulation exists in ASD, it is clear that OXT is far from explaining the variety of ASD symptoms and properties. In T*ASD, the main downstream event is an impairment in postnatal plasticity due to reduced growth signaling by UCNs and GSTRDs. OXT is one of the main sites of damage.

Another idea is that ASD involves an increased excitation-inhibition (E/I) ratio during early development [111]. This is indeed a plausible outcome of impaired postnatal plasticity, but a detailed review concluded that although excitation and inhibition are altered in ASD, there is no real evidence for the increased E/I theory [218].

A hypothesis with some mechanistic basis is that of aberrant growth pathways such as Wnt, ERK, and Akt [219]. In this idea, ASD begins in prenatal life, with a disruption of proliferation and migration. This follows with a disrupted postnatal brain connectivity. There is an emphasis on risk genes. T*ASD agrees with this hypothesis in the importance of impaired growth pathways, but disagrees with it in their timing and concrete identity, and in the genetic emphasis. In addition, this theory does not include any mechanistic account of the specific symptoms of ASD.

Strengths and weaknesses. T*ASD presents a view of the etiology of ASD that is highly biologically plausible and consistent with the evidence. It mechanistically addresses basically all of the symptoms of ASD, and utilizes all of the salient data gathered about the disorder. It is supported by a substantial body of empirical evidence of different types and modalities. As such, it is a very strong theory. Its greatest weakness at present is that there is no supporting evidence showing that the putative pathways are indeed impaired during the relevant damage period. There is a lot of evidence for the involvement of CRH and sex steroids somewhat after (and before) this period, but not during the first 1-9 postnatal months. In addition, there is very little UCN data.

Genetics. Because ASD occurs due to stress during pregnancy or after birth, T*ASD does not predict meaningful DNA changes. The tendency for increased

CRH release (and/or for increased effect on its downstream paths) may be encoded genetically or epigenetically, but this most likely involves a large number of genes and a small effect in each of them. The damage occurs during development, and may not leave any genetic or epigenetic trace in the causal genes, although there is likely a persistent epigenetic change to the CRH system that causes chronic CRH1 activation. Indeed, there are different DNA methylation patterns between disease-discordant monozygotic twins, with a significant correlation between DNA methylation and ASD traits [220]. Overall, T*ASD generally does not expect supporting genetic evidence. There is some hypothesized genetic data pointing to CRH, CRH2 and UCN3 genes [221], but it is not strong.

Treatment. An exciting aspect of T*ASD is that it points to easy biomarkers (ACTH, ASTRDs, adrenal volume) and to a readily available preventive treatment that's quite easy to administer to babies. Although the definition of what constitutes 'excessive' CRH/ACTH would surely be blurry, many of the more severe cases of ASD most likely involve levels that would be classified as excessive without argument. The proposed treatment may alleviate these cases, while people with ASD traits will not be treated, allowing human diversity.

List of abbreviations

Terms introduced in this chapter are marked by a **bold** font.

ACTH: adrenocorticotropic hormone.
aMSH: alpha-melanocyte stimulating hormone.
ASD: autism spectrum disorder.
ASTRD: adrenal steroid.
BNST: bed nucleus of the stria terminalis.
C-CRH2: CRH-induced CRH2 receptor signaling.
cAMP: cyclic adenosine monophosphate.
CRH: corticotropin-releasing hormone (also CRF, factor).
DHT: dihydrotestosterone.
EW: Edinger-Westphal (nucleus).
GSTRD: gonadal steroid.
DHEA(S): dehydroepiandrosterone (sulfated).
GC: glucocorticoid.
MAPK: mitogen-activated protein kinase.
OXT: oxytocin.
PCOS: polycystic ovary syndrome.
POMC: proopiomelanocortin.
PPP: pentose phosphate pathway.
SNS: sympathetic nervous system.
STRD: steroid.
T*ASD: the theory of ASD presented here.
U-CRH2: UCN-induced CRH2 receptor signaling.

References

[1] C. Lord, T.S. Brugha, T. Charman, J. Cusack, G. Dumas, T. Frazier, et al., Autism spectrum disorder, Nature Reviews Disease Primers 6 (1) (2020) 1–23.

[2] T. Hirota, B.H. King, Autism spectrum disorder: A review, JAMA 329 (2) (2023) 157–168.

[3] M.J. Maenner, Prevalence and characteristics of autism spectrum disorder among children aged 8 years—Autism and Developmental Disabilities Monitoring Network, 11 sites, United States 2020, in: MMWR Surveillance Summaries, 2023, p. 72.

[4] T.L. Bale, W.W. Vale, CRF and CRF receptors: role in stress responsivity and other behaviors, Annual Review of Pharmacology and Toxicology 44 (2004) 525–557.

[5] J.M. Deussing, A. Chen, The corticotropin-releasing factor family: physiology of the stress response, Physiological Reviews 98 (4) (2018) 2225–2286.

[6] C. Li, P. Chen, J. Vaughan, A. Blount, A. Chen, P.M. Jamieson, et al., Urocortin III is expressed in pancreatic β-cells and stimulates insulin and glucagon secretion, Endocrinology 144 (7) (2003) 3216–3224.

[7] C. Li, P. Chen, J. Vaughan, K.F. Lee, W. Vale, Urocortin 3 regulates glucose-stimulated insulin secretion and energy homeostasis, Proceedings of the National Academy of Sciences 104 (10) (2007) 4206–4211.

[8] S.J. Simpson, L.I. Smith, P.M. Jones, J.E. Bowe, UCN2: a new candidate influencing pancreatic β-cell adaptations in pregnancy, Journal of Endocrinology 245 (2) (2020) 247–257.

[9] A. Chanalaris, K.M. Lawrence, P.A. Townsend, S. Davidson, Y. Jashmidi, A. Stephanou, et al., Hypertrophic effects of urocortin homologous peptides are mediated via activation of the Akt pathway, Biochemical and Biophysical Research Communications 328 (2) (2005) 442–448.

[10] D. Markovic, A. Punn, H. Lehnert, D.K. Grammatopoulos, Molecular determinants and feedback circuits regulating type 2 CRH receptor signal integration, Biochimica Et Biophysica Acta. Molecular Cell Research 1813 (5) (2011) 896–907.

[11] H.Y. Huang, D.D. Liu, H.F. Chang, W.F. Chen, H.R. Hsu, J.S. Kuo, et al., Histone deacetylase inhibition mediates urocortin-induced antiproliferation and neuronal differentiation in neural stem cells, Stem Cells 30 (12) (2012) 2760–2773.

[12] M.M. Roustit, J.M. Vaughan, P.M. Jamieson, M.E. Cleasby, Urocortin 3 activates AMPK and AKT pathways and enhances glucose disposal in rat skeletal muscle, Journal of Endocrinology 223 (2) (2014) 143.

[13] S. Walther, F. Pluteanu, S. Renz, Y. Nikonova, J.T. Maxwell, L.Z. Yang, et al., Urocortin 2 stimulates nitric oxide production in ventricular myocytes via Akt-and PKA-mediated phosphorylation of eNOS at serine 1177, American Journal of Physiology. Heart and Circulatory Physiology 307 (5) (2014) H689-700.

[14] M.H. Gao, D. Giamouridis, N.C. Lai, E. Walenta, V.A. Paschoal, Y.C. Kim, et al., One-time injection of AAV8 encoding urocortin 2 provides long-term resolution of insulin resistance, JCI Insight 1 (15) (2016).

[15] S. Kavalakatt, A. Khadir, D. Madhu, H.A. Koistinen, F. Al-Mulla, J. Tuomilehto, et al., Urocortin 3 overexpression reduces ER stress and heat shock response in 3T3-L1 adipocytes, Scientific Reports 11 (1) (2021) 15666.

[16] J. Meister, D.B. Bone, J.R. Knudsen, L.F. Barella, L. Liu, R. Lee, et al., In vivo metabolic effects after acute activation of skeletal muscle Gs signaling, Molecular Metabolism 55 (2022) 101415.

[17] N. Lautherbach, D.A. Gonçalves, W.A. Silveira, S. Paula-Gomes, R.R. Valentim, N.M. Zanon, et al., Urocortin 2 promotes hypertrophy and enhances skeletal muscle function through cAMP and insulin/IGF-1 signaling pathways, Molecular Metabolism 60 (2022) 101492.

[18] S.E. Flaherty III, O. Bezy, W. Zheng, D. Yan, X. Li, S. Jagarlapudi, et al., Chronic UCN2 treatment desensitizes CRHR2 and improves insulin sensitivity, Nature Communications 14 (1) (2023) 3953.
[19] R.J. McCrimmon, Z. Song, H. Cheng, E.C. McNay, C. Weikart-Yeckel, X. Fan, et al., Corticotrophin-releasing factor receptors within the ventromedial hypothalamus regulate hypoglycemia-induced hormonal counterregulation, The Journal of Clinical Investigation 116 (6) (2006) 1723–1730.
[20] R.L. Hauger, J.A. Olivares-Reyes, S. Braun, J. Hernandez-Aranda, C.C. Hudson, E. Gutknecht, et al., Desensitization of human CRF2 (a) receptor signaling governed by agonist potency and βarrestin2 recruitment, Regulatory Peptides 186 (2013) 62–76.
[21] L.A. Croen, O. Zerbo, Y. Qian, M.L. Massolo, S. Rich, S. Sidney, et al., The health status of adults on the autism spectrum, Autism 19 (7) (2015) 814–823.
[22] A. Turcu, J.M. Smith, R. Auchus, W.E. Rainey, Adrenal androgens and androgen precursors: definition, synthesis, regulation and physiologic actions, Comprehensive Physiology 4 (4) (2014) 1369.
[23] K. Kageyama, Regulation of gonadotropins by corticotropin-releasing factor and urocortin, Frontiers in Endocrinology 4 (2013) 12.
[24] A.W. Norman, M.T. Mizwicki, D.P. Norman, Steroid-hormone rapid actions, membrane receptors and a conformational ensemble model, Nature Reviews Drug Discovery 3 (1) (2004) 27–41.
[25] B.J. Clark, R.A. Prough, C.M. Klinge, Mechanisms of action of dehydroepiandrosterone, Vitamins and Hormones 108 (2018) 29–73.
[26] S. Saponaro, V. Guarnieri, G.P. Pescarmona, F. Silvagno, Long-term exposure to dehydroepiandrosterone affects the transcriptional activity of the glucocorticoid receptor, The Journal of Steroid Biochemistry and Molecular Biology 103 (2) (2007) 129–136.
[27] J.C. McNelis, K.N. Manolopoulos, L.L. Gathercole, I.J. Bujalska, P.M. Stewart, J.W. Tomlinson, et al., Dehydroepiandrosterone exerts antiglucocorticoid action on human preadipocyte proliferation, differentiation, and glucose uptake, American Journal of Physiology: Endocrinology and Metabolism 305 (9) (2013) E1134-44.
[28] S. Ben-David, N. Zuckerman-Levin, M. Epelman, Z. Shen-Orr, M. Levin, P. Sujov, et al., Parturition itself is the basis for fetal adrenal involution, The Journal of Clinical Endocrinology and Metabolism 92 (1) (2007) 93–97.
[29] N.A. Dhayat, B. Dick, B.M. Frey, C.H. d'Uscio, B. Vogt, C.E. Flück, Androgen biosynthesis during minipuberty favors the backdoor pathway over the classic pathway: Insights into enzyme activities and steroid fluxes in healthy infants during the first year of life from the urinary steroid metabolome, The Journal of Steroid Biochemistry and Molecular Biology 165 (2017) 312–322.
[30] C.S. Carter, Oxytocin pathways and the evolution of human behavior, Annual Review of Psychology 65 (2014) 17–39.
[31] L.M. Frankiensztajn, R. Gur-Pollack, S. Wagner, A combinatorial modulation of synaptic plasticity in the rat medial amygdala by oxytocin, urocortin3 and estrogen, Psychoneuroendocrinology 92 (2018) 95–102.
[32] S. Ohno, H. Hashimoto, H. Fujihara, N. Fujiki, M. Yoshimura, T. Maruyama, et al., Increased oxytocin-monomeric red fluorescent protein 1 fluorescent intensity with urocortin-like immunoreactivity in the hypothalamo-neurohypophysial system of aged transgenic rats, Neuroscience Research 128 (2018) 40–49.
[33] D. Dai, Q.C. Li, Q.B. Zhu, S.H. Hu, R. Balesar, D. Swaab, et al., Direct Involvement of Androgen Receptor in Oxytocin Gene Expression: Possible Relevance for Mood Disorders, Neuropsychopharmacology (2017).
[34] C.P. Chu, W.Z. Jin, Y.H. Bing, Q.H. Jin, H. Kannan, D.L. Qiu, Effects of stresscopin on rat hypothalamic paraventricular nucleus neurons in vitro, PLoS ONE 8 (1) (2013) e53863.
[35] O.J. Bosch, J. Dabrowska, M.E. Modi, Z.V. Johnson, A.C. Keebaugh, C.E. Barrett, et al., Oxytocin in the nucleus accumbens shell reverses CRFR2-evoked passive stress-coping after partner loss in monogamous male prairie voles, Psychoneuroendocrinology 64 (2016) 66–78.

[36] D. Martinon, J. Dabrowska, Corticotropin-releasing factor receptors modulate oxytocin release in the dorsolateral bed nucleus of the stria terminalis (BNST) in male rats, Frontiers in Neuroscience 12 (2018) 337055.
[37] Y. Takamatsu, T. Moroji, The effects of intracerebroventricularly injected corticotropin-releasing factor (CRF) on the central nervous system: behavioural and biochemical studies, Neuropeptides 13 (3) (1989) 147–155.
[38] E.M. Strome, G.T. Wheler, J.D. Higley, D.L. Loriaux, S.J. Suomi, D.J. Doudet, Intracerebroventricular corticotropin-releasing factor increases limbic glucose metabolism and has social context-dependent behavioral effects in nonhuman primates, Proceedings of the National Academy of Sciences 99 (24) (2002) 15749–15754.
[39] V.P. Bakshi, S.M. Newman, S. Smith-Roe, K.A. Jochman, N.H. Kalin, Stimulation of lateral septum CRF2 receptors promotes anorexia and stress-like behaviors: functional homology to CRF1 receptors in basolateral amygdala, The Journal of Neuroscience 27 (39) (2007) 10568–10577.
[40] R.E. Carpenter, M.J. Watt, G.L. Forster, Øverli Ø, C. Bockholt, K.J. Renner, et al., Corticotropin releasing factor induces anxiogenic locomotion in trout and alters serotonergic and dopaminergic activity, Hormones and Behavior 52 (5) (2007) 600–611.
[41] M. Ogino, A. Okumura, M.S.I. Khan, M.A. Cline, T. Tachibana, Comparison of brain urocortin-3 and corticotrophin-releasing factor for physiological responses in chicks, Physiology & Behavior 125 (2014) 57–61.
[42] A. Van Erp, M. Kruk, H. Van Oers, N. Hemmers, Differential effect of ACTH1–24 and α-MSH induced grooming in the paraventricular nucleus of the hypothalamus, Brain Research 603 (2) (1993) 296–301.
[43] J.E. Wikberg, R. Muceniece, I. Mandrika, P. Prusis, J. Lindblom, C. Post, et al., New aspects on the melanocortins and their receptors, Pharmacological Research 42 (5) (2000) 393–420.
[44] J.E. Sherman, N.H. Kalin, ICV-CRH potently affects behavior without altering antinociceptive responding, Life Sciences 39 (5) (1986) 433–441.
[45] A. Gesing, A. Bilang-Bleuel, S.K. Droste, A.C. Linthorst, F. Holsboer, J.M. Reul, Psychological stress increases hippocampal mineralocorticoid receptor levels: involvement of corticotropin-releasing hormone, The Journal of Neuroscience 21 (13) (2001) 4822–4829.
[46] D. Montigny, P. Hemsworth, Gender-specific effects of prenatal stress on emotional reactivity and stress physiology of goat kids, Hormones and Behavior 47 (3) (2005) 256–266.
[47] Y. Shemesh, O. Forkosh, M. Mahn, S. Anpilov, Y. Sztainberg, S. Manashirov, et al., Ucn3 and CRF-R2 in the medial amygdala regulate complex social dynamics, Nature Neuroscience 19 (11) (2016) 1489–1496.
[48] A.E. Takesian, T.K. Hensch, Balancing plasticity/stability across brain development, Progress in Brain Research 207 (2013) 3–34.
[49] K.B. Quast, K. Ung, E. Froudarakis, L. Huang, I. Herman, A.P. Addison, et al., Developmental broadening of inhibitory sensory maps, Nature Neuroscience 20 (2) (2017) 189–199.
[50] C. Steenfeldt-Kristensen, C.A. Jones, C. Richards, The prevalence of self-injurious behaviour in autism: a meta-analytic study, Journal of Autism and Developmental Disorders 50 (2020) 3857–3873.
[51] A. Yamamoto, Y. Sugimoto, Involvement of peripheral mu opioid receptors in scratching behavior in mice, European Journal of Pharmacology 649 (1–3) (2010) 336–341.
[52] S.O. Fetissov, J. Hallman, I. Nilsson, A.K. Lefvert, L. Oreland, T. Hökfelt, Aggressive behavior linked to corticotropin-reactive autoantibodies, Biological Psychiatry 60 (8) (2006) 799–802.
[53] A.H. Veenema, L. Torner, A. Blume, D.I. Beiderbeck, I.D. Neumann, Low inborn anxiety correlates with high intermale aggression: link to ACTH response and neuronal activation of the hypothalamic paraventricular nucleus, Hormones and Behavior 51 (1) (2007) 11–19.
[54] K. Pajer, R. Tabbah, W. Gardner, R.T. Rubin, R.K. Czambel, Y. Wang, Adrenal androgen and gonadal hormone levels in adolescent girls with conduct disorder, Psychoneuroendocrinology 31 (10) (2006) 1245–1256.

[55] K.K. Soma, N.M. Rendon, R. Boonstra, H.E. Albers, G.E. Demas, DHEA effects on brain and behavior: insights from comparative studies of aggression, The Journal of Steroid Biochemistry and Molecular Biology 145 (2015) 261–272.
[56] F. McGlone, J. Wessberg, H. Olausson, Discriminative and affective touch: sensing and feeling, Neuron 82 (4) (2014) 737–755.
[57] T. Kozicz, J.C. Bittencourt, P.J. May, A. Reiner, P.D. Gamlin, M. Palkovits, et al., The Edinger-Westphal nucleus: A historical, structural, and functional perspective on a dichotomous terminology, Journal of Comparative Neurology 519 (8) (2011) 1413–1434.
[58] A. Cservenka, E. Spangler, D.M. Cote, A.E. Ryabinin, Postnatal developmental profile of urocortin 1 and cocaine- and amphetamine-regulated transcript in the perioculomotor region of C57BL/6J mice, Brain Research 1319 (2010) 33–43.
[59] Y.H. Lim, M. Licari, A.J. Spittle, R.E. Watkins, J.G. Zwicker, J. Downs, et al., Early motor function of children with autism spectrum disorder: a systematic review, Pediatrics 147 (2) (2021).
[60] S. Samuelsson, J.S. Lange, R.T. Hinkle, M. Tarnopolsky, R.J. Isfort, Corticotropin-releasing factor 2 receptor localization in skeletal muscle, The Journal of Histochemistry and Cytochemistry 52 (7) (2004) 967–977.
[61] R.T. Hinkle, E. Donnelly, D.B. Cody, S. Samuelsson, J.S. Lange, M.B. Bauer, et al., Activation of the CRF 2 receptor modulates skeletal muscle mass under physiological and pathological conditions, American Journal of Physiology: Endocrinology and Metabolism 285 (4) (2003) E889–E898.
[62] P. Jamieson, M. Cleasby, N. Morton, P. Kelly, D. Brownstein, K. Mustard, et al., Urocortin 3 transgenic mice exhibit a metabolically favourable phenotype resisting obesity and hyperglycaemia on a high-fat diet, Diabetologia 54 (2011) 2392–2403.
[63] J. Reutenauer-Patte, F.X. Boittin, O. Patthey-Vuadens, U.T. Ruegg, O.M. Dorchies, Urocortins improve dystrophic skeletal muscle structure and function through both PKA- and Epac-dependent pathways, The American Journal of Pathology 180 (2) (2012) 749–762.
[64] I. Azcoitia, G.E. Barreto, L.M. Garcia-Segura, Molecular mechanisms and cellular events involved in the neuroprotective actions of estradiol. Analysis of sex differences, Frontiers in Neuroendocrinology 55 (2019) 100787.
[65] T. Kuiri-Hänninen, U. Sankilampi, L. Dunkel, Activation of the hypothalamic-pituitary-gonadal axis in infancy: minipuberty, Hormone Research in Paediatrics 82 (2) (2014) 73–80.
[66] N.M. Derks, B. Gaszner, E.W. Roubos, L.T. Kozicz, Sex differences in urocortin 1 dynamics in the non-preganglionic Edinger–Westphal nucleus of the rat, Neuroscience Research 66 (1) (2010) 117–123.
[67] D. Sharma, R.J. Handa, R.M. Uht, The ERβ ligand 5α-androstane, 3β, 17β-diol (3β-diol) regulates hypothalamic oxytocin (Oxt) gene expression, Endocrinology 153 (5) (2012) 2353–2361.
[68] R. Hiroi, A.F. Lacagnina, L.R. Hinds, D.G. Carbone, R.M. Uht, R.J. Handa, The androgen metabolite, 5α-androstane-3β, 17β-diol (3β-diol), activates the oxytocin promoter through an estrogen receptor-β pathway, Endocrinology 154 (5) (2013) 1802–1812.
[69] L. Zwaigenbaum, S. Bryson, T. Rogers, W. Roberts, J. Brian, P. Szatmari, Behavioral manifestations of autism in the first year of life, International Journal of Developmental Neuroscience 23 (2–3) (2005) 143–152.
[70] P. Hu, I. Maita, M.L. Phan, E. Gu, C. Kwok, A. Dieterich, et al., Early-life stress alters affective behaviors in adult mice through persistent activation of CRH-BDNF signaling in the oval bed nucleus of the stria terminalis, Translational Psychiatry 10 (1) (2020) 396.
[71] P. Howlin, S. Goode, J. Hutton, M. Rutter, Savant skills in autism: psychometric approaches and parental reports, Philosophical Transactions of the Royal Society B: Biological Sciences 364 (1522) (2009) 1359–1367.
[72] A.A.S. Meilleur, P. Jelenic, L. Mottron, Prevalence of clinically and empirically defined talents and strengths in autism, Journal of Autism and Developmental Disorders 45 (2015) 1354–1367.

[73] R.M. Gardner, C. Dalman, D. Rai, B.K. Lee, H. Karlsson, The association of paternal IQ with autism spectrum disorders and its comorbidities: a population-based cohort study, Journal of the American Academy of Child and Adolescent Psychiatry 59 (3) (2020) 410–421.

[74] B. Roozendaal, J.L. McGaugh, Memory modulation, Behavioral Neuroscience 125 (6) (2011) 797.

[75] J. Seale, S. Wood, H. Atkinson, E. Bate, S. Lightman, C. Ingram, et al., Gonadectomy reverses the sexually diergic patterns of circadian and stress-induced hypothalamic-pituitary-adrenal axis activity in male and female rats, Journal of Neuroendocrinology 16 (6) (2004) 516–524.

[76] H. Gardener, D. Spiegelman, S.L. Buka, Perinatal and neonatal risk factors for autism: a comprehensive meta-analysis, Pediatrics 128 (2) (2011) 344–355.

[77] M. Smallwood, A. Sareen, E. Baker, R. Hannusch, E. Kwessi, T. Williams, Increased risk of autism development in children whose mothers experienced birth complications or received labor and delivery drugs, ASN Neuro 8 (4) (2016) 1759091416659742.

[78] X. Wang, J. Li, D. Liu, Effects of epidural analgesia exposure during parturition on autism spectrum disorder in newborns: A systematic review and meta-analysis based on cohort study, Frontiers in Psychiatry 13 (2022) 974596.

[79] I.C. Lee, Y.H. Wang, J.Y. Chiou, J.C.C. Wei, Perinatal factors in newborn are insidious risk factors for childhood autism spectrum disorders: a population-based study, Journal of Autism and Developmental Disorders 52 (1) (2022) 52–60.

[80] T. Zhang, A. Sidorchuk, L. Sevilla-Cermeño, A. Vilaplana-Pérez, Z. Chang, H. Larsson, et al., Association of cesarean delivery with risk of neurodevelopmental and psychiatric disorders in the offspring: a systematic review and meta-analysis, JAMA Network Open 2 (8) (2019) e1910236.

[81] C. Crump, J. Sundquist, K. Sundquist, Preterm or early term birth and risk of autism, Pediatrics 148 (3) (2021).

[82] C.L. Herrera, K. Maiti, R. Smith, Preterm birth and corticotrophin-releasing hormone as a placental clock, Endocrinology 164 (2) (2023) bqac206.

[83] Elevated serum neurotensin and CRH levels in children with autistic spectrum disorders and tail-chasing Bull Terriers with a phenotype similar to autism, Translational Psychiatry 4 (10) (2014) e466.

[84] K. Iwata, H. Matsuzaki, T. Miyachi, C. Shimmura, S. Suda, K.J. Tsuchiya, et al., Investigation of the serum levels of anterior pituitary hormones in male children with autism, Molecular Autism 2 (2011) 1–6.

[85] S. Tordjman, P.A. McBride, M.E. Hertzig, M.E. Snow, G.M. Anderson, L.M. Hall, et al., Plasma β-endorphin, adrenocorticotropin hormone, and cortisol in autism, Journal of Child Psychology and Psychiatry 38 (6) (1997) 705–715.

[86] J.M. Ćurin, J. Terzić, Z.B. Petković, L. Zekan, I.M. Terzić, I.M. Šušnjara, Lower cortisol and higher ACTH levels in individuals with autism, Journal of Autism and Developmental Disorders 33 (2003) 443–448.

[87] R.T. Hamza, D.H. Hewedi, M.A. Ismail, Basal and adrenocorticotropic hormone stimulated plasma cortisol levels among Egyptian autistic children: relation to disease severity, Italian Journal of Pediatrics 36 (2010) 1–6.

[88] P. Tani, N. Lindberg, V. Matto, B. Appelberg, T. Nieminen-von Wendt, L. von Wendt, et al., Higher plasma ACTH levels in adults with Asperger syndrome, Journal of Psychosomatic Research 58 (6) (2005) 533–536.

[89] T. Eilam-Stock, P. Xu, M. Cao, X. Gu, E. Van Dam NT Anagnostou, et al., Abnormal autonomic and associated brain activities during rest in autism spectrum disorder, Brain 137 (1) (2014) 153–171.

[90] E. Neuhaus, R.A. Bernier, T.P. Beauchaine, Children with autism show altered autonomic adaptation to novel and familiar social partners, Autism Research 9 (5) (2016) 579–591.

[91] B.A. Ellenbroek, H.K. Sengul, Autism spectrum disorders: Autonomic alterations with a special focus on the heart, Heart and Mind 1 (2) (2017) 78–83.

[92] E.E. Condy, A. Scarpa, B.H. Friedman, Respiratory sinus arrhythmia predicts restricted repetitive behavior severity, Journal of Autism and Developmental Disorders 47 (2017) 2795–2804.
[93] T.C. Theoharides, R. Doyle, K. Francis, P. Conti, D. Kalogeromitros, Novel therapeutic targets for autism, Trends in Pharmacological Sciences 29 (8) (2008) 375–382.
[94] B. Gesundheit, J.P. Rosenzweig, D. Naor, B. Lerer, D.A. Zachor, V. Procházka, et al., Immunological and autoimmune considerations of Autism Spectrum Disorders, Journal of Autoimmunity 44 (2013) 1–7.
[95] Y.X. Dai, Y.H. Tai, Y.T. Chang, T.J. Chen, M.H. Chen, Increased risk of atopic diseases in the siblings of patients with autism spectrum disorder: a nationwide population-based cohort study, Journal of Autism and Developmental Disorders 49 (2019) 4626–4633.
[96] L.W. Wang, D.J. Tancredi, D.W. Thomas, The prevalence of gastrointestinal problems in children across the United States with autism spectrum disorders from families with multiple affected members, Journal of Developmental & Behavioral Pediatrics 32 (5) (2011) 351–360.
[97] A. Sadik, C. Dardani, P. Pagoni, A. Havdahl, E. Stergiakouli, iPSYCH Autism Spectrum Disorder Working Group Grove Jakob 14 15 16 17, et al., Parental inflammatory bowel disease and autism in children, Nature Medicine 28 (7) (2022) 1406–1411.
[98] Å.V.Keita, Corticotropin-releasing hormone (CRH) regulates macromolecular permeability via mast cells in normal human colonic biopsies in vitro, Gut 57 (1) (2008) 50–58.
[99] T. Kozicz, A. Korosi, C. Korsman, L. Groenink, J. Veening, J. van Der Gugten, et al., Urocortin expression in the Edinger-Westphal nucleus is down-regulated in transgenic mice overexpressing neuronal corticotropin-releasing factor, Neuroscience 123 (3) (2004) 589–594.
[100] J. Reaven, The treatment of anxiety symptoms in youth with high-functioning autism spectrum disorders: Developmental considerations for parents, Brain Research 1380 (2011) 255–263.
[101] A.L. Roberts, K.C. Koenen, K. Lyall, A. Ascherio, M.G. Weisskopf, Women's posttraumatic stress symptoms and autism spectrum disorder in their children, Research in Autism Spectrum Disorders 8 (6) (2014) 608–616.
[102] J. Marinović-Ćurin, I. Marinović-Terzić, Z. Bujas-Petković, L. Zekan, V. Škrabić, Z. Đogaš, et al., Slower cortisol response during ACTH stimulation test in autistic children, European Child & Adolescent Psychiatry 17 (2008) 39–43.
[103] C.J. Yang, H.P. Tan, F.Y. Yang, H.P. Wang, C.L. Liu, H.Z. He, et al., The cortisol, serotonin and oxytocin are associated with repetitive behavior in autism spectrum disorder, Research in Autism Spectrum Disorders 18 (2015) 12–20.
[104] S. Varala, R. George, L. Mathew, P. Russell, B. Koshy, S.P. Oommen, et al., The diagnostic value of congenital and nevoid cutaneous lesions associated with autism Spectrum disorders in Indian children-a case-control study, Indian Dermatology Online Journal 12 (1) (2021) 84–89.
[105] F. Sandru, M.C. Dumitrascu, S.E. Albu, M. Carsote, A. Valea, Hyperpigmentation and ACTH–an overview of literature, Romanian Medical Journal 66 (4) (2019) 309–312.
[106] T. Hirvikoski, E. Mittendorfer-Rutz, M. Boman, H. Larsson, P. Lichtenstein, S. Bölte, Premature mortality in autism spectrum disorder, British Journal of Psychiatry 208 (3) (2016) 232–238.
[107] R. Raghavan, B. Zuckerman, X. Hong, G. Wang, Y Ji, D. Paige, et al., Fetal and infancy growth pattern, cord and early childhood plasma leptin, and development of autism spectrum disorder in the Boston birth cohort, Autism Research 11 (10) (2018) 1416–1431.
[108] D. Yalnizoglu, G. Haliloglu, G. Turanli, A. Cila, M. Topcu, Neurologic outcome in patients with MRI pattern of damage typical for neonatal hypoglycemia, Brain and Development 29 (5) (2007) 285–292.
[109] P.D. Wadhwa, T.J. Garite, M. Porto, L. Glynn, A. Chicz-DeMet, C. Dunkel-Schetter, et al., Placental corticotropin-releasing hormone (CRH), spontaneous preterm birth, and fetal growth restriction: a prospective investigation, American Journal of Obstetrics and Gynecology 191 (4) (2004) 1063–1069.

[110] A. Imperatore, P. Florio, P.B. Torres, M. Torricelli, L. Galleri, P. Toti, et al., Urocortin 2 and urocortin 3 are expressed by the human placenta, deciduas, and fetal membranes, American Journal of Obstetrics and Gynecology 195 (1) (2006) 288–295.
[111] J. Rubenstein, M.M. Merzenich, Model of autism: increased ratio of excitation/inhibition in key neural systems, Genes, Brain and Behavior 2 (5) (2003) 255–267.
[112] M.F. Casanova, The minicolumnopathy of autism, in: Recent Advances on the Modular Organization of the Cortex, Springer, 2015, pp. 225–237.
[113] C. Karns, H. Davis, R. Ziccardi, R. Carper, Z. Tigue, H. Chisum, et al., Unusual brain growth patterns in early life in patients with autistic disorder: an MRI study, Neurology 57 (2) (2001) 245–254.
[114] E. Courchesne, R. Carper, N. Akshoomoff, Evidence of brain overgrowth in the first year of life in autism, JAMA 290 (3) (2003) 337–344.
[115] J.L. Mills, M.L. Hediger, C.A. Molloy, G.P. Chrousos, P. Manning-Courtney, K.F. Yu, et al., Elevated levels of growth-related hormones in autism and autism spectrum disorder, Clinical Endocrinology 67 (2) (2007) 230–237.
[116] K. Chawarska, D. Campbell, L. Chen, F. Shic, A. Klin, J. Chang, Early generalized overgrowth in boys with autism, Archives of General Psychiatry 68 (10) (2011) 1021–1031.
[117] C.C. Green, C. Dissanayake, D.Z. Loesch, M. Bui, J. Barbaro, Skeletal growth dysregulation in australian male infants and toddlers with autism spectrum disorder, Autism Research 11 (6) (2018) 846–856.
[118] I. Dinstein, S. Haar, S. Atsmon, H. Schtaerman, No evidence of early head circumference enlargements in children later diagnosed with autism in Israel, Molecular Autism 8 (1) (2017) 15.
[119] Q. Zhong, S. Sridhar, L. Ruan, K.H. Ding, D. Xie, K. Insogna, et al., Multiple melanocortin receptors are expressed in bone cells, Bone 36 (5) (2005) 820–831.
[120] M.K. Belmonte, G. Allen, A. Beckel-Mitchener, L.M. Boulanger, R.A. Carper, S.J. Webb, Autism and abnormal development of brain connectivity, Journal of Neuroscience 24 (42) (2004) 9228–9231.
[121] E. Conti, S. Calderoni, V. Marchi, F. Muratori, G. Cioni, A. Guzzetta, The first 1000 days of the autistic brain: a systematic review of diffusion imaging studies, Frontiers in Human Neuroscience 9 (2015) 159.
[122] J.P. Pillion, D. Boatman-Reich, B. Gordon, Auditory brainstem pathology in autism spectrum disorder: a review, Cognitive and Behavioral Neurology 31 (2) (2018) 53–78.
[123] Z.B. Kaplan, E.N. Pearce, S.Y. Lee, H.M. Shin, R.J. Schmidt, Maternal Thyroid Dysfunction During Pregnancy as an Etiologic Factor in Autism Spectrum Disorder: Challenges and Opportunities for Research, Thyroid 34 (2) (2024) 144–157.
[124] J. Rowland, C.A. Wilson, The association between gestational diabetes and ASD and ADHD: a systematic review and meta-analysis, Scientific Reports 11 (1) (2021) 5136.
[125] M.H. Chen, S.J. Tsai, Y.M. Bai, K.L. Huang, T.P. Su, T.J. Chen, et al., Type 1 diabetes mellitus and risks of major psychiatric disorders: A nationwide population-based cohort study, Diabetes & Metabolism 48 (1) (2022) 101319.
[126] S. Liu, R. Kuja-Halkola, H. Larsson, P. Lichtenstein, J.F. Ludvigsson, A.M. Svensson, et al., Poor glycaemic control is associated with increased risk of neurodevelopmental disorders in childhood-onset type 1 diabetes: a population-based cohort study, Diabetologia 64 (4) (2021) 767–777.
[127] M. Manco, S. Guerrera, L. Ravà, M. Ciofi degli Atti, S. Di Vara, G. Valeri, et al., Cross-sectional investigation of insulin resistance in youths with autism spectrum disorder. Any role for reduced brain glucose metabolism?, Translational Psychiatry 11 (1) (2021) 229.
[128] A.M. Sheikh, M. Malik, G. Wen, A. Chauhan, V. Chauhan, C.X. Gong, et al., BDNF-Akt-Bcl2 antiapoptotic signaling pathway is compromised in the brain of autistic subjects, Journal of Neuroscience Research 88 (12) (2010) 2641–2647.
[129] G. Tang, K. Gudsnuk, S.H. Kuo, M.L. Cotrina, G. Rosoklija, A. Sosunov, et al., Loss of mTOR-dependent macroautophagy causes autistic-like synaptic pruning deficits, Neuron 83 (5) (2014) 1131–1143.

[130] C. Nicolini, Y. Ahn, B. Michalski, J.M. Rho, M. Fahnestock, Decreased mTOR signaling pathway in human idiopathic autism and in rats exposed to valproic acid, Acta Neuropathologica Communications 3 (2015) 1–13.
[131] A.J. Russo, Decreased phosphorylated protein kinase B (Akt) in individuals with autism associated with high epidermal growth factor receptor (EGFR) and low gamma-aminobutyric acid (GABA), Biomarker Insights 10 (2015), BMI-S21946.
[132] V.H. Gazestani, T. Pramparo, S. Nalabolu, B.P. Kellman, S. Murray, L. Lopez, et al., A perturbed gene network containing PI3K–AKT, RAS–ERK and WNT–β-catenin pathways in leukocytes is linked to ASD genetics and symptom severity, Nature Neuroscience 22 (10) (2019) 1624–1634.
[133] G. Bjørklund, N.A. Meguid, M.A. El-Bana, A.A. Tinkov, K. Saad, M. Dadar, et al., Oxidative stress in autism spectrum disorder, Molecular Neurobiology 57 (2020) 2314–2332.
[134] R.D. Maimburg, M. Vaeth, D.E. Schendel, B.H. Bech, J. Olsen, P. Thorsen, Neonatal jaundice: a risk factor for infantile autism?, Paediatric and Perinatal Epidemiology 22 (6) (2008) 562–568.
[135] M.L. Kujabi, J.P. Petersen, M.V. Pedersen, E.T. Parner, T.B. Henriksen, Neonatal jaundice and autism spectrum disorder: a systematic review and meta-analysis, Pediatric Research 90 (5) (2021) 934–949.
[136] H.Y. Lee, A. Ithnin, R.Z. Azma, A. Othman, A. Salvador, F.C. Cheah, Glucose-6-Phosphate dehydrogenase deficiency and neonatal hyperbilirubinemia: Insights on pathophysiology, diagnosis, and gene variants in disease heterogeneity, Frontiers in Pediatrics 10 (2022) 875877.
[137] M.D. Majewska, M. Hill, E. Urbanowicz, P. Rok-Bujko, P. Bieńkowski, I. Namysłowska, et al., Marked elevation of adrenal steroids, especially androgens, in saliva of prepubertal autistic children, European Child & Adolescent Psychiatry 23 (2014) 485–498.
[138] F. El-Baz, R.T. Hamza, M.S. Ayad, N.H. Mahmoud, Hyperandrogenemia in male autistic children and adolescents: relation to disease severity, International Journal of Adolescent Medicine and Health 26 (1) (2014) 79–84.
[139] M.H. Hassan, T. Desoky, H.M. Sakhr, R.H. Gabra, A.H. Bakri, Possible metabolic alterations among autistic male children: clinical and biochemical approaches, Journal of Molecular Neuroscience 67 (2019) 204–216.
[140] K. Janšáková, M. Hill, D. Čelárová, H. Celušáková, G. Repiská, M. Bičíková, et al., Alteration of the steroidogenesis in boys with autism spectrum disorders, Translational Psychiatry 10 (1) (2020) 340.
[141] F.S. Al-Zaid, A.F.A. Alhader, L.Y. Al-Ayadhi, A potential role for the adrenal gland in autism, Scientific Reports 11 (1) (2021) 17743.
[142] D.A. Geier, M.R. Geier, A prospective assessment of androgen levels in patients with autistic spectrum disorders: biochemical underpinnings and suggested therapies, Neuroendocrinology Letters 28 (5) (2007) 565–574.
[143] E. Schmidtova, S. Kelemenova, P. Celec, A. Ficek, D. Ostatnikova, Polymorphisms in genes involved in testosterone metabolism in Slovak autistic boys, The Endocrinologist 20 (5) (2010) 245–249.
[144] L. Ruta, E. Ingudomnukul, K. Taylor, B. Chakrabarti, S. Baron-Cohen, Increased serum androstenedione in adults with autism spectrum conditions, Psychoneuroendocrinology 36 (8) (2011) 1154–1163.
[145] F.S. Al-Zaid, A.A. Alhader, L.Y. Al-Ayadhi, Altered ghrelin levels in boys with autism: a novel finding associated with hormonal dysregulation, Scientific Reports 4 (1) (2014) 6478.
[146] D. Ostatnikova, A. Kubranska, V. Marcincakova, A. Pivovarciova, J. Babkova-Durdiakova, Neuroendocrine contribution to autism etiology, Act Nerv Super Rediviva 58 (3) (2016) 65–68.
[147] T.L. Procyshyn, M.V. Lombardo, M.C. Lai, B. Auyeung, S.K. Crockford, S. Baron-Cohen, et al., Effects of oxytocin administration on salivary sex hormone levels in autistic and neurotypical women, Molecular Autism 11 (2020) 1–11.

[148] R.A. Muscatello, E. Rafatjoo, K.K. Mirpuri, A. Kim, S. Vandekar, B.A. Corbett, Salivary testosterone in male and female youth with and without autism spectrum disorder: considerations of development, sex, and diagnosis, Molecular Autism 13 (1) (2022) 37.
[149] J. Croonenberghs, S. Van Grieken, A. Wauters, D. Van West, L. Brouw, M. Maes, et al., Serum testosterone concentration in male autistic youngsters, Neuroendocrinology Letters 31 (4) (2010) 483.
[150] P. Krajmer, M. Spajdel, P. Celec, D. Ostatníková, Relationship between salivary testosterone levels and empathizing/systemizing in Slovak boys with Asperger syndrome, Studia Psychologica 53 (3) (2011) 293.
[151] C.F. Sharpley, V. Bitsika, N.M. Andronicos, L.L. Agnew, Age-Related Variations in Comparative Testosterone Concentrations Between Boys with Autism Spectrum Disorder and their typically-Developing Peers: A Challenge to the 'Extreme Male Brain' Hypothesis of ASD, Journal of Developmental and Physical Disabilities 29 (2) (2017) 353–367.
[152] N. Sriram, P. Madaan, P. Malhi, N. Sachdeva, S. Negi, J. Das, et al., Evaluation of Hyperandrogenism in Children with Autism Spectrum Disorder, Indian Journal of Pediatrics 89 (7) (2022) 717–719.
[153] S. Baron-Cohen, A. Tsompanidis, B. Auyeung, B. Nørgaard-Pedersen, D.M. Hougaard, M. Abdallah, et al., Foetal oestrogens and autism, Molecular Psychiatry 25 (11) (2020) 2970–2978.
[154] A.J. Whitehouse, E. Mattes, M.T. Maybery, C. Dissanayake, M. Sawyer, R.M. Jones, et al., Perinatal testosterone exposure and autistic-like traits in the general population: a longitudinal pregnancy-cohort study, Journal of Neurodevelopmental Disorders 4 (2012) 1–12.
[155] K.T. Kung, D. Spencer, V. Pasterski, S. Neufeld, V. Glover, T.G.O'Connor, et al., No relationship between prenatal androgen exposure and autistic traits: convergent evidence from studies of children with congenital adrenal hyperplasia and of amniotic testosterone concentrations in typically developing children, Journal of Child Psychology and Psychiatry 57 (12) (2016) 1455–1462.
[156] B. Auyeung, J. Ahluwalia, L. Thomson, K. Taylor, G. Hackett, K.J.O'Donnell, et al., Prenatal versus postnatal sex steroid hormone effects on autistic traits in children at 18 to 24 months of age, Molecular Autism 3 (1) (2012) 17.
[157] J. Saenz, G.M. Alexander, Postnatal testosterone levels and disorder relevant behavior in the second year of life, Biological Psychology 94 (1) (2013) 152–159.
[158] K.T. Kung, M. Constantinescu, W.V. Browne, R.M. Noorderhaven, M. Hines, No relationship between early postnatal testosterone concentrations and autistic traits in 18 to 30-month-old children, Molecular Autism 7 (1) (2016) 15.
[159] F.M. Metwally, H. Rashad, H.M. Zeidan, A.F. Hashish, Impact of bisphenol A on gonadotropic hormone levels in children with autism spectrum disorders, Indian Journal of Clinical Biochemistry 35 (2020) 205–210.
[160] K. Kosidou, C. Dalman, L. Widman, S. Arver, B. Lee, C. Magnusson, et al., Maternal polycystic ovary syndrome and the risk of autism spectrum disorders in the offspring: a population-based nationwide study in Sweden, Molecular Psychiatry 21 (10) (2016) 1441.
[161] R.S. Rotem, V.T. Nguyen, G. Chodick, M. Davidovitch, V. Shalev, R. Hauser, et al., Associations of maternal androgen-related conditions with risk of autism spectrum disorder in progeny and mediation by cardiovascular, metabolic, and fertility factors, American Journal of Epidemiology 190 (4) (2021) 600–610.
[162] X.J. Xu, X.J. Shou, J. Li, M.X. Jia, J.S. Zhang, Y. Guo, et al., Mothers of autistic children: lower plasma levels of oxytocin and Arg-vasopressin and a higher level of testosterone, PLoS ONE 8 (9) (2013) e74849.
[163] K.J. Varcin, G.A. Alvares, M. Uljarević, A.J. Whitehouse, Prenatal maternal stress events and phenotypic outcomes in Autism Spectrum Disorder, Autism Research 10 (11) (2017) 1866–1877.
[164] J. Seebeck, K.K. Sznajder, K.H. Kjerulff, The association between prenatal psychosocial factors and autism spectrum disorder in offspring at 3 years: a prospective cohort study, Social Psychiatry and Psychiatric Epidemiology (2023) 1–11.

[165] H.Ó. Atladóttir, P. Thorsen, L. Østergaard, D.E. Schendel, S. Lemcke, M. Abdallah, et al., Maternal infection requiring hospitalization during pregnancy and autism spectrum disorders, Journal of Autism and Developmental Disorders 40 (2010) 1423–1430.
[166] D.J. Walder, D.P. Laplante, A. Sousa-Pires, F. Veru, A. Brunet, S. King, Prenatal maternal stress predicts autism traits in 61/2 year-old children: Project Ice Storm, Psychiatry Research 219 (2) (2014) 353–360.
[167] E.S. Barrett, L.E. Parlett, S. Sathyanarayana, F. Liu, J.B. Redmon, C. Wang, et al., Prenatal exposure to stressful life events is associated with masculinized anogenital distance (AGD) in female infants, Physiology & Behavior 114 (2013) 14–20.
[168] D. Glidden, W.P. Bouman, B.A. Jones, J. Arcelus, Gender dysphoria and autism spectrum disorder: A systematic review of the literature, Sexual Medicine Reviews 4 (1) (2016) 3–14.
[169] E. Weir, C. Allison, S. Baron-Cohen, The sexual health, orientation, and activity of autistic adolescents and adults, Autism Research 14 (11) (2021) 2342–2354.
[170] C.E. Rudolph, A. Lundin, J.W. Åhs, C. Dalman, K. Kosidou, Brief report: Sexual orientation in individuals with autistic traits: Population based study of 47,000 adults in Stockholm County, Journal of Autism and Developmental Disorders 48 (2018) 619–624.
[171] S. Bejerot, J.M. Eriksson, S. Bonde, K. Carlström, M.B. Humble, E. Eriksson, The extreme male brain revisited: gender coherence in adults with autism spectrum disorder, British Journal of Psychiatry 201 (2) (2012) 116–123.
[172] S.Z. Gilani, D.W. Tan, S.N. Russell-Smith, M.T. Maybery, A. Mian, P.R. Eastwood, et al., Sexually dimorphic facial features vary according to level of autistic-like traits in the general population, Journal of Neurodevelopmental Disorders 7 (1) (2015) 14.
[173] D.W. Tan, S.Z. Gilani, M.T. Maybery, A. Mian, A. Hunt, M. Walters, et al., Hypermasculinised facial morphology in boys and girls with Autism Spectrum Disorder and its association with symptomatology, Scientific Reports 7 (1) (2017) 9348.
[174] A.E. Calogero, N. Burrello, P. Negri-Cesi, L. Papale, M.A. Palumbo, A. Cianci, et al., Effects of corticotropin-releasing hormone on ovarian estrogen production in vitro, Endocrinology 137 (10) (1996) 4161–4166.
[175] M. De Cock, Y.G. Maas, M. Van De Bor, Does perinatal exposure to endocrine disruptors induce autism spectrum and attention deficit hyperactivity disorders? Review, Acta Pædiatrica 101 (8) (2012) 811–818.
[176] J.B. Hansen, N. Bilenberg, C.A.G. Timmermann, R.C. Jensen, H. Frederiksen, A.M. Andersson, et al., Prenatal exposure to bisphenol A and autistic- and ADHD-related symptoms in children aged 2 and5 years from the Odense Child Cohort, Environmental Health 20 (2021) 1–12.
[177] C. Phumsatitpong, S.M. Moenter, Estradiol-dependent stimulation and suppression of gonadotropin-releasing hormone neuron firing activity by corticotropin-releasing hormone in female mice, Endocrinology 159 (1) (2018) 414–425.
[178] D. Schöttle, P. Briken, O. Tüscher, D. Turner, Sexuality in autism: hypersexual and paraphilic behavior in women and men with high-functioning autism spectrum disorder, Dialogues in Clinical Neuroscience 19 (4) (2017) 381–393.
[179] R. Feldman, O. Golan, Y. Hirschler-Guttenberg, S. Ostfeld-Etzion, O. Zagoory-Sharon, Parent–child interaction and oxytocin production in pre-schoolers with autism spectrum disorder, British Journal of Psychiatry 205 (2) (2014) 107–112.
[180] S. John, A.V. Jaeggi, Oxytocin levels tend to be lower in autistic children: A meta-analysis of 31 studies, Autism 25 (8) (2021) 2152–2161.
[181] S. Yang, X. Dong, X. Guo, Y. Han, H. Song, L. Gao, et al., Serum oxytocin levels and an oxytocin receptor gene polymorphism (rs2254298) indicate social deficits in children and adolescents with autism spectrum disorders, Frontiers in Neuroscience 11 (2017) 230653.
[182] S. Phaneuf, G. Asboth, M. Carrasco, G. Europe-Finner, F. Saji, T. Kimura, et al., The desensitization of oxytocin receptors in human myometrial cells is accompanied by down-regulation of oxytocin receptor messenger RNA, Journal of Endocrinology 154 (1) (1997) 7–18.

[183] E. Friedlander, O. Feldstein, D. Mankuta, M. Yaari, A. Harel-Gadassi, R.P. Ebstein, et al., Social impairments among children perinatally exposed to oxytocin or oxytocin receptor antagonist, Early Human Development 106 (2017) 13–18.
[184] O. Boucher, J. Julvez, M. Guxens, E. Arranz, J. Ibarluzea, M. Sanchez de Miguel, et al., Association between breastfeeding duration and cognitive development, autistic traits and ADHD symptoms: a multicenter study in Spain, Pediatric Research 81 (3) (2017) 434–442.
[185] P.T. Tseng, Y.W. Chen, B. Stubbs, A.F. Carvalho, P. Whiteley, C.H. Tang, et al., Maternal breastfeeding and autism spectrum disorder in children: A systematic review and meta-analysis, Nutritional Neuroscience 22 (5) (2019) 354–362.
[186] G.N. Soke, M. Maenner, G. Windham, E. Moody, J. Kaczaniuk, C. DiGuiseppi, et al., Association between breastfeeding initiation and duration and autism spectrum disorder in preschool children enrolled in the study to explore early development, Autism Research 12 (5) (2019) 816–829.
[187] J. Chen, E. Strodl, L.H. Huang, J.Y. Chen, X.C. Liu, J.H. Yang, et al., Associations between prenatal education, breastfeeding and autistic-like behaviors in pre-schoolers, Children 8 (2) (2021) 124.
[188] M.S. Abd Elmaksoud, O. Aly, M. Abd Elfatah, A. Mahfouz, Breastfeeding and autism spectrum disorder: a cross-sectional study from Egypt, Alexandria Journal of Pediatrics 35 (1) (2022) 59–66.
[189] X. Xiang, T. Yang, J. Chen, L. Chen, Y. Dai, J. Zhang, et al., Association of feeding patterns in infancy with later autism symptoms and neurodevelopment: a national multicentre survey, BMC Psychiatry 23 (1) (2023) 174.
[190] X.L. Zhan, N. Pan, S. Karatela, L. Shi, X. Wang, Z.Y. Liu, et al., Infant feeding practices and autism spectrum disorder in US children aged 2–5 years: the national survey of children's health (NSCH) 2016–2020, International Breastfeeding Journal 18 (1) (2023) 41.
[191] P.M. Plotsky, M.J. Meaney, Early postnatal experience alters hypothalamic corticotropin-releasing factor (CRF) mRNA, median eminence CRF content and stress-induced release in adult rats, Molecular Brain Research 18 (3) (1993) 195–200.
[192] S. Avishai-Eliner, M. Eghbal-Ahmadi, E. Tabachnik, K.L. Brunson, T.Z. Baram, Down-regulation of hypothalamic corticotropin-releasing hormone messenger ribonucleic acid (mRNA) precedes early-life experience-induced changes in hippocampal glucocorticoid receptor mRNA, Endocrinology 142 (1) (2001) 89–97.
[193] M.D. Kaiser, D.Y.J. Yang, A.C. Voos, R.H. Bennett, I. Gordon, C. Pretzsch, et al., Brain mechanisms for processing affective (and nonaffective) touch are atypical in autism, Cerebral Cortex 26 (6) (2016) 2705–2714.
[194] R.F. Lucas, A. Cutler, Dysregulated breastfeeding behaviors in children later diagnosed with autism, The Journal of Perinatal Education 24 (3) (2015) 171.
[195] T. Kara, Ö. Alpgan, Nursing personality and features in children with autism spectrum disorder aged 0–2: an exploratory case-control study, Nutritional Neuroscience 25 (6) (2022) 1200–1208.
[196] M. Peries, F. Duhr, M.C. Picot, B. Heude, J.Y. Bernard, A. Baghdadli, Breastfeeding is not a risk factor for clinical severity in Autism spectrum disorder in children from the ELENA cohort, Scientific Reports 13 (1) (2023) 816.
[197] C. Varma, N. de Souza, Feeding behaviours in infancy of children later diagnosed with autism spectrum disorder, International Journal of Contemporary Pediatrics 10 (8) (2023) 1280.
[198] M. van't Hof, W.A. Ester, I. van Berckelaer-Onnes, M.H. Hillegers, H.W. Hoek, P.W. Jansen, Do early-life eating habits predict later autistic traits? Results from a population-based study, Appetite 156 (2021) 104976.
[199] A. Klockars, A.S. Levine, P.K. Olszewski, Central oxytocin and food intake: focus on macronutrient-driven reward, Frontiers in Neuroendocrinology 6 (2015) 136509.
[200] G.L. Wallace, C. Llewellyn, A. Fildes, A. Ronald, Autism spectrum disorder and food neophobia: clinical and subclinical links, The American Journal of Clinical Nutrition 108 (4) (2018) 701–707.

[201] J.M. Yabut, J.D. Crane, A.E. Green, D.J. Keating, W.I. Khan, G.R. Steinberg, Emerging roles for serotonin in regulating metabolism: new implications for an ancient molecule, Endocrine Reviews 40 (4) (2019) 1092–1107.
[202] The serotonin system in autism spectrum disorder: From biomarker to animal models, Neuroscience 321 (2016) 24–41.
[203] J. Lin, M.A. Costa, V.L. Rezende, R.R. Nascimento, P.G. Ambrósio, K. Madeira, et al., Risk factors and clinical profile of autism spectrum disorder in southern Brazil, Journal of Psychiatric Research 169 (2024) 105–112.
[204] E. Lazo-Wasem, Pituitary ACTH levels during adrenal involution following thiouracil, Proceedings of the Society for Experimental Biology and Medicine 103 (2) (1960) 300–302.
[205] B. Miśkowiak, A. Kasprzak, L. Malendowicz, Comparative stereological studies on the effects of long term CRF and ACTH treatment on the cortex of the suprarenal gland, Journal of Anatomy 146 (1986) 167.
[206] A.K. Hannerfors, C. Hellgren, D. Schijven, S.I. Iliadis, E. Comasco, A. Skalkidou, et al., Treatment with serotonin reuptake inhibitors during pregnancy is associated with elevated corticotropin-releasing hormone levels, Psychoneuroendocrinology 58 (2015) 104–113.
[207] M. Sandbank, K. Bottema-Beutel, S. Crowley, M. Cassidy, K. Dunham, J.I. Feldman, et al., Project AIM: Autism intervention meta-analysis for studies of young children, Psychological Bulletin 146 (1) (2020) 1.
[208] H.S. Futch, K.N. McFarland, B.D. Moore, M.Z. Kuhn, B.I. Giasson, T.B. Ladd, et al., An anti-CRF antibody suppresses the HPA axis and reverses stress-induced phenotypes, Journal of Experimental Medicine 216 (11) (2019) 2479–2491.
[209] A. Biason-Lauber, W.L. Miller, A.V. Pandey, C.E. Flück, Of marsupials and men: 'Backdoor' dihydrotestosterone synthesis in male sexual differentiation, Molecular and Cellular Endocrinology 371 (1–2) (2013) 124–132.
[210] T.D. Lund, L.R. Hinds, R.J. Handa, The androgen 5α-dihydrotestosterone and its metabolite 5α-androstan-3β, 17β-diol inhibit the hypothalamo–pituitary–adrenal response to stress by acting through estrogen receptor β-expressing neurons in the hypothalamus, The Journal of Neuroscience 26 (5) (2006) 1448–1456.
[211] R.J. Handa, A.E. Kudwa, N.C. Donner, R.F. McGivern, R. Brown, Central 5-alpha reduction of testosterone is required for testosterone's inhibition of the hypothalamo-pituitary–adrenal axis response to restraint stress in adult male rats, Brain Research (1529) (2013) 74–82.
[212] Kitay Ji, M.D. Coyne, N.H. Swygert, Effects of hypophysectomy and administration of cortisone or ACTH on adrenal 5α-reductase activity and steroid production, Endocrinology 89 (2) (1971) 432–438.
[213] M. Lee, T. Shnitko, S. Blue, A. Kaucher, A. Winchell, D. Erikson, et al., Labeled oxytocin administered via the intranasal route reaches the brain in rhesus macaques, Nature Communications 11 (1) (2020) 2783.
[214] W. Pan, A.J. Kastin, Urocortin and the brain, Progress in Neurobiology 84 (2) (2008) 148–156.
[215] K. Yenkoyan, A. Grigoryan, K. Fereshetyan, D. Yepremyan, Advances in understanding the pathophysiology of autism spectrum disorders, Behavioural Brain Research 331 (2017) 92–101.
[216] S. Baron-Cohen, Empathizing, systemizing, and the extreme male brain theory of autism, Progress in Brain Research 186 (2010) 167–175.
[217] C.S. Carter, Sex differences in oxytocin and vasopressin: implications for autism spectrum disorders?, Behavioural Brain Research 176 (1) (2007) 170–186.
[218] A. Dickinson, M. Jones, E. Milne, Measuring neural excitation and inhibition in autism: Different approaches, different findings and different interpretations, Brain Research (1648) (2016) 277–289.
[219] E. Courchesne, V.H. Gazestani, N.E. Lewis, Prenatal origins of ASD: the when, what, and how of ASD development, Trends in Neurosciences 43 (5) (2020) 326–342.

[220] C. Wong, T. Price, L. Schalkwyk, R. Plomin, J. Mill, Methylomic analysis of monozygotic twins discordant for autism spectrum disorder and related behavioural traits, Molecular Psychiatry 19 (4) (2014) 495–503.
[221] M.G. Frasch, B.J. Yoon, D.L. Helbing, G. Snir, M.C. Antonelli, R. Bauer, Autism spectrum disorder: a neuro-immunometabolic hypothesis of the developmental origins, Biology 12 (7) (2023) 914.

Chapter 2

A CRH2-CRH1 theory of anorexia and bulimia

2.1 Introduction

Anorexia nervosa (AN) and bulimia nervosa (BN) are the two major eating disorders [1,2]. The diagnostic criteria for AN include reduced food intake that leads to significant low body weight, "intense fear of gaining weight" or behaviors that oppose weight gain, mainly purging (intentional vomiting, usage of laxatives and diuretics) and excessive exercise, and "disturbed perception of body weight" (e.g., lack of insight on current low weight). The criteria for BN include recurrent binge eating episodes (eating larger amounts than normal in a short time, with a sense of lack of control over eating), and purging behavior, exercise, or fasting. Many AN patients also show binge eating.

Like almost all psychiatric disorders, the etiology of AN and BN is currently not understood [1–4]. Patient behavior is known to be influenced by biological factors rather than being a personal choice [3], but there is no theory explaining what these factors are.

Here I present the first theory that explains AN and BN (T*AB). The theory is complete is the sense that it explains their etiology, symptoms, and pathophysiology. T*AB is supported by strong empirical biological evidence, and implies several novel treatment directions.

Theory overview. AN and BN result from chronic stress-induced release of corticotropin-releasing hormone (CRH). This can be due to stress experienced by the patient, or to (epi)genetic parental transmission of the effects of past stress. Moderate levels of CRH activate the CRH1 receptor, whole main role is to respond to energy-deficient states by increasing blood glucose and food intake and stimulating the sympathetic nervous system (SNS). High CRH levels activate the CRH2 receptor, whose role is to support energy excess states by reducing food intake, storing glucose in tissue, and restraining the SNS. CRH2 recruits serotonin (SER) to achieve its function, mainly for suppressing gut motility and food intake.

The effects of CRH on food intake trivially explain the food intake aspects of AN and BN. Regarding purging behavior, it is done in order to reduce the nausea induced by excessive gut SER and CRH2. Excessive exercise in AN is done in order to recruit epinephrine (EPI) and norepinephrine (NEP), both suppressed by CRH2. Patients claim to be too fat because they feel that something is wrong

The Science of the Brain. https://doi.org/10.1016/B978-0-44-345008-2.00008-4

with their adipose tissue, which stems from excessive SER and CRH activity that mimics inflammatory responses. T*AB is supported by strong evidence regarding CRH, SER, and the autonomic nervous system in animal models and patients, and by established patient data.

2.2 Theory

2.2.1 CRH, CRH1, CRH2, serotonin

General. CRH is best known for its role in the hypothalamic-pituitary-adrenal (HPA) axis, where stress induces CRH release from the hypothalamus paraventricular nucleus (PVH), CRH acts on CRH1 receptors in the pituitary to stimulate ACTH release, which induces glucocorticoid (GC, cortisol in humans) release from the adrenals. CRH is also synthesized in other body tissues, including the skin, gut, the reproductive and immune systems [5], brain [6], and adipose tissue [7].

CRH acts via two G protein-coupled receptors, CRH1 and CRH2, which both bind Gs (to stimulate cAMP, PKA) and also Gi/o and Gq [8]. The affinity of CRH to CRH1 is greater. Following ligand binding, the receptors show sustained signaling from endosomes, allowing chronic signaling beyond the original release event [8]. CRH2 is also activated by urocortins, a family of ligands that do not have a major role in AN and BN.

CRH1. The role of CRH1 is well known. Besides its stimulation of GC release, it activates the SNS [9], to increase blood glucose, promote food intake, and induce other sympathetic responses (e.g., increased heart rate, lipolysis, thermogenesis). Note that it is not accurate to view CRH1 as triggering the response to all types of stress, but as responding to *deficiency* states, including low glucose, low temperature (cold), and low oxygen (hypoxia) [10]. Acute social stress increases the metabolic demands from the body, creating a deficiency stress state.

CRH2. CRH2 is known to oppose many CRH1-induced effects, including appetite, anxiety, and depression [9]. In particular, its food intake suppression function is overwhelmingly supported [11]. It also suppresses adrenal EPI release done as part of the counter-regulatory responses to insulin-induced hypoglycemia [12], opposes thermogenesis [13], and promotes glucose uptake by tissue, including skeletal muscle [14] (at least partly insulin-independently), heart [15], brain [16], and adipose tissue [17]. This effect occurs mainly in high glucose levels, and can utilize insulin via direct action on beta cells [18]. In the gut, CRH2 slows gastric transit [19].

Serotonin. SER is present in most body tissues, including the gut, brain, heart, lung, skeletal muscle, adipose tissue, and the reproduction system [20]. The SER system is complex, and for our purposes it suffices to highlight the following facts. First, CRH2 recruits SER, promoting its synthesis [21] and release from dorsal raphe neurons [22] and gut enterochromaffin cells [23]. SER reciprocally activates PVH CRH neurons, via SER2c [24]. Second, SER is well-known to suppress food intake, an effect mediated by SER2c [25]. Eating carbohydrates enhances the synthesis and release of hypothalamus SER, which suppresses carbohydrate intake [26]. Third, the food intake suppression function of CRH2 is done, at least in part, via SER2c [27].

Fourth, SER is a major gut agent. The gut contains most of the body's SER, and SER is present in both mucosal enterochromaffin cells and in the enteric nervous system [28]. The former support reflexes that increase local motility to enhance absorption after feeding [29], while the latter slow gastric emptying and suppress intestinal motility [28] in response to glucose [30]. Gut glucose induces gut SER release via SER3 on gut vagal sensory neurons [31].

Finally, SER promotes insulin-independent glucose uptake by tissue [32], including adipose tissue [33], skeletal muscle [34] and liver, where it promotes glycogen synthesis [35]. Plasma SER and blood glucose levels show a positive correlation [36], and raphe obscurus and raphe pallidus SER activity diminish following insulin-induced hypoglycemia [37]. Most relevant to AN, SER promotes lipogenesis in white adipose tissue (WAT) and opposes its browning and thermogenesis [38–40].

SER has 14 different receptors, and can also produce results in the opposite direction to the above, depending on conditions [41]. What is important for our purposes here is that it is clearly recruited by and cooperates with CRH2 in fulfilling its function. A full theory of SER function will be presented elsewhere.

Summary. T*AB posits that *the role of CRH2 is to trigger responses to excess stress*, including high glucose and heat, but also prolonged social stress. As part of this role, it suppresses the responses to deficiency stress, including EPI release, thermogenesis, and food intake. This account of the role of CRH2 is a novel contribution of the present chapter. To achieve its role, CRH2 recruits SER, which suppresses food intake, slows gut motility, responds to high glucose, and promotes its gut absorption and storage in tissue. In particular, SER promotes the growth of white adipose tissue but opposes brown adipose tissue.

2.2.2 Anorexia nervosa (AN)

According to T*AB, *AN is caused by excessive CRH release that chronically activates CRH2 in the brain and other tissues*. Since the affinity of CRH1 to CRH is higher than that of CRH2, there would be tissues in which CRH1 is chronically activated as well. The symptoms induced by these fundamental biological effects are most likely enhanced by modern cultural and media influences. This section explains how stress, including social stress, can cause this state, and shows that this simple premise can explain the defining characteristics of the disorder. Other data are presented in the evidence section.

AN core cause: stress. As described above, CRH is recruited in states of metabolic deficiency or excess. This includes social stress (e.g., maternal separation, conspecific aggression, social defeat, sexual trauma), which produces a deficiency state because the organism initially needs more energy to address the situation, and is well-known to induce CRH release [42]. If the problem is not quickly resolved, CRH release continues and can chronically activate the lower affinity receptor CRH2.

Stress that occurs during sensitive developmental periods, such as early life and adolescence, can yield persistent changes in protein expression via epigenetic marks [43]. Moreover, epigenetic changes can be multigenerational, passed from parents to offspring [44]. It is well-supported that early life stress can persistently increase CRH, e.g., CSF CRH in non-human primates [45], and mRNA in rodents [46].

Thus, prolonged social stress (and other types of stress), especially during early life or adolescence, can create the optimal conditions for AN. Indeed, social pressure and stress are known to be precipitating factors for AN, and social difficulties are very common [4]. Traumatic experiences are common in moderate-severe AN patients, with 50% being at the cutoff threshold for PTSD (without being diagnosed) [47]. In one report, almost half of AN patients have suffered childhood sexual abuse [48].

Food intake. Suppression of food intake is one of the major functions of CRH2, cooperating with SER2c. The AN patient's brain receives a strong signal of nutrient excess, even if the real state is that of deficiency. CRH2 opposes the main agents that promote food intake, GCs and EPI, and CRH opposes neuropeptide Y, which is elevated in AN but whose effect is not that strong [2]. Adiponectin reflects the status of adipose tissue and is indeed elevated in underweight AN patients, but it is not a strong appetite stimulator [2]. Thus, there is no strong physiological biological signal that can offset the erroneous message conveyed by excessive CRH2 in AN.

Purging behavior. Chronic CRH2 induces chronically high SER in AN. In the gut, SER is known to induce nausea and the vomiting reflex, mainly via SER3 but also via other receptors [49]. This is consistent with SER's role in suppressing food intake and gut motility. CRH itself has also been hypothesized to be responsible for the cyclic vomiting syndrome [50]. Thus, excessive CRH-induced gut SER explains the urge to vomit in AN.

CRH is produced by colon enterochromaffin cells [51], and triggers inflammation via mast cell activation [52]. Mast cells can uptake, store and secrete SER and CRH [53]. CRH2 specifically increases gut inflammation following stressors [54]. SER also promotes gut inflammation [28]. Since the state of the gut (as that of any other tissue) is continuously reported to the brain via sensory neurons, AN patients experience a constant feeling that there is something wrong in the gut. Since gut carbohydrates induce SER release, this uncomfortable feeling is relieved when the gut is empty. This explains general purging behaviors in AN, and provides another explanation for food avoidance.

Body image. White adipose tissue has a population of mast cells [55], whose activation promotes chronic low inflammation and macrophage accumulation [56].

Since CRH greatly potentiates mast cell activation [57], and mast cells secrete SER and CRH [53], AN adipose tissue involves a continuous inflammation-like state, as in the gut. This state is reported to the brain via interoception pathways [58], a feeling that patients verbalize as "I am too fat" (they could say "something is wrong with my fat stores", but this sounds strange, as opposed to the former, which is generally accepted by society). Even though patients are not too fat, some processes that make people fat, namely SER-induced glucose uptake and lipogenesis, are indeed chronically active in their WAT.

Binge-eating type. AN patients are defined to be either of the restricting type or the binge-eating/purging type, depending on whether they have engaged in recurrent binge eating or purging episodes during the last 3 months [1].

According to T*AB, the basic active AN state involves CRH levels that are high enough to activate the lower affinity receptor CRH2. If CRH levels diminish for any reason but do not get to full recovery level, or if CRH2 gets desensitized, CRH would strongly activate the CRH1 receptor, which promotes food intake. This, along with other signals stemming from the person's state of deficiency, explains binge eating episodes. Indeed, more than 40% of the restrictive type show binging and purging at some point [59].

2.2.3 Bulimia nervosa

According to T*AB, BN is caused by CRH release that chronically activates the CRH1 receptor. CRH1 strongly promotes food intake, explaining binge-eating episodes. Since the effects of CRH on mast cell inflammation and transit time in the gut can be promoted by both CRH1 and CRH2 [60], chronic CRH1 explains purging behavior in BN in the same manner as in AN.

2.3 Evidence

This section presents strong evidence supporting T*AB.

Sex differences. AN and BN show female dominance (10:1 and 3:1 respectively). This has two reasons. First, estrogen excites PVH CRH neurons [61], and increases CRH synthesis [62]. One reason for this is that CRH is needed for birth, and increases 100-1000x in maternal serum from the 2nd pregnancy trimester onwards [63]. Second, testosterone decreases PVH CRH expression via androgen response element [64], reducing CRH secretion [65].

The ratio in AN is higher than that in BN because estrogen mainly acts on CRH2 [66,67]. One reason for this is that the temperature of women is affected by the menstrual cycle, and estrogen serves to lower it [68].

Age of onset. AN usually erupts during early adolescence. This occurs because this is the period in which estrogen is dramatically increased, enhancing CRH secretion and CRH2 signaling as explained above. This biological reason is enhanced by the increased vulnerability to social stress during adolescence.

Heritability. AN and BN have a substantial heritable component [3]. As explained above, stress can yield transgenerational changes in protein expression via epigenetics [43,44].

Menstruation. Female amenorrhoea used to be a defining characteristic of AN. Currently, it is thought to be secondary to malnutrition. However, it can also be directly explained by the fact that CRH2 suppresses gonadotropin hormone-releasing hormone, and thus the hypothalamus-pituitary-gonadal (HPG) axis [67]. This account also explains why a substantial part of AN patients show prodromal menstrual issues [69].

Exercise. AN patients very commonly engage in excessive exercise, which is usually attributed to a desire to lose weight. In T*AB, excessive exercise is a form of self-treatment. Intense exercise stimulates the release of EPI and NEP [70], which are suppressed by CRH2 and are important for real-world stress resilience [71]. In addition, exercise relieves social stress by reducing SER release [72]. Again, this AN behavior is a rational response to the biological problem, not a psychiatric obsession done in order to reduce weight.

HPA axis: CRH, GC. There is considerable direct evidence for increased CRH secretion in AN. CSF CRH was reported to be 1.6x higher in patients, with a blunted ACTH and GC response to a CRH challenge [73]. CSF CRH was elevated in underweight AN patients with hyper cortisol, and normalized following recovery [74]. The HPA axis is hyperactive in AN, and this is due to CRH [75]. Patients show basally higher cortisol levels, with a blunted ACTH response to CRH [76] and a blunted GC response to social stress [77].

AN and BN are highly comorbid with depression and anxiety, both of which known to be associated with high CRH [78]. In particular, the central amygdala contains a large population of CRH-releasing neurons whose activity is associated with threat-induced stress and anxiety [79].

CRH2 genetics. An association between AN and a single nucleotide variant in the CRH2 gene has been reported [80]. Recall, however, that according to T*AB, most of the genomic effects would be via epigenetics.

Comorbidities. There is high comorbidity of AN with psychiatric conditions such as anxiety disorders (especially obsessive-compulsive disorder) [81] and autism [82], both known to be associated with stress. This can explain obsessions (including perfectionism) and social impairment in AN.

Serotonin. Higher plasma SER [83], higher CSF 5-HIAA (SER metabolite) [84], decreased SER2a PET binding [85,86], increased SER1a (suppressive autoreceptor) binding in many cortical areas [87], and decreased SER transporter (SERT) PET binding in parietal cortex [88] all indicate elevated SER activity in AN. Importantly, tryptophan depletion, which decreases the amount of synthesized SER, has been reported to reduce anxiety in patients [89], giving rise to the idea that starvation is done in order to reduce SER activity [90].

Some genetic alterations in AN were initially reported regarding SER2a and SERT, but they have not been replicated in more recent GWAS [91].

Drugs that antagonize some SER receptors are commonly given as treatment in AN, see Treatment below.

NEP, EPI levels. T*AB predicts reduced levels of EPI and NEP, due to direct inhibition by CRH2. Indeed, low plasma NEP has been reported [83,92], even in remitted weight-recovered patients [93]. Lower levels of the NEP metabolite MHPG were also reported, more significantly in AN than BN [94]. One of these papers reported somewhat higher EPI levels [83], which is most likely due to the fact that their cohort had more binge-eating than restrictive AN patients. Desensitization of the NEP system (via orthostatic tests) has been reported in BN patients with normal weight [95], and blunted cardiovascular EPI responses to mental stress has been reported in women with BN [96].

Heart rate. Low heart rate is probably the most consistent physical finding in underweight patients [97]. This is readily explained via CRH2 suppression of EPI and NEP.

Heat responses. Half of AN patients were reported to engage in intentional exposure to extreme cold at least monthly [98]. The authors attribute this behavior to a desire to control shape and/or weight. According to T*AB, this behavior is, like exercise, a form of self-treatment done in order to increase EPI/NEP release. Patient hands, face, and feet temperature is lower than in controls [99], and they have lower cold-activated brown adipose tissue [100], indicating an impaired sympathetic thermogenesis response.

Glucose, insulin. AN patients show chronic prolonged mild hypoglycemia (with normal fasting glucose) [101], and higher insulin sensitivity [102]. Hypoglycemia in AN can be explained via adipose tissue depletion, but also by reduced function of the SNS. Indeed, patients show a markedly decreased plasma EPI response to insulin-induced hypoglycemia [103].

Growth hormone (GRH). AN patients show increased levels of GRH, coupled with decreased levels of its target, IGF1 [2]. These data are consistent with desensitization of the GRH receptors. GRH release is stimulated by mild hypoglycemia and by ghrelin, whose release is stimulated by an empty stomach. Both of these occur in AN and explain the GRH data.

Gut. AN patients show decreased gastrointestinal tract motility [1]. This is not always due to starvation, because 20% of AN patients turned to get treatment for prodromal gut symptoms [69].

Skin. CRH activates mast cells, which are strongly present in human skin [55]. Hence, T*AB predicts that AN patients would show skin sensitivity. Indeed, patients suffer from itch, and engage in scratching and self-injury [104].

2.4 Treatment

This section discusses possible pharmacological treatments for AN and BN. Psychological treatments can certainly help, and are not discussed here.

CRH. The best treatment for both AN and BN would be to normalize brain and peripheral CRH levels. However, there are currently no approved drugs that directly induce this effect. Note that antagonizing CRH2 (for AN) or CRH1 (for BN) may switch patients to the other disorder.

CRH can be used in tests for the disorder. The combined DEX-CRH test, and the ACTH response to CRH, can both indicate chronically high CRH release.

Somatostatin (SST). SST directly opposes CRH receptor-mediated stress responses and CRH2 suppression of food intake [105], and stimulates food intake in animal models. It also suppresses growth hormone release. SST inhibits gut secretory responses induced by SER [106], and opposes insulin secretion [107], which may be good in AN because it would allow blood glucose to increase.

Several SST analogs (including octreotide, lanreotide, and pasireotide) are currently approved for treating various conditions, including acromegaly (excessive GRH), pancreatitis, diabetic retinopathy, diabetic nephropathy, pain, inflammation, and cancer [107]. Octreotide's brain penetration is not high, but there are methods to enhance it [108]. SST drugs should still suppresses CRH and SER in the periphery, including in the gut, pituitary, adrenal gland, adipose tissue, and pancreas, and they may act on some hypothalamic nuclei.

SST drugs reduce adrenal EPI release, so in AN there may be a risk of reducing heart rate even more than the usual slow rate. However, SST drugs are reported to stimulate NEP release [109], which should compensate for EPI. In any case, heart rate is easy to monitor and handle (e.g., via small NEP or EPI doses augmenting SST).

In light of these data, treatment of acute AN using SST needs to be seriously examined.

Tryptophan hydroxylase inhibitors. Another promising direction, alone or in combination with SST, is to use tryptophan hydroxylase (TPH) inhibitors [110]. Telotristat etiprate suppresses peripheral SER synthesis by inhibiting TPH1, the rate limiting enzyme for peripheral SER synthesis. It is approved for humans in combination with SST analogs for treating cancer-related diarrhea. This drug might be very helpful in AN, because it is highly possible that the main factor in the fear of eating exhibited by patients is SER-induced negative events starting at the gut, more than central effects.

It is also possible that ondansetron (Zofran), a SER3 antagonist routinely used to relieve nausea and vomiting [49], would help in AN.

Atypical antipsychotics. Atypical antipsychotics are SER2a antagonists, and can be expected to alleviate some of the symptoms of AN. Indeed, a UK survey found that olanzapine is the most common drug treatment for AN [111]. However, because these drugs do not act on the important targets, their effects are quite limited [112].

SSRIs. Selective SER reuptake inhibitors (SSRIs) increase brain SER levels. Some SSRIs may be helpful in BN, because SER opposes the CRH1 mode. Because this SSRI effect can include decreased CRH production, SSRIs might also help in AN under some conditions. SER is a major promoter of the disorder, but its main effect is in the gut and adipose tissue, which are less affected by SSRIs. Due to the causative involvement of SER in AN, care should be taken in the usage of SSRIs for treatment.

2.5 Discussion

This chapter presented the first complete biological theory of AN and BN. T*AB is complete in the sense that it explains the etiology, symptoms, and pathology of these disorders. A complete theory does not have to be correct, but being complete is the minimal requirement from a theory.

AN and CRH. It is widely acknowledged that AN is currently not understood, and no biological theory has been formulated to fully explain it. T*AB focuses on stress (mainly social stress) and CRH. Given the well-known link of AN and BN with both of these, and given that the food intake suppression effects of CRH2 have been well-known for more than 20 years [9], it is surprising that a CRH2-based AN theory has not been proposed yet. CRH has been discussed in AN, but this has virtually always been in the context of HPA activity.

A possible explanation for this might be the general view of CRH2 as being anxiolytic, as opposed to the anxiogenic CRH1. Thus, it was perhaps not natural to link CRH2 with AN, which clearly involves anxiety. The new theory of CRH2 presented in this chapter resolves this apparent paradox, by noting that deficiency stress is different from excess stress, and by assigning CRH2 to the latter. CRH1 is assigned to the former, and this provides an immediate parallel theory for BN.

The evidence. This chapter has brought evidence supporting every aspect of T*AB (CRH, SER, EPI, NEP, gut, skin, epidemiology, various properties) except direct evidence for SER- and/or CRH-induced adipose tissue inflammation. The evidence for AN is larger than that for BN, reflecting the relative interest of researchers in the two disorders.

Other eating disorders. AN and BN are the major eating disorders, but there are additional ones, including binge-eating disorder (BED), pica, rumination, and avoidant/restrictive food intake disorder. These disorders were not dealt with here in order to keep the presentation simple. BED is defined via binge-eating episodes without purging behaviors (as in BN). BED can be explained via chronic activation of CRH1 in areas that control feeding (mainly the brain), without strong activation in the gut. That this can happen is natural, in light of the fact that TPH2 controls SER synthesis in the enteric nervous system and brain, while TPH1 controls it in enterochromaffin cells [28]. These are two different systems.

Serotonin. Depression is treated today by SSRIs, which increase brain SER levels. As a result, SER is commonly associated with positive emotions. Thus, readers may question the negative role SER has in T*AB. The T*AB answer is that SSRIs improve depressive symptoms because they mimic a state of healthy excess in which the organism's needs (food, sex) have been met. Hence, they reduce deficiency-related stress responses, including CRH activation of CRH1. However, in AN, SER is associated with excess-related stress and CRH2, and is a negative factor. Indeed, SSRIs are known to induce a large variety of gut side effects when used for treating depression.

The negative role of SER in AN has been recognized a long time ago, yielding a proposal that starvation is done in order to decrease SER activity [90]. T*AB agrees with this insight and shows how it fits within a complete theory.

Behavior is rational. According to T*AB, the major drivers for eating and purging behaviors in AN and BN are molecular, not psychological. While sociocultural constructs such as "being thin is better than being fat" and social media-promoted body image probably promote pathogenesis by increasing social stress, only a minor fraction of people are ill with AN. The parsimonious account is that the fundamental cause is biological.

The T*AB account is that metabolic body signals erroneously convey the message that the person has eaten too much, even if the objective state is that of deficiency. The major causal factor in the "intense fear of eating" in AN is not fear of gaining weight. The cause is the stress-inducing activations in the brain, gut and adipose tissue that are exacerbated by eating and by a non-empty stomach. Reduced eating and purging behaviors are a form of self-treatment meant to reduce the highly uncomfortable feeling accompanying these activations. Patient behavior is a rational response to their biological situation. This view can by itself reduce patient stress, and can serve as a basis for novel pharmacological treatments.

List of abbreviations

ACTH: adrenocorticotropic hormone.
AN: anorexia nervosa.
BED: binge-eating disorder.
BN: bulimia nervosa.
CRH: corticotropin-releasing hormone.
CRH1, CRH2: CRH receptors 1 and 2.
EPI: epinephrine.
GC: glucocorticoid.
GRH: growth hormone.
HPA: hypothalamic-pituitary-adrenal (axis).
NEP: norepinephrine.
PVH: hypothalamus paraventricular nucleus.
SER: serotonin.

SER1a, SER2a, SER2c, SER3: SER receptors 1a, 2a, 2c, 3.
SERT: SER transporter.
SNS: sympathetic nervous system.
SSRI: selective serotonin reuptake inhibitor.
SST: somatostatin.
T*AB: The theory of AN and BN presented here.
TPH: tryptophan hydroxylase.
WAT: white adipose tissue.

References

[1] D.R. Glasofer, E. Attia, B. Timothy Walsh, Feeding and eating disorders, Psychiatry (2015).

[2] I. Kowalska, M. Karczewska-Kupczewska, M. Straczkowski, R.T. Rubin, Anorexia nervosa, bulimia nervosa, and other eating disorders, Endocrinology: Adult and Pediatric (2016).

[3] K. Schaumberg, E. Welch, L. Breithaupt, C. Hübel, J.H. Baker, M.A. Munn-Chernoff, et al., The science behind the academy for eating disorders' nine truths about eating disorders, European Eating Disorders Review 25 (6) (2017) 432–450.

[4] J. Treasure, S. Zipfel, N. Micali, T. Wade, E. Stice, A. de Medeiros Claudino, et al., Anorexia nervosa, Nature Reviews Disease Primers (2015).

[5] R.M. Slominski, R.C. Tuckey, P.R. Manna, A.M. Jetten, A. Postlethwaite, C. Raman, et al., Extra-adrenal glucocorticoid biosynthesis: implications for autoimmune and inflammatory disorders, Genes and Immunity 21 (3) (2020) 150–168.

[6] J.M. Deussing, A. Chen, The corticotropin-releasing factor family: physiology of the stress response, Physiological Reviews 98 (4) (2018) 2225–2286.

[7] B. Lu, Y. Diz-Chaves, A. Contarino, F. Fanelli, S. Clark, D. Cota, et al., The corticotrophin-releasing factor/urocortin system regulates white fat browning in mice through paracrine mechanisms, International Journal of Obesity 39 (3) (2015) 408–417.

[8] C. Inda, N.G. Armando, P.A. dos Santos Claro, S. Silberstein, Endocrinology and the brain: corticotropin-releasing hormone signaling, Endocrine Connections 6 (6) (2017) R99–R120.

[9] T.L. Bale, W.W. Vale, CRF and CRF receptors: role in stress responsivity and other behaviors, Annual Review of Pharmacology and Toxicology 44 (2004) 525–557.

[10] R.W. O'Rourke, K.A. Meyer, G. Gaston, A.E. White, C.N. Lumeng, D.L. Marks, Hexosamine biosynthesis is a possible mechanism underlying hypoxia's effects on lipid metabolism in human adipocytes, PLoS ONE 8 (8) (2013) e71165.

[11] A. Stengel, Y. Taché, CRF and urocortin peptides as modulators of energy balance and feeding behavior during stress, Frontiers in Neuroscience 8 (2014) 52.

[12] R.J. McCrimmon, Z. Song, H. Cheng, E.C. McNay, C. Weikart-Yeckel, X. Fan, et al., Corticotrophin-releasing factor receptors within the ventromedial hypothalamus regulate hypoglycemia-induced hormonal counterregulation, The Journal of Clinical Investigation 116 (6) (2006) 1723–1730.

[13] K.M. Carlin, W.W. Vale, T.L. Bale, Vital functions of corticotropin-releasing factor (CRF) pathways in maintenance and regulation of energy homeostasis, Proceedings of the National Academy of Sciences 103 (9) (2006) 3462–3467.

[14] P. Jamieson, M. Cleasby, N. Morton, P. Kelly, D. Brownstein, K. Mustard, et al., Urocortin 3 transgenic mice exhibit a metabolically favourable phenotype resisting obesity and hyperglycaemia on a high-fat diet, Diabetologia 54 (2011) 2392–2403.

[15] J. Li, D. Qi, H. Cheng, X. Hu, E.J. Miller, X. Wu, et al., Urocortin 2 autocrine/paracrine and pharmacologic effects to activate AMP-activated protein kinase in the heart, Proceedings of the National Academy of Sciences 110 (40) (2013) 16133–16138.

[16] G. Warnock, D. Moechars, X. Langlois, T. Steckler, In vivo evidence for ligand-specific receptor activation in the central CRF system, as measured by local cerebral glucose utilization, Peptides 30 (5) (2009) 947–954.

[17] S. Kavalakatt, A. Khadir, D. Madhu, H.A. Koistinen, F. Al-Mulla, J. Tuomilehto, et al., Urocortin 3 overexpression reduces ER stress and heat shock response in 3T3-L1 adipocytes, Scientific Reports 11 (1) (2021) 15666.
[18] C. Li, P. Chen, J. Vaughan, K.F. Lee, W. Vale, Urocortin 3 regulates glucose-stimulated insulin secretion and energy homeostasis, Proceedings of the National Academy of Sciences 104 (10) (2007) 4206–4211.
[19] V. Martínez, L. Wang, J. Rivier, D. Grigoriadis, Y. Taché, Central CRF, urocortins and stress increase colonic transit via CRF1 receptors while activation of CRF2 receptors delays gastric transit in mice, The Journal of Physiology 556 (1) (2004) 221–234.
[20] M. Berger, J.A. Gray, B.L. Roth, The expanded biology of serotonin, Annual Review of Medicine 60 (1) (2009) 355–366.
[21] N.C. Donner, P.H. Siebler, D.T. Johnson, M.D. Villarreal, S. Mani, A.J. Matti, et al., Serotonergic systems in the balance: CRHR1 and CRHR2 differentially control stress-induced serotonin synthesis, Psychoneuroendocrinology 63 (2016) 178–190.
[22] G.L. Forster, E.M. Anderson, J.L. Scholl, J.L. Lukkes, M.J. Watt, Negative consequences of early-life adversity on substance use as mediated by corticotropin-releasing factor modulation of serotonin activity, Neurobiology of Stress 9 (2018) 29–39.
[23] S.V. Wu, P.Q. Yuan, J. Lai, K. Wong, M.C. Chen, G.V. Ohning, et al., Activation of Type 1 CRH receptor isoforms induces serotonin release from human carcinoid BON-1N cells: an enterochromaffin cell model, Endocrinology 152 (1) (2011) 126–137.
[24] L.K. Heisler, N. Pronchuk, K. Nonogaki, L. Zhou, J. Raber, L. Tung, et al., Serotonin activates the hypothalamic–pituitary–adrenal axis via serotonin 2C receptor stimulation, The Journal of Neuroscience 27 (26) (2007) 6956–6964.
[25] P. Gorwood, L. Lanfumey, O. Viltart, N. Ramoz, 5-HT 2A receptors in eating disorders, 5-HT2A Receptors in the Central Nervous System (2018) 353–373.
[26] S.F. Leibowitz, J.T. Alexander, Hypothalamic serotonin in control of eating behavior, meal size, and body weight, Biological Psychiatry 44 (9) (1998) 851–864.
[27] Y. Harada, K. Takayama, S. Ro, M. Ochiai, M. Noguchi, S. Iizuka, et al., Urocortin1-induced anorexia is regulated by activation of the serotonin 2C receptor in the brain, Peptides 51 (2014) 139–144.
[28] M.D. Gershon, Serotonin is a sword and a shield of the bowel: serotonin plays offense and defense, Transactions of the American Clinical and Climatological Association 123 (2012) 268.
[29] J.M. Yabut, J.D. Crane, A.E. Green, D.J. Keating, W.I. Khan, G.R. Steinberg, Emerging roles for serotonin in regulating metabolism: new implications for an ancient molecule, Endocrine Reviews 40 (4) (2019) 1092–1107.
[30] D. Gentilcore, T.J. Little, C. Feinle-Bisset, M. Samsom, A.J. Smout, M. Horowitz, et al., Role of 5-hydroxytryptamine mechanisms in mediating the effects of small intestinal glucose on blood pressure and antropyloroduodenal motility in older subjects, American Journal of Physiology: Gastrointestinal and Liver Physiology 293 (4) (2007) G692.
[31] T. Babic, A. Troy, S. Fortna, K. Browning, Glucose-dependent trafficking of 5-HT3 receptors in rat gastrointestinal vagal afferent neurons, Neurogastroenterology and Motility 24 (10) (2012) e476.
[32] V.L. Pszczolkowski, M.K. Connelly, A.D. Beard, A.D. Benn, J. Laporta, L.L. Hernandez, et al., Serotonin alters the response to a glucose challenge in lactating cows, Journal of Endocrinology 257 (3) (2023).
[33] Q. Li, T. Hosaka, N. Harada, Y. Nakaya, M. Funaki, Activation of Akt through 5-HT2A receptor ameliorates serotonin-induced degradation of insulin receptor substrate-1 in adipocytes, Molecular and Cellular Endocrinology 365 (1) (2013) 25–35.
[34] E. Hajduch, F. Rencurel, A. Balendran, I.H. Batty, C.P. Downes, H.S. Hundal, Serotonin (5-hydroxytryptamine), a novel regulator of glucose transport in rat skeletal muscle, Journal of Biological Chemistry 274 (19) (1999) 13563–13568.

[35] S.J. Tudhope, C.C. Wang, J.L. Petrie, L. Potts, F. Malcomson, J. Kieswich, et al., A novel mechanism for regulating hepatic glycogen synthesis involving serotonin and cyclin-dependent kinase-5, Diabetes 61 (1) (2012) 49–60.
[36] A.M. Martin, R.L. Young, L. Leong, G.B. Rogers, N.J. Spencer, C.F. Jessup, et al., The diverse metabolic roles of peripheral serotonin, Endocrinology 158 (5) (2017) 1049–1063.
[37] F.J. Martín-Cora, C.A. Fornal, C.W. Metzler, B.L. Jacobs, Insulin-induced hypoglycemia decreases single-unit activity of serotonergic medullary raphe neurons in freely moving cats: relationship to sympathetic and motor output, European Journal of Neuroscience 16 (4) (2002) 722–734.
[38] C.M. Oh, J. Namkung, Y. Go, K.E. Shong, K.Kim, H.Kim, et al., Regulation of systemic energy homeostasis by serotonin in adipose tissues, Nature Communications 6 (1) (2015) 6794.
[39] J.D. Crane, R. Palanivel, E.P. Mottillo, A.L. Bujak, H. Wang, R.J. Ford, et al., Inhibiting peripheral serotonin synthesis reduces obesity and metabolic dysfunction by promoting brown adipose tissue thermogenesis, Nature Medicine 21 (2) (2015) 166–172.
[40] K.E. Shong, C.M. Oh, J. Namkung, S. Park, H. Kim, Serotonin regulates de novo lipogenesis in adipose tissues through serotonin receptor 2A, Endocrinology and Metabolism 35 (2) (2020) 470–479.
[41] I.P. Voronova, 5-HT receptors and temperature homeostasis, Biomolecules 11 (12) (2021) 1914.
[42] C.M. Hostetler, A.E. Ryabinin, The CRF system and social behavior: a review, Frontiers in Neuroscience 7 (2013) 92.
[43] V. Reshetnikov, P. Kisaretova, N. Ershov, T. Merkulova, N. Bondar, Social defeat stress in adult mice causes alterations in gene expression, alternative splicing, and the epigenetic landscape of H3K4me3 in the prefrontal cortex: an impact of early-life stress, Progress in Neuro-Psychopharmacology and Biological Psychiatry 106 (2021) 110068.
[44] M. Szyf, Nongenetic inheritance and transgenerational epigenetics, Trends in Molecular Medicine 21 (2) (2015) 134–144.
[45] J. Coplan, M. Andrews, L. Rosenblum, M. Owens, S. Friedman, J. Gorman, et al., Persistent elevations of cerebrospinal fluid concentrations of corticotropin-releasing factor in adult nonhuman primates exposed to early-life stressors: implications for the pathophysiology of mood and anxiety disorders, Proceedings of the National Academy of Sciences 93 (4) (1996) 1619–1623.
[46] S. Avishai-Eliner, M. Eghbal-Ahmadi, E. Tabachnik, K.L. Brunson, T.Z. Baram, Down-regulation of hypothalamic corticotropin-releasing hormone messenger ribonucleic acid (mRNA) precedes early-life experience-induced changes in hippocampal glucocorticoid receptor mRNA, Endocrinology 142 (1) (2001) 89–97.
[47] M. Sjögren, M.B. Lichtenstein, R.K. Støving, Trauma experiences are common in anorexia nervosa and related to eating disorder pathology but do not influence weight-gain during the start of treatment, Journal of Personalized Medicine 13 (5) (2023) 709.
[48] J.C. Carter, C. Bewell, E. Blackmore, D.B. Woodside, The impact of childhood sexual abuse in anorexia nervosa, Child Abuse and Neglect 30 (3) (2006) 257–269.
[49] K.D. Johnston, Z. Lu, J.A. Rudd, Looking beyond 5-HT3 receptors: A review of the wider role of serotonin in the pharmacology of nausea and vomiting, European Journal of Pharmacology 722 (2014) 13–25.
[50] Y. Tache, Cyclic vomiting syndrome: the corticotropin-releasing-factor hypothesis, Digestive Diseases and Sciences 44 (8 Suppl) (1999) 79S–86S.
[51] Y. Kawahito, H. Sano, M. Kawata, K. Yuri, S. Mukai, Y. Yamamura, et al., Local secretion of corticotropin-releasing hormone by enterochromaffin cells in human colon, Gastroenterology 106 (4) (1994) 859–865.
[52] P. Yang, Psychological stress induces eosinophils to produce corticotrophin releasing hormone in the intestine, Gut 58 (11) (2009) 1473–1479.

[53] T.C. Theoharides, Neuroendocrinology of mast cells: Challenges and controversies, Experimental Dermatology 26 (9) (2017) 751–759.
[54] E. Kokkotou, D. Torres, A.C. Moss, M. O'Brien, D.E. Grigoriadis, K. Karalis, et al., Corticotropin-releasing hormone receptor 2-deficient mice have reduced intestinal inflammatory responses, The Journal of Immunology 177 (5) (2006) 3355–3361.
[55] S. Poglio, F. De Toni-Costes, E. Arnaud, P. Laharrague, E. Espinosa, L. Casteilla, et al., Adipose tissue as a dedicated reservoir of functional mast cell progenitors, Stem Cells 28 (11) (2010) 2065–2072.
[56] A. Divoux, S. Moutel, C. Poitou, D. Lacasa, N. Veyrie, A. Aissat, et al., Mast cells in human adipose tissue: link with morbid obesity, inflammatory status, and diabetes, The Journal of Clinical Endocrinology and Metabolism 97 (9) (2012) E1677.
[57] S. Ayyadurai, A.J. Gibson, S. D'Costa, E.L. Overman, L.J. Sommerville, A.C. Poopal, et al., Frontline science: corticotropin-releasing factor receptor subtype 1 is a critical modulator of mast cell degranulation and stress-induced pathophysiology, Journal of Leukocyte Biology 102 (6) (2017) 1299–1312.
[58] G. Mishra, K.L. Townsend, The metabolic and functional roles of sensory nerves in adipose tissues, Nature Metabolism 5 (9) (2023) 1461–1474.
[59] R. Serra, C. Di Nicolantonio, R. Di Febo, F. De Crescenzo, J. Vanderlinden, E. Vrieze, et al., The transition from restrictive anorexia nervosa to binging and purging: a systematic review and meta-analysis. Eating and Weight Disorders-Studies on Anorexia, Bulimia and Obesity 27 (3) (2021) 857–865.
[60] M. Yamanaka-Takaichi, Y. Mizukami, K. Sugawara, K. Sunami, Y. Teranishi, Y. Kira, et al., Stress and nasal allergy: corticotropin-releasing hormone stimulates mast cell degranulation and proliferation in human nasal mucosa, International Journal of Molecular Sciences 22 (5) (2021) 2773.
[61] P. Hu, J. Liu, A. Yasrebi, J.D. Gotthardt, N.T. Bello, Z.P. Pang, et al., Gq protein-coupled membrane-initiated estrogen signaling rapidly excites corticotropin-releasing hormone neurons in the hypothalamic paraventricular nucleus in female mice, Endocrinology 157 (9) (2016) 3604–3620.
[62] X.N. Chen, H. Zhu, Q.Y. Meng, J.N. Zhou, Estrogen receptor-α and-β regulate the human corticotropin-releasing hormone gene through similar pathways, Brain Research 1223 (2008) 1–10.
[63] A.K. Hannerfors, C. Hellgren, D. Schijven, S.I. Iliadis, E. Comasco, A. Skalkidou, et al., Treatment with serotonin reuptake inhibitors during pregnancy is associated with elevated corticotropin-releasing hormone levels, Psychoneuroendocrinology 58 (2015) 104–113.
[64] A. Bao, D. Fischer, Y. Wu, E. Hol, R. Balesar, U. Unmehopa, et al., A direct androgenic involvement in the expression of human corticotropin-releasing hormone, Molecular Psychiatry 11 (6) (2006) 567–576.
[65] M.R. Green, M. Zeidan, T.E. Hodges, C.M. McCormick, Age-dependent regulation by androgens of gene expression in the anterior hypothalamus and stress-induced release of adrenal hormones in adolescent and adult male rats, Journal of Neuroendocrinology 31 (6) (2019) e12714.
[66] B. Cong, X. Zhu, B. Cao, J. Xiao, Z. Wang, X. Ni, Estrogens protect myocardium against ischemia/reperfusion insult by up-regulation of CRH receptor type 2 in female rats, International Journal of Cardiology (2013) 5:4755–60.
[67] J.S. Kinsey-Jones, X.F. Li, J.E. Bowe, S.L. Lightman, K.T. O'Byrne, Corticotrophin-releasing factor type 2 receptor-mediated suppression of gonadotrophin-releasing hormone mRNA expression in GT1-7 cells, Stress 9 (2006) 215–222.
[68] F.C. Baker, F. Siboza, A. Fuller, Temperature regulation in women: effects of the menstrual cycle, Temperature 7 (3) (2020) 226–262.
[69] A. Gomez Del Barrio, F. Ruiz Guerrero, P. Benito Gonzalez, M. Perez Fernandez, L. Sanchez Blanco, E. Losa Mugica, et al., A retrospective investigation of the prodromal stages of eating disorders and use of health services in young patients the year prior to the diagnosis, Early Intervention in Psychiatry 16 (2) (2022) 162–167.

[70] M. Kjær, K. Lange, Adrenergic regulation of energy metabolism, in: Endocrinology of Physical Activity and Sport, Second Edition, 2013, pp. 167–174.
[71] M. Grueschow, N. Stenz, H. Thörn, U. Ehlert, J. Breckwoldt, M. Brodmann Maeder, et al., Real-world stress resilience is associated with the responsivity of the locus coeruleus, Nature Communications 12 (1) (2021) 2275.
[72] T.W. Kim, B.V. Lim, K. Kim, J.H. Seo, C.J. Kim, Treadmill exercise alleviates stress-induced impairment of social interaction through 5-hydroxytryptamine 1A receptor activation in rats, Journal of Exercise Rehabilitation 11 (4) (2015) 192.
[73] M. Hotta, T. Shibasaki, A. Masuda, T. Imaki, H. Demura, N. Ling, et al., The responses of plasma adrenocorticotropin and cortisol to corticotropin-releasing hormone (CRH) and cerebrospinal fluid immunoreactive CRH in anorexia nervosa patients, The Journal of Clinical Endocrinology and Metabolism 62 (2) (1986) 319–324.
[74] W.H. Kaye, H.E. Gwirtsman, D.T. George, M.H. Ebert, D.C. Jimerson, T.P. Tomai, et al., Elevated cerebrospinal fluid levels of immunoreactive corticotropin-releasing hormone in anorexia nervosa: relation to state of nutrition, adrenal function, and intensity of depression, The Journal of Clinical Endocrinology and Metabolism 64 (2) (1987) 203–208.
[75] F. Connan, S.L. Lightman, S. Landau, M. Wheeler, J. Treasure, I.C. Campbell, An investigation of hypothalamic-pituitary-adrenal axis hyperactivity in anorexia nervosa: the role of CRH and AVP, Journal of Psychiatric Research 41 (1–2) (2007) 131–143.
[76] P.W. Gold, H. Gwirtsman, P.C. Avgerinos, L.K. Nieman, W.T. Gallucci, W. Kaye, et al., Abnormal hypothalamic–pituitary–adrenal function in anorexia nervosa, The New England Journal of Medicine 314 (21) (1986) 1335–1342.
[77] I. Schmalbach, B. Herhaus, S. Pässler, S. Runst, H. Berth, S. Wolff-Stephan, et al., Cortisol reactivity in patients with anorexia nervosa after stress induction, Translational Psychiatry 10 (1) (2020) 275.
[78] F. Holsboer, The corticosteroid receptor hypothesis of depression, Neuropsychopharmacology 23 (5) (2000) 477–501.
[79] L. Regev, M. Tsoory, S. Gil, A. Chen, Site-specific genetic manipulation of amygdala corticotropin-releasing factor reveals its imperative role in mediating behavioral response to challenge, Biological Psychiatry 71 (4) (2012) 317–326.
[80] A. Oka, S. Hadano, M.T. Ueda, S. Nakagawa, G. Komaki, T. Ando, Rare CRHR2 and GRM8 variants identified as candidate factors associated with eating disorders in Japanese patients by whole exome sequencing, Heliyon 10 (8) (2024).
[81] L. Mandelli, S. Draghetti, U. Albert, D. De Ronchi, A.R. Atti, Rates of comorbid obsessive-compulsive disorder in eating disorders: a meta-analysis of the literature, Journal of Affective Disorders 277 (2020) 927–939.
[82] T. Inoue, R. Otani, T. Iguchi, R. Ishii, S. Uchida, A. Okada, et al., Prevalence of autism spectrum disorder and autistic traits in children with anorexia nervosa and avoidant/restrictive food intake disorder, BioPsychoSocial Medicine (2021) 15.
[83] F. Lechin, B. van der Dijs, B. Pardey-Maldonado, J.E. Rivera, S. Baez, M.E. Lechin, Anorexia nervosa depends on adrenal sympathetic hyperactivity: opposite neuroautonomic profile of hyperinsulinism syndrome, Diabetes Metabolic Syndrome and Obesity: Targets and Therapy (2010) 311–317.
[84] W.H. Kaye, H.E. Gwirtsman, D.T. George, M.H. Ebert, Altered serotonin activity in anorexia nervosa after long-term weight restoration: does elevated cerebrospinal fluid 5-hydroxyindoleacetic acid level correlate with rigid and obsessive behavior?, Archives of General Psychiatry 48 (6) (1991) 556–562.
[85] G.K. Frank, W.H. Kaye, C.C. Meltzer, J.C. Price, P. Greer, C. McConaha, et al., Reduced 5-HT2A receptor binding after recovery from anorexia nervosa, Biological Psychiatry 52 (9) (2002) 896–906.
[86] K. Audenaert, K. Van Laere, F. Dumont, M. Vervaet, I. Goethals, G. Slegers, et al., Decreased 5-HT2a receptor binding in patients with anorexia nervosa, Journal of Nuclear Medicine 44 (2) (2003) 163–169.

[87] U.F. Bailer, G.K. Frank, S.E. Henry, J.C. Price, C.C. Meltzer, C.A. Mathis, et al., Exaggerated 5-HT1A but normal 5-HT2A receptor activity in individuals ill with anorexia nervosa, Biological Psychiatry 61 (9) (2007) 1090–1099.

[88] M. Yokokura, T. Terada, T. Bunai, K. Nakaizumi, Y. Kato, E. Yoshikawa, et al., Alterations in serotonin transporter and body image-related cognition in anorexia nervosa, NeuroImage: Clinical 23 (2019) 101928.

[89] W.H. Kaye, N.C. Barbarich, K. Putnam, K.A. Gendall, J. Fernstrom, M. Fernstrom, et al., Anxiolytic effects of acute tryptophan depletion in anorexia nervosa, The International Journal of Eating Disorders 33 (3) (2003) 257–267.

[90] W.H. Kaye, J.L. Fudge, M. Paulus, New insights into symptoms and neurocircuit function of anorexia nervosa, Nature Reviews. Neuroscience 10 (8) (2009) 573–584.

[91] J.H. Baker, K. Schaumberg, M.A. Munn-Chernoff, Genetics of anorexia nervosa, Current Psychiatry Reports 19 (2017) 1–8.

[92] P. Luck, P. Mikhailidis, M. Dashwood, M. Barradas, P. Sever, P. Dandona, et al., Platelet hyperaggregability and increased α-adrenoceptor density in anorexia nervosa, The Journal of Clinical Endocrinology and Metabolism 57 (5) (1983) 911–914.

[93] K.M. Pirke, M. Kellner, E. Philipp, R. Laessle, J.C. Krieg, M.M. Fichter, Plasma norepinephrine after a standardized test meal in acute and remitted patients with anorexia nervosa and in healthy controls, Biological Psychiatry 31 (10) (1992) 1074–1077.

[94] E. Philipp, M. Eckert, R.J. Tuschl, M.M. Fichter, Pirke KM. MHPG in urine of patients with anorexia nervosa and bulimia and of healthy controls, The International Journal of Eating Disorders 9 (3) (1990) 323–328.

[95] A. Heufelder, M. Warnhoff, K. Pirke, Platelet α2-adrenoceptor and adenylate cyclase in patients with anorexia nervosa and bulimia, The Journal of Clinical Endocrinology and Metabolism 61 (6) (1985) 1053–1060.

[96] J.H. Koo-Loeb, C. Pedersen, S.S. Girdler, Blunted cardiovascular and catecholamine stress reactivity in women with bulimia nervosa, Psychiatry Research 80 (1) (1998) 13–27.

[97] K.V. Sachs, B. Harnke, P.S. Mehler, M.J. Krantz, Cardiovascular complications of anorexia nervosa: a systematic review, The International Journal of Eating Disorders 49 (3) (2016) 238–248.

[98] D.L. Reas, C. Dahlgren Lindvall, J. Wonderlich, Ø. Rø, Intentional Exposure to Extreme Cold Temperature to Influence Shape and/or Weight and Its Association to Eating Disorder Pathology, Frontiers in Psychology 10 (2019) 2539.

[99] C.M. Belizer, J. Vagedes, High-resolution infrared body surface temperature and self-perceived warmth distribution in adolescent anorexia nervosa patients, Journal of Psychophysiology 33 (3) (2019).

[100] M.A. Bredella, P.K. Fazeli, L.M. Freedman, G. Calder, H. Lee, C.J. Rosen, et al., Young women with cold-activated brown adipose tissue have higher bone mineral density and lower Pref-1 than women without brown adipose tissue: a study in women with anorexia nervosa, women recovered from anorexia nervosa, and normal-weight women, The Journal of Clinical Endocrinology and Metabolism 97 (4) (2012) E584.

[101] N. Germain, C.D. Genteuil, G. Belleton, T.L. Da Silva, C. Exbrayat, F. Degas, et al., Continuous glucose monitoring assessment in patients suffering from anorexia nervosa reveals chronic prolonged mild hypoglycemia all over the nycthemeron, European Eating Disorders Review 31 (3) (2023) 402–412.

[102] A. Ilyas, C. Hübel, D. Stahl, M. Stadler, K. Ismail, G. Breen, et al., The metabolic underpinning of eating disorders: A systematic review and meta-analysis of insulin sensitivity, Molecular and Cellular Endocrinology 497 (2019) 110307.

[103] K. Nakagawa, M. Matsubara, T. Obara, M. Kubo, K. Akikawa, Responses of pituitary and adrenal medulla to insulin-induced hypoglycemia in patients with anorexia nervosa, Endocrinologia Japonica 32 (5) (1985) 719–724.

[104] M.A. Gupta, A.K. Gupta, J.J. Voorhees, Starvation-associated pruritus: a clinical feature of eating disorders, Journal of the American Academy of Dermatology 27 (1) (1992) 118–120.

[105] A. Stengel, Y.F. Taché, Activation of brain somatostatin signaling suppresses CRF receptor-mediated stress response, Frontiers in Neuroscience 11 (2017) 231.
[106] J. Fassler, T. O'Dorisio, H. Mekhjian, T. Gaginella, Octreotide inhibits increases in short-circuit current induced in rat colon by VIP, substance P, serotonin and aminophylline, Regulatory Peptides 29 (2–3) (1990) 189–197.
[107] U. Rai, T.R. Thrimawithana, C. Valery, S.A. Young, Therapeutic uses of somatostatin and its analogues: current view and potential applications, Pharmacology & Therapeutics 152 (2015) 98–110.
[108] E.N. Lerner, E.H. van Zanten, G.R. Stewart, Enhanced delivery of octreotide to the brain via transnasal iontophoretic administration, Journal of Drug Targeting 12 (5) (2004) 273–280.
[109] A. Tsujimoto, S. Tanaka, Stimulatory effect of somatostatin on norepineprhine release from rat brain cortex slices, Life Sciences 28 (8) (1981) 903–910.
[110] Q. Liu, Q. Yang, W. Sun, P. Vogel, W. Heydorn, X.Q. Yu, et al., Discovery and characterization of novel tryptophan hydroxylase inhibitors that selectively inhibit serotonin synthesis in the gastrointestinal tract, The Journal of Pharmacology and Experimental Therapeutics 325 (1) (2008) 47–55.
[111] M.Y. Beykloo, D. Nicholls, M. Simic, R. Brauer, E. Mills, I.C. Wong, Survey on self-reported psychotropic drug prescribing practices of eating disorder psychiatrists for the treatment of young people with anorexia nervosa, BMJ Open 9 (9) (2019) e031707.
[112] S. Thorey, C. Blanchet, S.B. Guessoum, M.R. Moro, M. Ludot, É. Carretier, Efficacy and tolerance of second-generation antipsychotics in anorexia nervosa: A systematic scoping review, PLoS ONE (2023) 18.

Chapter 3

A polyunsaturated fatty acid (PUFA) theory of schizophrenia

3.1 Introduction

Schizophrenia (SZ) is one of the truly major psychiatric disorders, involving hallucinations, delusions (positive symptoms), reduced motivation, activity, speech, affect, sociality, and pleasure (negative symptoms), impaired cognition, and mood symptoms [1]. It has a strong heritable component. SZ is typically diagnosed at late adolescence, with prodromal non-positive symptoms. It affects dozens of millions of people, and has a strong devastating impact throughout the person's life. Treatment is generally effective only against positive symptoms. Suicide and relatively early death are common.

At present, there is no theory that explains SZ. Several hypotheses have been formulated [2], but each of them addresses only a partial subset of the data, and none of them provides a mechanistic account of the disorder. The standard hypothesis, motivated by the effects of dopamine (DA) agonists and antagonists on psychosis, is that SZ is caused by DA imbalance. However, this hypothesis is neither fully explanatory nor supported by strong evidence [3]. Endocannabinoids (ECBs) [4] and polyunsaturated fatty acids (PUFAs) [5] are thought to be involved in SZ, but there is no specific proposal for exactly how.

This chapter presents the **PUFA Theory of Schizophrenia (P*SZ)**, a theory of SZ that addresses all of the salient data known about the disorder. Briefly, P*SZ posits that *schizophrenia is caused by chronic synthesis and signaling of PUFAs and PUFA products associated with stress-induced plasticity, including ECBs, due to stress experienced at sensitive periods that yields persistent and heritable changes. The chronic presence of these processes can mechanistically explain the full range of SZ symptoms and data.*

P*SZ is conceptually simple, differing from previous SZ hypotheses in two major ways. First, it is a complete theory, not a hypothesis, providing a detailed mechanistic account of the disorder, including its etiology, symptoms, pathophysiology, and treatment. Second, it unifies virtually all of the existing SZ evidence into a single coherent story. This includes the two largest bodies of evidence in SZ, lipids and ECBs, as well as evidence related to immunity, pain, neuromodulators, hormones, neurotransmitters, symptoms, and cortical parameters.

Below, I present the theory, explain the mechanisms and roles of PUFAs and ECBs in health and stress, and detail extensive evidence supporting the theory. I then discuss possible treatments implied by the theory, some of which not requiring new drug development.

The Science of the Brain. https://doi.org/10.1016/B978-0-44-345008-2.00009-6

3.2 PUFA theory of schizophrenia (P*SZ)

Motivation. Examination of strong risk factors and their inter-relationships is a good starting point when trying to understand a disorder. The following four pieces of data are well-known and supported by overwhelming evidence (further detailed below).

First, cannabis use can acutely induce psychosis similar to the positive symptoms of SZ [6,7], and greatly increases the risk of SZ, with a 4-fold and 2-fold increase in heavy and average users, respectively [8]. Second, acute stress induces ECB synthesis, release and signaling, and chronic stress induces chronic ECB synthesis [9]. Third, schizophrenia is strongly associated with parental, prenatal, perinatal, and early life stress [10,11]. Finally, both acute and chronic stress can induce long-term epigenetic changes to the ECB system [12], which can be heritable [13].

These data provide a clear motivation for examining the hypothesis that stress-induced chronic ECB synthesis and/or signaling is the core cause of schizophrenia.

PUFAs. We will see right below that chronic ECBs can indeed explain the symptoms of SZ. However, before concluding that ECBs are the culprits in SZ, it should be asked whether the problem might be upstream of ECBs.

The main ECB linked to SZ is N-arachidonoylethanolamine (AEA), whose synthesis requires the omega-6 (om6) PUFA arachidonic acid (ARA). A study of the literature quickly reveals a large body of evidence showing the involvement of ARA in SZ (see below). ARA is released from membranes by phospholipase A2 (PLA2), which also releases omega-3 (om3) PUFAs, mainly docosahexanoic acid (DHA), which are also known to be involved in SZ. Moreover, PLA2 is recruited by stress and inflammation, and induces the synthesis of the other major ECB, 2-arachidonoylglycerol (2AG).

ECB, ARA, and DHA mechanisms. The main mechanistic effects of ECBs are well-known and supported by vast evidence (see Section 3.3). First, ECBs disconnect the synthesizing cell from the neural network by suppressing presynaptic inputs (both GABAergic and glutamatergic). Second, ECBs disconnect the cell from the extracellular environment by suppressing ion channels (calcium, potassium, cholinergic, serotonergic, others). Third, ECBs increase the cell's intrinsic excitability via elevated intracellular Ca^{2+}, reduced GABAergic inputs, and oscillating currents. Finally, many of these effects are receptor-independent, requiring only ECB synthesis. Importantly, like ECBs, both ARA and DHA (and its precursor eicosapentaenoic acid (EPA)) suppress external cellular inputs, and ARA increases intracellular calcium and intrinsic excitability. Thus,

- ARA, ECBs and DHA decrease coordinated network activation, and ARA and ECBs increase spontaneous activation.

In light of the shared effects of ECBs, ARA, and DHA, our initial hypothesis can be revised to assume that chronic stress-induced PUFAs are the cause of SZ.

Explaining the SZ symptoms. Given these accepted mechanisms of action, can chronic PUFAs explain the symptoms of schizophrenia? It turns out that they can do so in a straightforward manner. P*SZ explains SZ symptoms as follows.

- Positive symptoms occur due to spontaneous activation of neurons representing sensory experience (e.g., in the case of audition, in auditory and frontal cortices and hippocampus), which then activate others to form sensory sequences (e.g., voiced sentences). Since cells are disconnected from the network, this activation is not restrained by neurons representing the spatial and temporal context or by neurons supporting executive function. Instead, it is guided by the probability of spontaneous activation, which is higher in the ECB-rich threat areas. This explains why psychosis is commonly accompanied by a feeling of threat and by paranoid delusions.
  Note that perception with a sense of reality in the absence of external sensory inputs is quite common. This is what happens when dreaming, and stimulation of the superior temporal gyrus readily induces auditory hallucinations [14].
- Negative symptoms occur because neurons that support volitional movement and social interaction are disconnected and are difficult to activate in a controlled manner. More specifically, ECBs and ARA directly oppose acetylcholine (ACh) signaling, which is crucial for movement. Opposition to ACh also explains eye pursuit abnormalities, a known marker of SZ. In addition, DA and norepinephrine (NEP) neurons are also disconnected and hyperexcitable, impairing vigorous volitional movement and arousal.
- Cognitive symptoms occur because cognition depends on coordinated network activity.
- Mood symptoms can occur prodromally simply because the person feels that their cognitive, motor and social performance is impaired. Such symptoms are naturally exacerbated following psychosis. However, they can also occur due to excessive spontaneous excitability of neurons in stress areas. Mood symptoms combined with hyperactive threat inputs and decreased cognitive control also explain occassional violence and suicidality.

Since the released PUFAs, especially ECBs, have a role in brain plasticity, their chronic activation constitutes a dysfunction that impairs brain development and plasticity.

I-PUFAs: the final hypothesis. ARA is the substrate for prostaglandins (PGs), thromboxanes (Tbxs), and leukotrienes (Lkts), in addition to being a substrate for ECBs. DHA is a substrate for a family of derivatives known as specialized pro-resolving mediators (SPMs) (mainly lipoxins, resolvins, protectins) [15]. We need to consider the involvement of these families in SZ.

Examining the evidence, three data points stand out. First, SZ patients show a decreased niacin skin flush response, which is known to be induced by PGs.

Second, many autoimmune diseases, including those linked to Lkts, are associated with increased risk of SZ, but rheumatoid arthritis (RA), which is strongly linked to PGs, is associated with decreased risk. Third, there is considerable evidence showing decreased PG synthesis in SZ. Based on these and other data (see below), I hypothesize that PGs are not involved in SZ, while Lkts probably are.

What is the factor that determines whether an agent has a role in SZ? A common distinction is that between pro-inflammation and anti-inflammation agents. However, both PGs and Lkts can show both effects, depending on context. I propose that the important distinction is the nature of stimulation by calcium, which coincides with the family's role in the stress response.

I distinguish PUFAs and PUFA products into three types, those stimulated by extracellular Ca^{2+} influx (E-PUFAs), those stimulated by intracellular Ca^{2+} (I-PUFAs), and those suppressing the other two (SPMs). E-PUFAs are associated with the initial acute stage of stress, and I-PUFAs are associated with prolonged stress and stress-induced plasticity. SPMs terminate stress and its induced processes. I-PUFAs overlap to a large extent with the products stimulated by one particular enzyme, iPLA2.

Most PGs are E-PUFAs, and ECBs, Lkts and DHA are I-PUFAs. ARA belongs to both groups. E-PUFAs promote strong neural activity, so do not signal like ECBs. The effects of ARA, DHA and Lkts are similar to those of ECBs. Since the P*SZ account of SZ symptoms depends on the suppression of network activity, it is valid for I-PUFAs but not for E-PUFAs. Thus, P*SZ posits the following:

- *SZ is caused by chronic upregulation of I-PUFAs, including ARA, DHA, ECBs, and LKts. The core cause is an upregulation of their synthesis by iPLA2, induced by prolonged stress during sensitive periods.*

We will see below that ARA accumulation, rather than ECB signaling, may be the specific trigger of initial psychosis.

I-PUFAs increase intracellular Ca^{2+}, thereby stimulating 2AG (and AEA) synthesis. However, AEA decreases 2AG synthesis [16]. These conflicting effects may explain why 2AG is not as strongly linked with SZ as AEA.

Evidence. Is there evidence supporting this theory in addition to the stress- and cannabis-related data mentioned above? A study of the literature provides a definite affirmative answer (detailed in Section 3.5).

- There is very strong lipid-based evidence, consistently reported over decades, for chronically increased release of ARA and DHA in SZ.
- There is very strong evidence for chronic ECB synthesis and signaling in SZ.
- There is clear evidence for reduced coordinated network activity and neural hyperexcitability in SZ, affecting neuromodulators, hormones, and neurotransmitters.
- There is lipid- and immunity-based evidence that E-PUFA responses are blunted in SZ.

Other triggers of psychosis. Psychosis is a relatively common condition and can be induced by several agents, most sharing mechanisms of action with ECBs. DA (e.g., amphetamines) can induce psychosis by activating dopamine D2 receptors [17]. DA induces AEA release, and its the brain distribution of D2 and its signaling cascade substantially overlap with that of the type 1 cannabinoid receptor (CB1), so the effect of activating D2 is partially similar to that of ECBs. Muscarinic ACh antagonists such as scopolamine induce psychosis by opposing ACh, which is also strongly opposed by ECBs. Salvinorin A is the primary psychoactive component of the hallucinogenic plant salvia divinorum. It is a selective agonist of the kappa opioid receptor, whose distribution and mechanism of action partially overlap those of CB1 [18]. NMDAR antagonists such as PCP and ketamine can induce psychosis [19]. NMDARs are the main receptors supporting prolonged Ca^{2+}-mediated execution, and their antagonism disconnects the network. Glucocorticoids (GCs) are routinely given during surgery to reduce post-surgery nausea and vomiting and to relieve pain, but can cause psychosis in almost 20% of cases [20]. This happens because GCs recruit ECBs.

Agonists of the serotonin receptor type 2a (SER2a) such as LSD are known psychedelics. SER2a cooperates with CB1 as well, but can facilitate psychosis via an additional route. It is present on thalamocortical inputs [21] (which also produce 2AG [22]), and its strong activation can induce cortical activations similar to that induced by real sensory inputs. In addition, SER2a excites pyramidal neurons, mainly in prefrontal cortex (PFC) [23], and increases intracellular Ca^{2+}, which can recruit ECBs.

See below for psychosis induction in epilepsy and by NSAIDs and antimalaria drugs.

Antipsychotics. P*SZ explains the mechanisms and deficiencies of existing SZ medication as follows. All current antipsychotics are D2 antagonists, and atypical antipsychotics are also SER2a antagonists. D2 and SER2a can promote psychosis via the mechanisms described above. Antagonizing D2 suppresses its induction of AEA release, while antagonizing SER2a reduces the drive for sensory hallucinations by suppressing thalamocortical inputs. However, these drugs are not effective against other symptoms, because I-PUFAs affect many neurons not expressing D2 or SER2a. D2 antagonism can also lead to desensitization of the ACh system to induce tardive dyskinesia, and both types of antagonists may exacerbate chronic I-PUFAs in the longer term by increasing PUFA release.

Summary. Stress normally recruits PUFAs and their products. Prolonged stress recruits I-PUFAs. In some cases, e.g., when prolonged stress occurs at sensitive periods, this recruitment can become chronic. Chronic I-PUFAs can explain SZ symptoms and pathophysiological data. The stress-induced alterations include epigenetic changes that are heritable, explaining the familial association data of SZ.

3.3 PUFAs and PUFA derivatives in health

General. The major membrane lipids are glycerophospholipids, sphingolipids, and sterols. In mammals, the most abundant glycerophospholipids are phosphatidylcholine (PC), phosphatidylethanolamine (PE) and phosphatidylinositol (PI). PC and PE contain a choline or ethanolamine head group (respectively) and fatty acids, usually one saturated and one unsaturated. The latter is commonly a polyunsaturated fatty acid (PUFA), with both omega 6 (om6) and omega 3 (om3) PUFA being common [24]. The most abundant PUFAs are ARA (om6) and DHA (om3), both located at the sn-2 position of phospholipids. ARA and DHA are produced by elongation and desaturation from linoleic acid (LA) and alpha-LA (ALA) (respectively), which must be procured from the diet. PEs usually contain more ARA and DHA than PCs.

PLA2. The PLA2 family is comprised of calcium-dependent (cPLA2), secreted (sPLA2), calcium-independent (iPLA2), and other less major members [25]. All PLA2s hydrolyze the fatty acid at the sn-2 position of phospholipids (mainly ARA and DHA), releasing free fatty acids and lysophospholipids. iPLA2 induces both ARA and DHA release, while cPLA2 mainly releases ARA for PG synthesis [25]. While iPLA2 activity is mainly associated with PE, it also hydrolizes PC [26] and PI [27].

The activation of cPLA2 and sPLA2 is triggered by extracellular Ca^{2+}, while reduced endoplasmic reticulum Ca^{2+} (associated with increased intracellular Ca^{2+} or with calcium depletion) activates iPLA2 [28]. Thus, iPLA2 is an I-PUFA enzyme. GCs stimulate cPLA2 expression when signaling via cAMP (i.e., at the initial stage of GC signaling), and downregulate it otherwise [29], freeing ARA to be used by iPLA2. iPLA2 transcription is stimulated by sterol regulatory element-binding proteins (SREBPs) [30].

ECBs. The ECB system comprises a family of signaling lipids, their synthesis and degradation enzymes, and receptors [31]. Most research focuses on two ECBs, AEA and 2AG, and on the brain's CB1 receptor. CB2 is mainly expressed by immune cells.

The synthesis of AEA and 2AG is stimulated by intracellular Ca^{2+} [31] and by factors that increase it, including stress (see below), and requires ARA. PE and ARA form N-arachidonoyl phosphatidylethanolamine (NAPE), which serves as a substrate for direct AEA synthesis via NAPE phospholipase D (NAPE-PLD), or indirect synthesis via PLA2 [32] or phospholipase C (PLC) [33]. AEA is hydrolized by fatty acid amide hydrolase (FAAH). Importantly, FAAH also induces the reverse reaction, producing AEA from ARA and ethanolamine at larger substrate concentrations [34]. 2AG contains ARA and glycerol, and is formed from diacylglycerol (DAG) by diacylglycerol lipase (DAGL). PLC mediates the production of DAG from phosphatidylinositol 4,5-bisphosphate (PIP2). 2AG is hydrolized by monoacylglycerol lipase (MAGL).

CB1 is mainly located in presynaptic axons, although it also exhibits postsynaptic and mitochondria localization [35]. In axons, it is mainly expressed by GABAergic inhibitory interneurons (IINs). However, ECBs directly affect pyramidal neurons as well [36].

The brain areas involved in stress and memory, including the amygdala, hippocampus, and PFC, are especially enriched in ECBs.

Other ARA products. As mentioned above, ARA is a substrate for ECBs, PGs, Tbxs, and Lkts. PGs and Tbxs are produced via cyclooxygenases (COX), mainly using cPLA2-released ARA, and most of them promote acute inflammation. The key PG enzymes COX1 and COX2 can also produce PG from AEA and 2AG. ECB and PG synthesis seem to compete for ARA, with GCs pushing ARA utilization towards AEA [37], most likely via destabilization of COX2 mRNA [38]. Non-steroidal anti-inflammatory drugs (NSAIDs) such as aspirin and ibuprofen suppress COX2, thereby increasing the utilization of ARA by iPLA2. PGE2 opposes CB1 [39], while 2AG opposes COX2 expression [40]. Thus, the inflammatory PGs and Tbxs are E-PUFAs.

Lkts are produced from ARA by lipoxygenases (LOX, mainly LOX5), and can both promote and oppose inflammation. Lkt synthesis is usually described as being stimulated by cPLA2. However, Lkt production requires Ca^{2+} influx via calcium release activated channels [41,42], whose activation in turn requires iPLA2 [43]. Thus, Lkts are I-PUFAs. LOX5 is also activated by substrate availability [44].

DHA. The om3 PUFA DHA is used by lipoxygenases (LOX, mainly LOX15 but also LOX12) to produce a family of derivatives known as specialized pro-resolving mediators (SPMs) (e.g., lipoxins, resolvins, protectins) [15], which actively terminate inflammation and stress. Most DHA is used for beta-oxidation or reesterified into membranes [24].

Mechanistic effect. Most aspects of ECB signaling are well-known. ECBs are mainly retrograde messengers, acting on receptors located presynaptically to the releasing cell. They can also act on the cell itself in an autocrine manner. They have both receptor-dependent and receptor-independent effects.

CB1 is a G protein-coupled receptor (GPCR) mainly bound to Gi/o. When activated, it inhibits adenylate cyclase to decrease cAMP and neurotransmission release, and increases G protein-coupled inwardly rectifying K^+ (GIRK) channels [35]. Since CB1 is mainly expressed on presynaptic axons, its activation serves to disconnect neurons from their inputs. Since it is mainly expressed on IIN axons, its net effect is to reduce external inhibition.

ECBs also have direct receptor-independent effects. They directly suppress ion channels, including calcium, nicotinic ACh, serotonin, and some potassium channels [45]. AEA and a related molecule bind muscarinic ACh receptors, and inhibit agonist binding to it at high doses (with facilitation at low doses) [46]. ECBs also act on DA, NEP, ACh and SER neurons (see under evidence below).

The transient receptor potential vanilloid 1 (TRPV1) channel is a general cation channel mainly expressed in sensory input paths (e.g., dorsal root ganglia). AEA is a TRPV1 ligand that induces rapid channel desensitization, resulting in a relatively small increase of intracellular Ca^{2+} and autocrine cellular excitation [47]. ECBs can also utilize the GPR55 receptor to increase intracellular Ca^{2+} [48], and increase intrinsic postsynaptic excitability via Ih currents [36].

Both ARA and DHA inhibit voltage-gated calcium and sodium channels [49,50], nicotinic ACh receptors [51], and GABA currents (DHA at chronic doses) [52]. Both trigger Ca^{2+} release from intracellular stores [28,53], and DHA directly activates TRPV1 and other TRP channels [54].

LktC4 increases the potassium M-currents in hippocampus pyramid neurons, thereby hyperpolarizing them and directly opposing muscarinic ACh signaling [55]. Both LktC4 [56] and LktB4 [57] promote itch via neural circuits, including TRPV1 [57].

SPMs reduce brain activity during strong stress [58] and increased ECB levels in a pain model [59], but are different from other I-PUFAs in that they reduce intrinsic excitability by suppressing TRP channels, including TRPV1 [60].

In summary,

- I-PUFAs and SPMs disconnect cells from network inputs and from the extracellular environment, and I-PUFAs increase intrinsic neural excitability.

Function. The possible roles of ECBs have been widely discussed, with the leading candidates being plasticity, neuroprotection, and energy homeostasis [61]. For the purpose of this paper, we only need their established role in synaptic plasticity. Plasticity processes involve massive DNA access, which is dangerous with extracellular Ca^{2+} influx and the activation of various signaling cascades triggered by inputs from other neurons. ECBs disconnect cells from the environment in order to minimize this risk, and promote intracellular Ca^{2+} (and thus spontaneous excitability) to streamline ATP production and protein synthesis activities in mitochondria and the endoplasmic reticulum.

Other I-PUFAs are also involved in stress-induced plasticity. Inhibition of iPLA2 prevents plasticity, which can be rescued by ARA or DHA [62]. LOX5 knockout mice exhibit motor deficits associated with abnormal cortical and hippocampal synapses [63]. The DHA metabolite synaptamide stimulates neurite growth and synaptogenesis [64]. SPMs were investigated mainly in the context of inflammation resolution, but there is some evidence that they promote brain plasticity [65,66].

The functional difference between AEA and 2AG has been widely discussed, but for our purposes it suffices to note that 2AG release is rapid while AEA release is slower and of longer duration. Thus, it is natural to assume that 2AG and AEA support the initial and later phases of plasticity, respectively. Indeed, the triggering phase of stress involves suppression of FAAH and reduction of amygdala AEA [67].

3.4 PUFAs and PUFA derivatives and stress

The interaction between stress and the ECB system is very well-known, and is summarized here. The term 'stress' describes the states induced by threatening inputs or internal danger to cells (e.g., due to radiation, energy deficiency, calcium overload, immunity-inducing pathogens). These are the major states that trigger plasticity processes, whose role is to ensure that the organism is better prepared to execute a response the next time that the threat or danger occur.

Threat inputs trigger two types of stress responses, early and late. The early response, mediated by NEP, recruits energy and neural resources to support quick and vigorous execution. The late response, mediated by glucocorticoids (GCs, cortisol in humans), is meant to occur after execution termination, and its goal is to implement the plasticity changes that follow execution. In both cases, the appropriate agents (NEP and GC) are recruited by corticotropin-releasing hormone (CRH). CRH represses AEA (as noted above), and GC recruits it (see below).

Internal cellular stress recruits and signals via oxidative species, mainly superoxide and hydrogen peroxide (H2O2).

The relevant facts for SZ are:

- *Stress recruits ECBs* [68,69]. GCs can increase intracellular calcium [70] and directly stimulate PLA2 expression [29]. As noted above, they shift ARA utilization from PGs to ECBs. H2O2 increases cytosolic calcium [71], upregulates CB1 expression, and downregulates FAAH expression [72].
- *Stress can have long-term effects, mainly when it occurs in sensitive developmental periods* such as pregnancy, perinatal, early life, and adolescence [73–77]. The induced effects include increased risk for many disorders, and alterations in the stress system itself.
- *The long-term effects of stress can involve epigenetic alterations and be heritable* [78,79].
- *Stress can have long-term effects on the ECB system* [9,80–82]. In this sense, exposure to cannabis is a stress state [83].
- *The ECB system can be affected by epigenetics*, including after stress [12,39, 84–86].
- *Stress and cannabis effects on ECBs can be heritable* [13,84].

The major long-term change induced by stress is increased excitability of circuits involved in stress responses, which may seem to imply an upregulation of all stress system components. However, the CRH-GC axis suppresses itself via negative feedback, and chronic activation of GC and ECB receptors can desensitize them [87,88]. As a result, chronic stress usually results in increased agent levels (GC, ECBs), but can induce both increased and decreased receptor density and signaling. Indeed, stress has been reported to upregulate all of the components of the ECB system [82,89–94], but also to downregulate CB1 expression [9,84,90,91].

SPMs have not been investigated to the same extent as ECBs, but seem to show similar properties. SPMs are recruited by acute inflammation (immune stress) and by GCs (external stress) [95], their alteration during pregnancy affects the newborn [96], and their paths are affected by epigenetic mechanisms [97].

3.5 Evidence for P*SZ

In addition to the cannabis and stress evidence summarized above, P*SZ is supported by large bodies of evidence with respect to lipids, immunity, pain, the ECB system, neuromodulators, hormones, neurotransmitters, and cortical activity in SZ.

3.5.1 PUFAs

There is overwhelming evidence showing lipid dysregulation in SZ. Here I show that the vast majority of this evidence points to increased liberation of ARA and DHA in SZ. The main evidence is presented below.[1]

PLA2. Increased PLA2 activity was directly measured and reported in many papers [98–110]. Increased protein [107] and mRNA [108] were reported as well. Measurements were in plasma or serum [98,99,101,107,108], platelets [100,109], red blood cells [110], or brain [102]. The results pertained to SZ but not other psychiatric disorders [100,102] or occurred in several disorders [99]. Results were not due to medication [98,102,103], in some cases only occurring in first-episode psychosis (FEP), medicated or not [104–106]. They were also reported for people at ultra-high risk [109]. Most papers reported increased iPLA2 [101,102,104–107,109]. Two of these reported also increased [109] or decreased [102] cPLA2. One paper found higher plasma cPLA2 with no clear iPLA2 changes [108]. One paper reported normal activity in drug-naive patients [111].

Two additional facts support the involvement of iPLA2 in psychosis. First, the prevalence of psychosis in epilepsy, especially temporal lobe epilepsy, is much higher than in the general population [112]. Indeed, there is increased hippocampus iPLA2 (but not sPLA2 or cPLA2) in patients with vs. without psychosis [113]. In many cases, epilepsy psychosis involves an ongoing small seizure activity [114], which would increase non-acute intracellular Ca^{2+}. Second, NSAIDs, which suppress COX2 and thereby increase the utilization of ARA by iPLA2, can induce psychosis [115].

A little-known epidemiological fact supports a role for higher PLA2 activity in SZ. Anti-malaria drugs such as chloroquine and quinacrine are non-selective PLA2 inhibitors [116], and some of the lowest mean SZ prevalence rates are in sub-Saharan Africa, where anti-malaria drugs are highly used [117].[2]

ARA. Decreased membrane ARA was reported in many papers [118–131]. Measurements were in blood [118,119,121–124,126,127,129–132] and brain

---

[1] A large number of papers reported lipid-related measurements in SZ, so it can be assumed that for each change listed here there are several papers that have not detected it. Explicitly opposite results and some of the null results are reported here.

[2] However, similarly low rates were reported for North Africa and the Middle East.

[120,125,128]. Reports included FEP or drug-free patients [121,123,125,131, 132] and people at ultra-high risk [127,130]. This result was also reported in meta-reviews [5]. Significantly increased ARA metabolism and turnover were reported in two papers [133,134]. Plasma showed higher cPLA2 activity, with unchanged ARA membrane incorporation enzyme [108]. Moreover, red blood cell ARA and LA were inversely correlated with symptom severity [135]. These results point to increased ARA release and utilization in SZ.

One paper reported CSF ARA, and as expected, it was negatively correlated with symptoms [136]. This paper reported no ARA differences in red blood cells. Normal ARA in skin fibroblasts was also reported [137].

Increased levels of red blood cell LA (the ARA precursor) were associated with increased conversion of people at ultra-high risk [138]. Red blood cell ARA was positively correlated with total intracellular PLA2 activity in people at ultra-high risk who converted to psychosis, and negatively in non-converters [139]. Both patients and their siblings show increased red blood cell ARA, DHA and DPA [140]. Increased ARA vs. om3 PUFA was reported to correlate with hostility symptoms [141,142]. These results indicate that increased availability of ARA increases SZ risk.

Prostaglandin. PG data in SZ were reported in several papers, many reporting decreased levels. In the brain, significantly decreased frontal cortex PGE synthase was reported, with no COX changes [143]. However, this was shown by depression and bipolar patients as well. Dorsolateral PFC COX1 was decreased (41%) in SZ brain but not in depression [144]. Blood antibodies from patients trigger PGE2 production and induce COX1 mRNA in rat frontal cortex [145].

In blood, PGE1 synthesis in platelets can be stimulated in controls and patients with depression, but not in SZ patients, especially acute ones [146,147]. Decreased COX2 mRNA was reported, but only in patients older than 40 years old [148]. Plasma COX2 and PGE2 were reported higher in chronic medicated patients vs. controls and bipolar patients, while COX1 was higher in both SZ and bipolar [149]. Serum COX-produced PGs were decreased in FEP [129]. Serum PGE2, 15d-PGJ, and inflammation marker CRP were reported significantly lower [150]. Serum COX- produced PGs and LOX12 metabolites were reported lower, while EPA and LOX15 metabolites were higher in pre-medication SZ [129]. Plasma COX2 and TbxA synthase were reported reduced in SZ, while COX1 (and cPLA2) mRNA was higher [108].

One paper reported unchanged COX2 mRNA in frontal cortex and blood mononuclear cells [151].

Several papers reported increased PGs, all in blood. Patients had increased plasma PGE2, with patients with higher levels having more hallucinations [152]. The higher ARA metabolism in FEP platelets was attributed to PG [134] (but this has not been directly shown). SZ patients had higher plasma PGE2 and decreased 15d-PGJ2 and its nuclear receptor PPARg in red blood cells [153]. Higher COX1 and PG3 receptor mRNA was reported along with the decreased COX2 mRNA in patients older than 40 years old cited above [148]. FEP blood mononuclear cells showed increased COX2 (PGE2 only trend), and decreased 15d-PGJ2 [154]. PGE2 and COX2 were increased with (very large variability of PGE2), and PGJ2 decreased, in FEP blood [155]. Plasma PGE2 and thromboxane B2 were higher in ultra-high risk, and correlate with negative and positive symptoms respectively [156].

Niacin (also known as nicotinic acid and vitamin B3) normally induces PG and a skin flush response [157]. This response has been consistently shown to be reduced in SZ [108,157], indicating either reduced PGs or desensitized receptors (PG receptors are GPCRs). In one paper, the decrease was associated with increased PLA2 activity [103].

As mentioned above, GCs (and thus prolonged stress) push ARA utilization towards AEA rather than PGE2. This explains the generally decreased PGs in SZ. Nonetheless, precursor availability by itself most likely stimulates PG synthesis [158], explaining the reports of increased PGs in SZ. It is also possible that both paths are enhanced, with the I-PUFA more strongly so.

DHA, om3. Brain membrane DHA levels were reported unchanged in 9 papers [159] and decreased in one [125]. Several papers reported decreased blood DHA, in drug-native FEP (including a meta-review) [5,121–123,126,129,160, 161], ultra-high risk [130], and in general [118,121,124,132,136,162,163]. Significantly decreased DHA, total om3 PUFAs, and lower utilization of PEA into DHA were reported in FEP skin fibroblasts [137,164].

Decreased DHA, and a high om6/om3 ratio, are associated with symptoms [132,135,141,142,165]. Treatment that improved symptoms also increased the reduced om3 and om6 levels [132]. However, the om3 index was decreased after treatment. One paper reported increased red blood cell DHA and ARA in patients and their siblings [140]. One paper reported no om3 changes in ultra-high risk [127].

These data indicate higher release and utilization of DHA in blood, and a protective association of higher om3 or om3/om6 ratio, in blood but not brain. This might show that the underlying PUFA problem is manifested more strongly in blood, and that symptoms are directly related to ARA but not to DHA.

ARA precursors and metabolites. Membrane PE and PC (mainly PE) are widely reported to be decreased in SZ [120,130,161,166–176], and phosphodiesters (ARA metabolites) are reported to be increased [110,166,169,170,175–177]. These results were reported in brain (dorsolateral PFC, caudate, thalamus) [120,166,169,173], blood [110,130,161,167,170–172,174–177], and skin fibroblasts [168], including in early and drug-free stages [161,169,174,177] and ultra-high risk [130]. One group reported decreased serum lysoPC [175,176]. One paper reported significant depletion of om3 and om6 PUFAs from internal PE (recall that iPLA2 activity is internal), with increased PE in the external membrane leaflet of red bloow cells [178].

These results strongly support increased ARA release in patient brain and blood cells, including in prodromal and early drug-free stages.

Inositol. Increased PI turnover was reported in patient brain [179–181] (but also in depression [179]), blood [119,182–185], and skin fibroblasts [168]. PI enzymes were altered in postmortem brain in SZ [186]. This may indicate that 2AG is also hyperactive in SZ, not just AEA. Indeed, there is an iPLA2 variant that hydrolizes PI [27].

LOX products (Lkts, SPMs). There is almost no data about LOX products in SZ. With respect to Lkts, One paper reported decreased serum LOX5 products [129], and another reported reduced LOX5 activating protein in SZ vs. neural degeneration disorders [187]. With respect to SPMs, decreased LOX12 products but increased LOX15 products [129], increased LOX12 products [119], down-regulated LOX15b in three repositories [188], and an association with LOX12 mutations [189] were reported. No conclusions can be drawn from these results. In a mouse model, chronic social defeat stress increased basal ganglia LOX12 metabolites after one week (but not after a day), significantly more in resilient mice [190]. This is not a validated model for SZ, but it does show that prolonged social stress recruits SPMs.

Genetic data. Genetic associations of iPLA2 with SZ have been reported, all of them relatively weak [191–193]. A combined iPLA2-cPLA2 heterozygosity was associated with a 2x higher risk [194]. Five SREBP1 and two SREBP2 genetic markers were associated with SZ in German, Danish, and Norwegian samples of total size of about 1500 people [195] (recall that SREBPs, mainly SREBP1, stimulate iPLA2 transcription [30]). Seven positive and five negative results were reported for cPLA2 [193,196,197].

It should be noted that weak genetic associations of this kind have been reported for a large number of other genes, so this data does not provide strong support for the theory.

Obesity, diet. SZ patients tend to be more obese than controls [198]. This is widely attributed to the effect of antipsychotics, but is commonly (not always) reported also in FEP [198,199]. A review found that patients exhibit higher caloric intake, without preference to any particular category [200]. These data support P*SZ, since ECBs promote food intake and obesity [61].

Obesity can also be attributed to patient diet, as the natural diet of people with SZ seems to include a high consumption of fats [201,202]. However, the situation here is more complex. Mammals cannot synthesize most PUFAs so must obtain them from the diet, mainly linoleic acid (LA) as the om6 precursor and alpha-LA (ALA) as the om3 one. The synthesis of om3 and om6 precursor-derived fatty acids competes for the same enzymes, so increasing intake of one of them can reduce the other to change the om6/om3 ratio [24]. The common view is that increased om6 vs. om3 PUFA increases risk. People at ultra-high risk who convert to psychosis, and FEP patients, showed a higher intake of om6 PUFA than controls [203,204], and significantly lower om3 intake in patients has been found [205]. Normal red blood cell LA in FEP drug-naive patients, coupled with lower ARA, were reported in 5/6 papers [206], which indicates higher LA (om6) intake. In addition, in several clinical trials, om3 supplementation was modestly beneficial during the initial stages of the disorder [207] or in patients with a low om3 baseline [208]. These data generally support P*SZ, because ARA products (mainly ECBs) have a stronger I-PUFA effect on the brain than DHA products. Indeed, om3 supplementation reduces total intracellular PLA2 activity [139], and decreases tissue levels of AEA and 2AG [209]. Thus, high om6 and/or low om3 intake (e.g., due to economic conditions) can increase risk.

However, both om3 and om6 intake reduced risk in a large Swedish cohort [210], and higher om3 intake in FEP patients vs. controls was also found [204]. In addition, a negative correlation between SZ incidence and average om6 and ARA intake was found in 24 countries [211].

P*SZ explains these data by noting that intake patterns can also be compensatory. SZ involves excessive release of ARA and DHA from membranes, and this can promote higher PUFA intake (especially om6) to replace them. Ethanolamine, which is used by FAAH to produce AEA when ARA is excessive, must be obtained from the diet and is 3x more abundant in meat than fish [212]. Hence, meat consumption opposes its depletion. In this view, patients consume higher amounts of fat because their cells need fat. The risk to the organism posed by complete collapse of cell membranes due to lack of PUFA is higher than the risk resulting from the symptoms of SZ.

Summary. PLA2 (usually iPLA2) activity is definitely increased in SZ, accompanied by increased freeing of ARA and DHA. This activity is not due to medication. The freed ARA is most likely used for AEA and not PG (a conclusion strengthened by the immunity and pain data below). All this indicates that increased I-PUFA synthesis capacity is a core property of the disorder. The fact that the phenomenon occurs in both blood and brain supports an immune and/or epigenetic origin. Patients try to compensate for reduced membrane PUFA via their diet.

3.5.2 Immunity and pain

Meta-reviews show evidence for immune involvement in SZ, including activation of brain microglia [213], increased levels of CSF and blood inflammation cytokines in FEP [214], and plasma biomarkers possibly predicting transition to psychosis in high risk [215].

More specific information can be derived from immunity-related diseases. SZ is positively associated with psoriasis, atopic dermatitis, asthma, lupus, and some other diseases [216–220]. There is a strong negative association with rheumatoid arthritis (RA) [216,221] (although a recent positive association in an all-Taiwan cohort was also reported [217]). It has long ago been noted that patients are less likely to have allergies and show decreased responses to histamine injections [222,223].

Importantly, PGs are known to promote RA [224] and allergies [225], while Lkts promote asthma, psoriasis, and atopic dermatitis [226,227]. This implies reduced PGs in SZ, which supports the distinction made in P*SZ between E-PUFAs and I-PUFAs, and the P*SZ hypothesis that the excessive ARA in SZ is used for ECB and Lkt, rather than PG, production.

SZ patients show decreased pain sensitivity [223,228,229]. This can be explained in two ways, both supporting P*SZ. First, the TRPV1 channel is an important conveyor of pain, and is desensitized by I-PUFAs. Second, PGE2 is a major pain-inducing agent, and decreased pain accords with it being reduced in SZ.

3.5.3 ECB system

All of the components of the ECB system are dysregulated in SZ, with the evidence pointing to a chronic increase.

ECB levels. Plasma and CSF ECB levels (mainly AEA but also 2AG) were reported to be dramatically increased in many papers [129,230–241], including a systematic review and meta-analysis [242]. These reports include FEP, drug-naive [232,233], prodromal [235], and drug-free [129,236] patients, and patients evaluated in psychiatric emergency [238]. Cannabis use has been accounted for in some papers. Increased blood AEA was also reported in people at high-risk with childhood trauma (vs. high-risk without trauma), with significant correlation of NAPE with symptoms [243].

Lower AEA in some brain areas was reported too, with the same paper reporting higher 2AG [236]. Decreased serum 2AG was reported in a paper reporting increased N-acylethanolamines (which are ECB-like) [240]. Lower blood AEA and 2AG was reported in ultra-high risks vs. controls [244]. This is the only result in which both AEA and 2AG were reduced. Note that it is in blood, not CSF.

Ethanolamine is markedly decreased in patient plasma and platelets [163]. This indicates higher AEA synthesis, which is stimulated by abudance of ARA and ethanolamine via the FAAH reverse reaction [34].

Thus, AEA (and 2AG) levels are increased in SZ, which supports P*SZ. Further support is provided by papers from Leweke and colleagues reporting dramatically higher CSF (but not serum) AEA in disorder states, but with higher AEA correlating with better, not worse, prognosis. The papers compared FEP drug-naive patients vs. controls [232], FEP drug-naive patients with low frequency of cannabis use vs. high frequency use or controls [233], initial prodromal state vs. controls [235], and discordant twins vs. healthy twins [237]. In two papers, AEA negatively correlated with psychotic symptoms [232,233], and in the other two, higher AEA was associated with reduced conversion to psychosis [235,237]. The authors interpret their results as AEA being protective in SZ. In their view, AEA is high in risk states as a protective mechanism, and risk may transform to psychosis when it is not high enough [4].

The P*SZ interpretation is different. AEA is high in risk states due to chronic ARA release, which is the major problem in SZ. When ARA release becomes excessive, it overwhelms the capacity of AEA synthesis enzymes (FAAH reverse reaction, NAPE-PLD, others), and possibly of ARA release due to depletion, leading to a small decrease. At the same time, excessive ARA clogs the membrane and severely impairs its channels and receptors. It is this event that induces a conversion to full psychosis in the reported cases.

Some support for this view is given by the decreased NAPE-PLD in FEP blood (see below).

FAAH. FAAH activity is significantly increased in patient brains [245] (without mRNA changes), with clinical remission associated with significantly decreased FAAH mRNA [231]. In addition, FEP patients show increased FAAH after controlling for cannabis use [246] (here there was a negative correlation between FAAH and symptoms before controlling for cannabis, which can be explained by the fact that exogenous cannabis reduces the activity of the ECB system [247].) These data accord with increased AEA, which is produced by FAAH via the reverse reaction when ARA levels are high.

An association of SZ with NAPE-PLD and FAAH mutations has also been reported [248].

NAPE, NAPE-PLD. Increased frontal cortex NAPE and decreased NAPE metabolites (N-acylethanolamines) were reported [249]. Accordingly, significantly decreased NAPE-PLD (the direct AEA synthesis enzyme) was reported in blood mononuclear cells in FEP [246].

DAGL, MAGL. One paper reported decreased DAGL (2AG synthesis) in FEP blood cells (before and after controlling for cannabis use), and increased MAGL (2AG degradation, only after controlling for cannabis) [246]. One paper reported no MAGL mRNA changes [245].

CB1 expression. Higher CB1 expression was reported in several papers, mainly using postmortem brain autoradiography but also PET and blood [250–259]. CB1 PET binding was higher in unmedicated than medicated patients (10% vs 5%) [255]. One paper reported higher CB1 PET binding in paranoid SZ but not other SZ types [260]. An increase was reported only in patients who commited suicide, with a decrease in others [258].

As predicted by P*SZ, downregulated CB1 (protein, mRNA, or ligand binding), which is a natural result of chronic signaling, is also frequently reported [245,258,259,261–265]. Decreased PFC CB1 was seen only in medicated patients [262], supporting desensitization. CB1 was significantly higher in excitatory boutons, but lower in IINs [259], again supporting desensitization, which is expected to be faster in IINs due to their higher activation level. A greater decrease was somewhat associated with higher symptom severity in males [265]. Two papers reported no changes in superior temporal gyrus [266] and anterior cingulate cortex [267].

Recall that many of the negative effects of chronic ECB synthesis are independent of the CB1 receptor, made via direct I-PUFA effects on ion channels, intracellular Ca^{2+}, and membranes. Thus, chronic I-PUFAs can promote symptoms even when CB1 is downregulated.

Gi/o. CB1 is coupled to Gi/o. Increased GPCR Go activation was reported in SZ [181,268]. A trend for higher basal CB1 coupling to Gi/o, indicating chronic activation, was also reported [245].

Genetic data. Patient blood shows decreased DNA methylation of the CB1 promoter, with a trend for increased expression [269]. As mentioned above, an association of SZ with NAPE-PLD and FAAH mutations was found [248]. There is considerable data on CB1 mutations and SZ, but a recent thorough review found no consistent pattern [270].

Summary. ECB synthesis, signaling, and turnover are chronically increased in SZ.

3.5.4 Hyperexcitability: neuromodulators, hormones, neurotransmitters

Neuromodulators: DA, NEP, SER, ACh. The important neuromodulators of the brain, DA, NEP, SER, and ACh (which is also a neurotransmitter) are released by neurons located in specific nuclei. DA, NEP and SER neurons are regulated by ECBs [271–273], which increases spontaneous firing and agent release. Thus, the effects of ECBs on neuromodulator release is similar to their effects in general. Indeed, there is direct evidence for slightly increased DA and NEP levels in SZ [241,274]. With respect to SER, there is only indirect evidence. The loudness dependence of auditory evoked potentials (LDAEP) is a measure of amplitude changes of auditory evoked electroencephalogram potentials in primary auditory cortex, and is known to be reduced by SER [275]. LDAEP is reduced in SZ patients, which indicates higher cortical SER levels [275].

The situation regarding ACh is more complex. On one hand, axonal inputs to basal forebrain ACh neurons express some CB1, and ACh neurons express FAAH [276]. On the other hand, CB1 agonists induce a prolonged inhibition of ACh release [277], and ECBs clearly oppose ACh receptor signaling (see above). This makes sense, since there is substantial co-release of ACh and GABA [278], and ECBs inhibit GABAergic neurons to suppress coordinated network activity.

Three ACh-related facts support P*SZ. First, there is widespread reduction in ACh receptor expression and signaling in SZ [279]. Second, CB1 agonists induce cognitive deficits via decreased ACh [280,281]. Third, SZ patients show increased prevalence of smoking [1], which is most likely a form of self-treatment.

Hormones: prolactin (PRL), cortisol. PRL levels are increased in SZ, and this has been traditionally viewed as being due to the anti-DA effect of antipsychotic medication. However, PRL levels are also greatly increased in first-episode, drug-naive patients [282] and in high-risk people who converted to psychosis [283]. This PRL increase supports P*SZ, because PLA2 increases PRL secretion [284,285]. In fact, many known agents that stimulate PRL release, such as thyrotropin-releasing hormone, neurotensin, and angiotensin II, do so via PLA2 [284,285].

Cortisol levels are also moderately increased in SZ, along with dysregulation of release rhythms [283,286]. This can be part of the epigenetic changes induced by stress, or more specifically be due to hyperexcitability of neurons recruits GCs.

Neurotransmitters: GABA, glutamate. The two main brain neurotransmitters, glutamate and GABA, are both affected in SZ, in the directions predicted by P*SZ. GABAergic IINs support coordinated and synchronous activity, and are normally suppressed by ECBs as part of their suppression of network activity. Chronic ECBs are predicted to induce a lasting decrease in GABA pathways. Indeed, CSF GABA is decreased in SZ [241], and GABA synthesis enzymes, GABA transporters, and several GABAA subunits are decreased in patient postmortem dorsolateral PFC [287]. These effects were not due to medication, since they did not occur in monkeys given chronic antipsychotics.

Glutamate is the brain's main excitatory neurotransmitter, and predicted to be increased due to hyperexcitability. Indeed, chronic spillover of glutamate from the synaptic cleft has been shown [288]. This glutamate activates extrasynaptic receptors, producing a positive feedback loop that increases excitability. There is a well-known NMDAR hypofunction hypothesis of SZ [289], but it is based on the psychosis-inducing effects of NMDARs antagonists.

Motor symptoms. In addition to classical negative symptoms, which show decreased motor activity, SZ patients show motor symptoms that involve increased activity. In fact, catatonia in FEP patients mainly involves hyperkinesia, much more than hypokinesia [290]. Akathisia has been shown to be associated with worse prognosis [291].

Neural excitability. Patients with active paranoia show significantly increased resting cerebral blood flow activity in left amygdala (and a trend in the right amygdala) vs. other SZ patients or controls) [292]. SZ patients show higher tonic activity in right ventral striatum and bilateral amygdala [293]. A metareview found increased PET or fMRI activation in response to neutral stimuli in 20 out of 29 reports, including in the amygdala (10), PFC (14), anterior cingulate cortex (6), and hippocampal formation (6) [294].

Medicated SZ patients exhibit faster (and accurate) imagery, despite their working memory deficit [295]. This supports priming (increased excitability) of high-level sensory experience paths.

3.5.5 Coordinated network activity

There are several accepted measures of coordinated network activity, and all are reduced in SZ.

Event-related potentials (ERPs). ERPs measure the electroencephalography or magnetoencephalography responses to stimuli. ERPs include negativities and positivities at relatively fixed post-stimulus delays (e.g., the P300, N400), and some composite measures (e.g., the mismatch negativity). Shorter-term ERPs measure the brain's immediate responses to sensory inputs, while longer-term ERPs are a standard measure for the capacity of the brain to engage in coordinated top-down activity.

ERPs, especially top-down ones, are reduced in SZ [296,297]. Anticipatory ERPs such as the contingent negative variation and the stimulus preceding negativity are reduced as well [298].

Oscillations. Normal cortical execution involves electroencephalography oscillations at various frequency bands. Oscillations and synchrony are disrupted in SZ [299,300].

Cortical activity. In addition to these measures, a well-known result in SZ, sometimes termed hypofrontality, is that of decreased PFC activity in resting and cognitive challenge conditions [1]. In addition, there is hypoperfusion in wide brain areas [301].

Synapses. Synapses are essential for brain execution. There is clear evidence for reduced synaptic density and for synaptic dysfunction in SZ, including in ion channels, exocytosis, glutamate receptors, postsynaptic density, and adhesion molecules [302].

Brain volume. Another well-supported result in SZ is reduced total brain volume, with larger third and lateral ventricular spaces [1]. This is not a direct index of coordinated activity, but it indicates impaired plasticity and development.

3.5.6 Summary

P*SZ enjoys overwhelming support from virtually all bodies of evidence gathered about SZ in the last 50 years. On the agent side, there is increased I-PUFA and decreased E-PUFA synthesis and signaling, increased ECB (especially AEA) synthesis, and increased CB1 activation and desensitization. On the effect side, there is clear neural hyperexcitability coupled with decreased coordinated cortical activity. These effects induce the symptoms of SZ as explained above.

3.6 Treatment

Here I discuss novel and existing treatment directions, including iPLA2 suppression, dietary om3, CB1 antagonism, NAC, and antipsychotics. I explain the mechanisms of antipsychotics and discuss their upsides and downsides.

Reducing iPLA2. According to P*SZ, SZ involves excessive PLA2 activity, mainly iPLA2. Hence, the most promising drug-based direction is to reduce iPLA2 activity. Several families of potent and highly selective small molecule iPLA2 inhibitors have been designed [303–305]. None of them has been tested on humans. The published papers provide extensive explanations of design considerations and techniques.

Alternatively, there are non-selective PLA2 inhibitors that are readily available for treating humans. Anti-malaria drugs such as chloroquine, quinacrine, hydroxychloroquine, and quinine have been used by many millions of people for decades, and are PLA2 inhibitors, with efficacy ranking at this order [116]. These drugs cross the blood-brain barrier [306], and are widely available and inexpensive. SZ prevalence is indeed lowest in areas where anti-malaria drugs are used [117] (although this datum is not strong). Thus, anti-malaria drugs are candidates for treating SZ.

This proposal might seem paradoxical, because quinacrine and related drugs can induce psychosis [307]. This is not surprising, since, in addition to its effect on PLA2, quinacrine inhibits muscarinic [308] and nicotinic [309] ACh receptors. In addition, when given to people with normal PLA2 activity (i.e., people without SZ), quinacrine can induce excessive I-PUFA suppression, which can cause excessive activation of the ACh system, followed by its desensitization. This can disconnect the neural network and increase spontaneous spiking to induce psychosis in the same manner as ECBs and muscarinic antagonists do.

In spite of this, there are arguments to support the usage of anti-malaria drugs for treating SZ. First, psychosis is a rare adverse event. Among 30,000 soldiers treated for malaria, psychosis occurred in only 0.1-0.4% [310]. Second, psychosis overwhelmingly occurred when using high drug doses, higher than those used for normal treatment [311]. Doses resulting in plasma levels of less than 18 microgram per 100 cubic cm did not yield any in mental or intellectual impairment [310]. Since the PLA2 upregulation in SZ is a small-scale phenomenon, relatively small inhibitor doses would be needed in SZ, which almost completely avoids risk. Third, the reports of anti-malaria drugs causing psychosis are with people without SZ. As explained above, P*SZ predicts that PLA2 inhibition could yield psychosis in healthy people, but when used with people with SZ, their effect would be to normalize an impaired state, not impair a healthy state. Finally, quinacrine is a structural antecedent of the phenothiazines, and its structure is similar to that of chlorpromazine [312], the first antipsychotic drug.[3] Chlorpromazine is effective against positive symptoms, but has undesired side effects. The fact that a highly similar molecule has been shown to be effective in SZ provides some validation with respect to PLA2 inhibitors and quinacrine.

---

[3] In light of P*SZ, it is hypothesized here that the benefits of chlorpromazine are due to a PLA2 effect more than to other discussed mechanisms. Indeed, it is a highly potent inhibitor of cPLA2 [313].

Even if not used directly, non-selective iPLA2 inhibitors constitute a promising direction to pursue at present, since it is possible that relatively small modifications could oppose their ACh suppression and make them more selective towards iPLA2 than to cPLA2.

Dietary PUFA. According to P*SZ, ARA's role in SZ is most likely much larger than that of DHA. As a result, reducing the om6/om3 ratio via diet is probably a good idea, certainly for patients who show om3 deficiency. Indeed, the evidence section above summarized evidence that om3 may have a protective effect, and that dietary om3 supplementation might be beneficial at the initial stages of the disease. The lack of benefit at later stages may be related to the supplementation being adjunctive to antipsychotics.

CB1 antagonists. Rimonabant and other related CB1 antagonists were tested in long trials for reducing obesity. They turned out to be moderately effective for weight loss, but to increase the risk of depression and anxiety [314]. For this reason, rimonabant was withdrawn from the market. Since ECBs are recruited to facilitate the early stages of stress termination, mood symptoms can be expected when ECB signaling is reduced in healthy people. In addition, CB1 antagonism may yield accumulation of ARA and increased spontaneous excitability.

Nonetheless, in SZ, the ECB system is hyperactive, and CB1 antagonism may normalize it to some extent, especially in patients with increased CB1 expression. Indeed, in a small clinical trial using rimonabant for the treatment of obesity in SZ, patients showed a significantly decreased psychiatric score and anxiety. There were no adverse effects [315], but the trial was terminated early due to the drug's withdrawal. In another trial, rimonabant had no effect on SZ symptoms and no adverse effects [316]. Similarly, a trial using co-treatment with the CB1 antagonist AVE1625 and atypical antipsychotics was terminated early due to insufficient benefit [317]. CB1 antagonism does not address the root problem of excessive ARA in SZ, since it can promote ARA accumulation. This might explain the lack of efficacy in these trials.

Cannabidiol is a cannabis component that counters the psychotic effects of cannabis, possibly by opposing CB1 signaling [318]. It can be expected to have effects in a similar direction to CB1 antagonists, but weaker.

N-acetylcysteine (NAC). Based on the assumption that NAC might be beneficial in SZ by reducing oxidative stress, several clinical trials have been conducted, with positive results. In a systematic review and network meta-analysis, adjunctive NAC, but not om3 PUFAs, folic acid, vitamin B12, or vitamin D, was found to significantly reduce symptoms vs. placebo [319]. In my view, the main mechanism here is not oxidative stress but PGs. Paracetamol reduces pain by suppressing COX, and NAC is routinely used against paracetamol overdose, with common skin rash, reddening, and itch side effects. This implies that NAC probably enhances PG synthesis, which should be beneficial in SZ due to channeling of ARA utilization away from I-PUFAs.

One paper reported that ultraviolet radiation stimulated cPLA2 synthesis, which was correlated with increased ARA and PGE2, and that this stimulation was prevented by NAC [320]. This result contradicts the PG assumption above, but suppression of cPLA2 synthesis could be independently beneficial in SZ.

Antipsychotics. Today, SZ is treated with so-called antipsychotics, which are all D2 antagonists. Atypical antipsychotics are also SER2a antagonists. Like CB1, D2 is a GPCR coupled to Gi/o, and their brain distributions have a moderate overlap, especially in the basal ganglia striatum, PFC [321] and amygdala [322]. D2 agonists greatly increase AEA release and suppress its degradation [323–325]. Thus, antagonizing D2 reduces the excessive AEA present in SZ.

SER2a is excitatory and has a wide brain distribution. In particular, it is presynaptically expressed in thelamocortical neurons, and postsynaptically expressed in layer 5 PFC pyramidal neurons [21], so antagonizing it reduces the excitability of many neurons participating in sensory perception. These data explain the benefit of these drugs on positive symptoms.

There is evidence that these drugs improve patient ECB and PUFA state. Olanzapine-induced remission was associated with decrease in blood AEA and FAAH mRNA [231]. Patients treated with typical (but not atypical) antipsychotics did not show the excessive CSF ARA shown in FEP and atypical medicated patients [232]. Eight week treatment reduced higher serum AEA and increased the lower serum COX products (PGE2 and others) [129]. Treatment partially normalized decreased membrane ARA and DHA [125,132], and decreased PLA2 activity [98,103]. The odds that treatment improves negative symptoms was higher with high basal iPLA2 activity [106]. Antipsychotics decrease iPLA2 gene expression in patients [326]. Clozapine upregulated COX2 mRNA in human astrocytes [327], which might be beneficial by channeling ARA to E-PUFAs rather than I-PUFAs. In addition, one preclinical study found that chronic clozapine decreased rat plasma ARA, brain COX and PGE2, and the incorporation of ARA into the brain [328]. Other studies found that D2 [329,330] and SER2 [331] potentiate PLA2, and that olanzapine decreases LOX5 activating protein [332].

However, there is also data showing that antipsychotics may exacerbate patient I-PUFA state. Antipsychotics activate SREBP genes [333], which stimulate iPLA2 mRNA and protein [30]. They also upregulate the desaturase enzymes that participate in the production of ARA and DHA from their precursors [334]. Chronic risperidone, olanzapine, and haloperidol increased ARA and DHA in red blood cells (quetiapine increased only DHA) [335]. 30 days of clozapine increased iPLA2 (but not other PLA2) mRNA, protein, and activity, and decreased COX activity and PGE2 in rats [336]. 30 days of olanzapine increased frontal cortex iPLA2 and COX1 mRNA, and decreased brain PGE2 and ARA brain incorporation [337]. Seizures are a frequent adverse event of antipsychotics [338], which can be explained via increased excitability or upregulated PG (recall that PGs are highly excitatory).

CB1-D2 heteromers are common, and co-stimulation of the receptors promote heteromer formation and reverses CB1 signaling to induce cAMP [339]. Since CB1 is chronically stimulated in SZ, stimulation of D2 should be beneficial in SZ by reversing CB1 signaling. In this view, antipsychotics may enhance chronic CB1 signaling. However, after treatment of cells expressing CB1 and D2 with a CB1 agonist, haloperidol switched CB1 to inducing cAMP [340]. These conflicting data do not allow firm conclusions.

SZ patients show increased CB1-SER2a heteromers and inhibition of cAMP (i.e., classic CB1 signaling) in the olfactory neuroepithelium, due to a switch of SER2a signaling from Gq to Gi [341]. Co-stimulation additively decreased cAMP in non-cannabis users treated with clozapine. Here, antipsychotics enhance CB1-like signaling, which would worsen patient state.

At the functional level, SER2a promotes active coping in stress and enhances learning and memory [342], so antagonizing it could be harmful if it does not directly target the disorder causes.

Importantly, atypical antipsychotics have strong anticholinergic properties [343], and many of the detrimental effects of ECBs in SZ are due to opposition to ACh. A very common adverse effect after months or years of treatment is a movement disorder called tardive dyskinesia (TD), which has many similarities with Parkinsonism [344]. TD is usually treated using muscarinic antagonists (although improvement after their discontinuation has also been reported) [344]. It has been shown in mice that catalepsy (the mouse parallel of TD) depends on D2 expression in cholinergic neurons and a subsequent excessive ACh in the striatum [345], probably leading to desensitization of ACh receptors. This may imply that ECB- and antipsychotic-induced ACh damage combine in SZ to exacerbate long-term patient state.

There is independent evidence that long-term usage of antipsychotics may be detrimental. A 20-year followup study found that patients not on drugs after the first two years have a higher chance of recovery [346]. However, a recent clinical trial reported that gradual antipsychotics dose reduction over two years increased the occurrence of adverse psychotic events without having any effect on other symptoms or general functioning [347].

Drugs probably get desensitized. The response to drugs, measured via phospholipids (PE, lysoPC) and neurosteroids, diminished after 6 months [170] or 5 years [348]. In a clinical trial, FEP patients improved similarly with drugs or placebo after the first 6 months [349].

In summary, P*SZ can explain the mechanisms through which antipsychotics yield beneficial results on positive symptoms, and why they have only a weak effect on other symtpoms. These drugs affect PLA2 and its products, with most of the short-term effects reported in SZ being positive. However, these reports are inconsistent, while negative long-term effects are also reported, implying that chronic antipsychotics might be detrimental via PLA2 for some patients.

AChR drugs. There are ongoing efforts to develop muscarinic agonists (positive allosteric modulators) for SZ (e.g., by Karuna, Cerevel, MapLight, and Neumora). As explained above, this direction is biologically valid, since ECBs suppress these receptors. However, such drugs address only part of the problem (and weakly so), so I do not expect them to provide substantial benefit to patients across the symptom spectrum when used alone.

Biomarkers. According to P*SZ, increased blood or brain iPLA2 (or any PLA2) activity, increased CSF ECB (mainly AEA) levels, and decreased membrane ARA and DHA in blood or brain cells, all indicate a high risk of SZ, especially when combined with reduced PGs (mainly PGE2). Indeed, AEA, ARA and oleoylethanolamine [129], and PE, PC, LA and some other lipids [177] allow very good classification accuracy. Since blood PLA2, ARA and PGs can easily be measured, this is the most promising biomarker for identifying high risk and for monitoring treatment effects.

3.7 Discussion

SZ is a major brain disorder and has been a mystery to humankind for a long time. This paper presented the PUFA theory of SZ (P*SZ), in which chronic synthesis of I-PUFAs (ARA, DHA, ECBs (mainly AEA), Lkts), usually stemming from stress occurring in sensitive periods, causes the symptoms of SZ. P*SZ is supported by a large body of evidence showing excessive I-PUFA synthesis, elevated ECB system activity, hyperexcitability of neuromodulators and neurotransmitters, and the effects of antipsychotics. The theory explains the benefits and limitations of current treatment and implies novel treatment directions.

Related theories. P*SZ is a complete theory, covering SZ etiology, symptoms, pathology, risk factors, and treatment. It seems to be the first theory of SZ that provides a mechanistic account of SZ symptoms.[4] It is also the first to recognize the connection between ECBs and the strong evidence involving PUFA in SZ.

The links between SZ and ECBs are well-known and have been extensively reviewed [4,350]. Such work highlights the effect of cannabis on SZ risk, the fact that cannabis can induce psychotic symptoms, and changes to the ECB system (mainly to CB1 density) in SZ. I found only one paper that goes further to propose that hyperactivity of the ECB system is involved in the pathogenesis of SZ [6]. However, even this paper does not propose any mechanistic account, and its authors justly present it as moving towards an ECB hypothesis of SZ rather than a theory.

Similarly, the link between SZ and PUFAs (including ARA and PLA2) has already been recognized, as attested by the clinical trials using om3 supplementation. However, I am not aware of any previous proposal for how PUFA

---

[4] Note: I used the word 'disconnect' when describing the effects of ECBs on the synthesizing cell. To prevent any confusion, it should be noted that P*SZ has absolutely no relationship with the 'dysconnection hypothesis of SZ', which discusses the effect of impaired DA on synapses [289].

alterations might induce the symptoms of SZ, nor of any recognition of the relationship between the PUFA and the ECB evidence in SZ.

One of the first hypotheses for the cause of SZ was that it is a PG deficiency disorder [228]. However, this hypothesis was based on a small set of observations, not on a mechanistic account. In sharp contrast to P*SZ, it concluded with the proposal that ARA should help patients.

Dopamine. The DA hypothesis figures prominently in all current reviews and textbooks of SZ. It is based on the perceived efficacy of D2 antagonists, the psychotic effects of amphetamine, and the moderately increased DA levels in SZ. However, no detailed proposal has been made as to how DA induces SZ symptoms. In P*SZ, increased DA levels are a consequence of the uncontrolled excitability induced by ECBs when acting on DA neurons. However, ECBs induce a similar effect on almost all other cell types in the brain as well. The effect of D2 antagonists can be explained via the partial overlap in distribution and signaling between D2 and CB1, while the effect of amphetamine can be explained via its action on D2. I conclude that dopamine does not have any special role in SZ.

The role of iPLA2. The ARA used for I-PUFA synthesis is mainly released by iPLA2. In this sense, this paper could have been titled "the iPLA2 theory of SZ". However, P*SZ does not claim that iPLA2 is the sole cause of SZ. At its root, SZ is caused by persistent expression changes following prolonged stress. These most likely lead to upregulated iPLA2, but can also involve a wide range of additional effects (e.g., suppression of PG pathway genes, enhancement of AEA and Lkt genes, increased constitutive CB1 activity, etc). iPLA2 upregulation itself can occur due to epigenetic alterations or mutations to its gene, but can also involve upstream genes (e.g., genes regulating store-operated calcium channels, calcium pumps, endoplasmic reticulum, mitochondria, etc). These alterations can be relatively small and difficult to identify, at least using current technology.

In the acronym 'iPLA2', the letter 'i' can conveniently denote 'intracellular' rather than 'independent'. The description 'intracellular calcium store-induced PLA2' is a more appropriate name for this enzyme than 'calcium-independent PLA2'.

Cannabis. P*SZ does not claim that SZ is directly caused by cannabis use. However, exogenous cannabis activates ECB signaling and hence greatly increases risk in susceptible individuals. Moreover, prolonged cannabis use mimics some aspects of chronic stress, so can induce prolonged symptoms, especially if the exposure occurs in sensitive developmental periods.

Symptoms. In P*SZ, positive symptoms are mainly due to excessive excitability, while non-positive symptoms are mainly due to network disconnect. This is one reason why drugs that counter the former are not beneficial for the latter.

It is not the case that 'lack of affect' negative symptoms in SZ occur because SZ patients do not experience emotions. On the contrary, their capacity for experiencing hedonic emotions is intact [351]. These symptoms occur because controlled access to emotion representations and responses is impaired [352]. The problem mainly manifests in emotion anticipation, and is not limited to hedonic emotions, occurring also with respect to losses [353]. Thus, affect symptoms can be viewed as a subtype of cognitive symptoms, both being due to network disconnect.

Age of onset. SZ is usually diagnosed during adolescence or some time later, with the eruption of psychosis. Juvenile psychosis exists, but it is rare (incidence less than 0.04% [354]), while the other types of symptoms can be present throughout the person's life and are commonly present prodromally.

The relatively late appearance of psychosis compared to other symptoms may be explained by the fact that adolescence is a period with massive cortical plasticity. In particular, GC (cortisol) is one of the major recruiters of ECBs, and adolescence is when the expression of the GC receptor is at its peak [355]. Thus, adolescence involves a strong enhancement of the ECB system, which drives it above the psychosis threshold in people who already exhibit the capacity for chronic ECB activity.

Sex differences. SZ is diagnosed earlier in males, and women show increased incidence following menopause [356]. This probably happens because estrogen, although it recruits ECBs [357], is neuroprotective via diverse mechanisms including mitochondria, anti-inflammation, anti-oxidative stress, synaptic plasticity, ACh, growth factors, the microvasculature, and the blood-brain barrier [358]. Estrogen is elevated earlier in females than testosterone in males, delaying disease onset.

Testosterone is neuroprotective as well, and indeed, the sex difference in SZ diminishes with age. Testosterone is reported decreased or unchanged in SZ [356], with the decrease most likely being due to increased PRL and to GC opposition of gonadal steroids.

Future work. Large parts of the discussion here apply to bipolar disorder and depression as well. Some of the analysis here can be used to improve our understanding of immunity-related diseases. The animal models used today for SZ are not valid, but it is possible to develop valid ones. These topics and others will be discussed elsewhere.

Theory predictions. The synthesis and signaling mechanisms of ARA and its products are well-known. This paper has amassed strong evidence for increased I-PUFAs, disconnected network, and hyperexcitability in SZ, and for their capacity of inducing SZ symptoms. Thus, most of the major aspects of P*SZ have already been validated. The areas that most lack evidence are the epigenetic or genetic mechanisms that upregulate the PLA2/ARA paths. A theory prediction is that such mechanisms exist. It might be difficult to find them, as noted above.

The ultimate theory prediction is that normalizing the I-PUFA synthesis paths would improve patient symptoms. Normalization might not be able to undo all of the brain damage done until treatment has started, but it might alleviate it, hopefully to practically unnoticeable levels.

List of abbreviations

Abbreviations introduced in this paper are marked by *** and boldface.

2AG: 2-arachidonoylglycerol.
ALA: alpha-linoleic acid.
ARA: arachidonic acid.
ACh: acetylcholine.
AEA: N-arachidonoylethanolamine.
CB1: type 1 cannabinoid receptor.
COX1, COX2: cyclooxygenase-1, -2.
cPLA2: calcium-dependent PLA2.
CRH (also known as CRF): corticotropin-releasing hormone (or factor).
CSF: cerebrospinal fluid.
D2, D2R: dopamine 2 receptor.
DA: dopamine.
DAG: diacylglycerol.
DAGL: diacylglycerol lipase.
DHA: docosahexaenoic acid.
ECB: endocannabinoid.
*****E-PUFA: PUFA derivates stimulated by extracellular Ca^{2+} (e.g., PGs).**
FAAH: fatty acid amide hydrolase.
FEP: first-episode psychosis.
GABA: gamma-aminobutyric acid.
GC: glucocorticoid.
GIRK channel: G protein-coupled inward rectifying potassium (K^+) channel.
GPCR: G protein-coupled receptor.
H2O2: hydrogen peroxide.
IIN: inhibitory interneuron.
iPLA2: calcium-independent PLA2.
*****I-PUFA: PUFA derivates stimulated by intracellular Ca^{2+} (e.g., AEA, Lkts).**
LA: linoleic acid.
*****Lkt: leukotriene.**
LOX: lipoxygenase.
LSD: lysergic acid diethylamide.
MAGL: monoacylglycerol lipase.
NAPE: N-arachidonoyl phosphatidylethanolamine.
NAPE-PLD: NAPE phospholipase D.
NEP: norepinephrine.
NMDAR: N-methyl-D-aspartate receptor.
NSAIDs: non-steroidal anti-inflammatory drugs.
om3: omega 3 (PUFA).

om6: omega 6 (PUFA).
*****P*SZ: PUFA theory of schizophrenia.**
PC: phosphatidylcholine.
PCP: phenylcyclohexyl piperidine.
PE: phosphatidylethanolamine.
PFC: prefrontal cortex.
PG: prostaglandin.
PI: phosphatidylinositol.
PLA2: phospholipase A2.
PLC: phospholipase C.
PUFA: polyunsaturated fatty acid.
RA: rheumatoid arthritis.
SER: serotonin (5-HT).
SER2a: 5-TH 2a receptor.
SPMs: specialized pro-resolving mediators.
SREBP: sterol regulatory element-binding protein.
SZ: schizophrenia.
TD: tardive dyskinesia.
TRPV1: transient receptor potential vanilloid 1 (channel).

References

[1] R. Tandon, M.S. Keshavan, H.A. Nasrallah, Schizophrenia "just the facts": what we know in 2008: Part 1: overview, Schizophrenia Research 100 (1–3) (2008) 4–19.

[2] Z. Fišar, Biological hypotheses, risk factors, and biomarkers of schizophrenia, Progress in Neuro-Psychopharmacology & Biological Psychiatry (2022) 110626.

[3] M.J. Owen, A. Sawa, P.B. Mortensen, Schizophrenia, The Lancet 388 (2016) 86–97.

[4] F.M. Leweke, C. Rohleder, Putative role of endocannabinoids in schizophrenia, in: The Endocannabinoid System, Elsevier, 2017, pp. 83–113.

[5] W.P. Hoen, J.G. Lijmer, M. Duran, R.J. Wanders, N.J. van Beveren, L. de Haan, Red blood cell polyunsaturated fatty acids measured in red blood cells and schizophrenia: a meta-analysis, Psychiatry Research 207 (1–2) (2013) 1–12.

[6] K.R. Müller-Vahl, H.M. Emrich, Cannabis and schizophrenia: towards a cannabinoid hypothesis of schizophrenia, Expert Review of Neurotherapeutics 8 (7) (2008) 1037–1048.

[7] J.A. Cortes-Briones, J.D. Cahill, P.D. Skosnik, D.H. Mathalon, A. Williams, R.A. Sewell, et al., The psychosis-like effects of Δ9-tetrahydrocannabinol are associated with increased cortical noise in healthy humans, Biological Psychiatry 78 (11) (2015) 805–813.

[8] A. Marconi, M. Di Forti, C.M. Lewis, R.M. Murray, E. Vassos, Meta-analysis of the association between the level of cannabis use and risk of psychosis, Schizophrenia Bulletin 42 (5) (2016) 1262–1269.

[9] K.M. Crosby, J.S. Bains, The intricate link between glucocorticoids and endocannabinoids at stress-relevant synapses in the hypothalamus, Neuroscience 204 (2012) 31–37.

[10] A.W. MacDonald, S.C. Schulz, What we know: findings that every theory of schizophrenia should explain, Schizophrenia Bulletin 35 (3) (2009) 493–508.

[11] F. Varese, F. Smeets, M. Drukker, R. Lieverse, T. Lataster, W. Viechtbauer, et al., Childhood adversities increase the risk of psychosis: a meta-analysis of patient-control, prospective- and cross-sectional cohort studies, Schizophrenia Bulletin 38 (4) (2012) 661–671.

[12] C. D'Addario, A. Di Francesco, M. Pucci, A. Finazzi Agrò, M. Maccarrone, Epigenetic mechanisms and endocannabinoid signalling, The FEBS Journal 280 (9) (2013) 1905–1917.

[13] R. Meccariello, A. Santoro, S. D'Angelo, R. Morrone, S. Fasano, A. Viggiano, et al., The epigenetics of the endocannabinoid system, International Journal of Molecular Sciences 21 (3) (2020) 1113.

[14] M.R. Scott, J.H. Meador-Woodruff, Intracellular compartment-specific proteasome dysfunction in postmortem cortex in schizophrenia subjects, Molecular Psychiatry 25 (4) (2020) 776–790.

[15] C.N. Serhan, Pro-resolving lipid mediators are leads for resolution physiology, Nature 510 (7503) (2014) 92–101.

[16] M. Maccarrone, S. Rossi, M. Bari, V. De Chiara, F. Fezza, A. Musella, et al., Anandamide inhibits metabolism and physiological actions of 2-arachidonoylglycerol in the striatum, Nature Neuroscience 11 (2) (2008) 152–159.

[17] S. Glasner-Edwards, L.J. Mooney, Methamphetamine psychosis: epidemiology and management, CNS Drugs 28 (2014) 1115–1126.

[18] D.M. Walentiny, R.E. Vann, J.A. Warner, L.S. King, H.H. Seltzman, H.A. Navarro, et al., Kappa opioid mediation of cannabinoid effects of the potent hallucinogen, salvinorin A, in rodents, Psychopharmacology 210 (2010) 275–284.

[19] W. Hu, M.L. MacDonald, D.E. Elswick, R.A. Sweet, The glutamate hypothesis of schizophrenia: evidence from human brain tissue studies, Annals of the New York Academy of Sciences 1338 (1) (2015) 38–57.

[20] D.A. Ross, J.S. Cetas, Steroid psychosis: a review for neurosurgeons, Journal of Neuro-Oncology 109 (2012) 439–447.

[21] A. Barre, C. Berthoux, D. De Bundel, E. Valjent, J. Bockaert, P. Marin, et al., Presynaptic serotonin 2A receptors modulate thalamocortical plasticity and associative learning, Proceedings of the National Academy of Sciences 113 (10) (2016) E1382.

[22] C.S. Wu, J. Zhu, J. Wager-Miller, S. Wang, D. O'Leary, K. Monory, et al., Requirement of cannabinoid CB1 receptors in cortical pyramidal neurons for appropriate development of corticothalamic and thalamocortical projections, European Journal of Neuroscience 32 (5) (2010) 693–706.

[23] R.L. Jakab, P.S. Goldman-Rakic, Segregation of serotonin 5-HT2A and 5-HT3 receptors in inhibitory circuits of the primate cerebral cortex, Journal of Comparative Neurology 417 (3) (2000) 337–348.

[24] R.P. Bazinet, S. Layé, Polyunsaturated fatty acids and their metabolites in brain function and disease, Nature Reviews. Neuroscience 15 (12) (2014) 771–785.

[25] W. Wilkins Iii, S. Barbour, et al., Group VI phospholipases A2: homeostatic phospholipases with significant potential as targets for novel therapeutics, Current Drug Targets 9 (8) (2008) 683–697.

[26] S.E. Barbour, A. Kapur, C.L. Deal, Regulation of phosphatidylcholine homeostasis by calcium-independent phospholipase A2, Biochimica et Biophysica Acta (BBA)-Molecular and Cell Biology of Lipids 1439 (1) (1999) 77–88.

[27] P. Nègre-Aminou, R.A. Nemenoff, M.R. Wood, B. de La Houssaye, K. Pfenninger, Characterization of phospholipase A2 activity enriched in the nerve growth cone, Journal of Neurochemistry 67 (1996) 2599–2608.

[28] A.O. Rosa, S.I. Rapoport, Intracellular- and extracellular-derived Ca2+ influence phospholipase A2-mediated fatty acid release from brain phospholipids, Biochimica et Biophysica Acta (BBA)-Molecular and Cell Biology of Lipids 1791 (8) (2009) 697–705.

[29] C. Guo, J. Li, L. Myatt, X. Zhu, K. Sun, Induction of Gαs contributes to the paradoxical stimulation of cytosolic phospholipase A2α expression by cortisol in human amnion fibroblasts, Molecular Endocrinology 24 (5) (2010) 1052–1061.

[30] S. Ramanadham, T. Ali, J.W. Ashley, R.N. Bone, W.D. Hancock, X. Lei, Calcium-independent phospholipases A2 and their roles in biological processes and diseases, Journal of Lipid Research 56 (9) (2015) 1643–1668.

[31] I. Katona, T.F. Freund, Multiple functions of endocannabinoid signaling in the brain, Annual Review of Neuroscience 35 (2012) 529–558.

[32] Y.X. Sun, K. Tsuboi, Y. Okamoto, T. Tonai, M. Murakami, I. Kudo, et al., Biosynthesis of anandamide and N-palmitoylethanolamine by sequential actions of phospholipase A2 and lysophospholipase D, Biochemical Journal 380 (3) (2004) 749–756.
[33] J. Liu, L. Wang, J. Harvey-White, D. Osei-Hyiaman, R. Razdan, Q. Gong, et al., A biosynthetic pathway for anandamide, Proceedings of the National Academy of Sciences 103 (36) (2006) 13345–13350.
[34] K. Tsuboi, T. Uyama, Y. Okamoto, N. Ueda, Endocannabinoids and related N-acylethanolamines: biological activities and metabolism, Inflammation and Regeneration 38 (2018) 1–10.
[35] A. Busquets-Garcia, J. Bains, G. Marsicano, CB1 receptor signaling in the brain: extracting specificity from ubiquity, Neuropsychopharmacology 43 (1) (2018) 4–20.
[36] M. Maroso, G.G. Szabo, H.K. Kim, A. Alexander, A.D. Bui, S.H. Lee, et al., Cannabinoid control of learning and memory through HCN channels, Neuron 89 (5) (2016) 1059–1073.
[37] M. Goppelt-Struebe, D. Wolter, K. Resch, Glucocorticoids inhibit prostaglandin synthesis not only at the level of phospholipase A2 but also at the level of cyclo-oxygenase/PGE isomerase, British Journal of Pharmacology 98 (4) (1989) 1287–1295.
[38] A. Ristimäki, K. Narko, T. Hla, Down-regulation of cytokine-induced cyclo-oxygenase-2 transcript isoforms by dexamethasone: evidence for post-transcriptional regulation, Biochemical Journal 318 (1) (1996) 325–331.
[39] D. Xia, D. Wang, S.H. Kim, H. Katoh, R.N. DuBois, Prostaglandin E2 promotes intestinal tumor growth via DNA methylation, Nature Medicine 18 (2) (2012) 224–226.
[40] J. Zhang, C. Chen, Endocannabinoid 2-arachidonoylglycerol protects neurons by limiting COX-2 elevation, Journal of Biological Chemistry 283 (33) (2008) 22601–22611.
[41] W.C. Chang, A.B. Parekh, Close functional coupling between Ca2+ release-activated Ca2+ channels, arachidonic acid release, and leukotriene C4 secretion, Journal of Biological Chemistry 279 (29) (2004) 29994–29999.
[42] T.K. Finney-Hayward, P. Bahra, S. Li, C.T. Poll, A.G. Nicholson, R.E. Russell, et al., Leukotriene B4 release by human lung macrophages via receptor-not voltage-operated Ca2+ channels, The European Respiratory Journal 33 (5) (2009) 1105–1112.
[43] T. Smani, S.I. Zakharov, E. Leno, P. Csutora, E.S. Trepakova, V.M. Bolotina, Ca2+-independent phospholipase A2 is a novel determinant of store-operated Ca2+ entry, Journal of Biological Chemistry 278 (14) (2003) 11909–11915.
[44] A.R. Brash, et al., Arachidonic acid as a bioactive molecule, The Journal of Clinical Investigation 107 (11) (2001) 1339–1345.
[45] M. Oz, Receptor-independent actions of cannabinoids on cell membranes: focus on endocannabinoids, Pharmacology & Therapeutics 111 (1) (2006) 114–144.
[46] S. Lagalwar, E.Z. Bordayo, K.L. Hoffmann, J.R. Fawcett, W.H. Frey, Anandamides inhibit binding to the muscarinic acetylcholine receptor, Journal of Molecular Neuroscience 13 (1999) 55–61.
[47] A. Varga, A. Jenes, T.H. Marczylo, J. Sousa-Valente, J. Chen, J. Austin, et al., Anandamide produced by Ca2+-insensitive enzymes induces excitation in primary sensory neurons, Pflügers Archiv-European Journal of Physiology 466 (2014) 1421–1435.
[48] H. Sharir, M.E. Abood, Pharmacological characterization of GPR55, a putative cannabinoid receptor, Pharmacology & Therapeutics 126 (3) (2010) 301–313.
[49] L.M. Boland, M.M. Drzewiecki, Polyunsaturated fatty acid modulation of voltage-gated ion channels, Cell Biochemistry and Biophysics 52 (2008) 59–84.
[50] M. Vreugdenhil, C. Bruehl, R. Voskuyl, J. Kang, A. Leaf, W. Wadman, Polyunsaturated fatty acids modulate sodium and calcium currents in CA1 neurons, Proceedings of the National Academy of Sciences 93 (22) (1996) 12559–12563.
[51] C. Bouzat, F. Barrantes, Effects of long-chain fatty acids on the channel activity of the nicotinic acetylcholine receptor, Receptors & Channels 1 (3) (1993) 251–258.
[52] J. Nabekura, K. Noguchi, M.R. Witt, M. Nielsen, N. Akaike, Functional modulation of human recombinant γ-aminobutyric acid type A receptor by docosahexaenoic acid, Journal of Biological Chemistry 273 (18) (1998) 11056–11061.

[53] H. Meves, Arachidonic acid and ion channels: an update, British Journal of Pharmacology 155 (1) (2008) 4–16.

[54] J.A. Matta, R.L. Miyares, G.P. Ahern, TRPV1 is a novel target for omega-3 polyunsaturated fatty acids, The Journal of Physiology 578 (2) (2007) 397–411.

[55] P. Schweitzer, S. Madamba, G.R. Siggins, Arachidonic acid metabolites as mediators of somatostatin-induced increase of neuronal M-current, Nature 346 (6283) (1990) 464–467.

[56] F. Wang, A.M. Trier, F. Li, S. Kim, Z. Chen, J.N. Chai, et al., A basophil-neuronal axis promotes itch, Cell 184 (2) (2021) 422–440.

[57] E.S. Fernandes, C.T. Vong, S. Quek, J. Cheong, S. Awal, C. Gentry, et al., Superoxide generation and leukocyte accumulation: key elements in the mediation of leukotriene B4-induced itch by transient receptor potential ankyrin 1 and transient receptor potential vanilloid 1, The FASEB Journal 27 (4) (2013) 1664–1673.

[58] N.G. Bazan, A.E. Musto, E.J. Knott, Endogenous signaling by omega-3 docosahexaenoic acid-derived mediators sustains homeostatic synaptic and circuitry integrity, Molecular Neurobiology 44 (2011) 216–222.

[59] I.A. Khasabova, M.Y. Golovko, S.A. Golovko, D.A. Simone, S.G. Khasabov, Intrathecal administration of Resolvin D1 and E1 decreases hyperalgesia in mice with bone cancer pain: Involvement of endocannabinoid signaling, Prostaglandins & Other Lipid Mediators 151 (2020) 106479.

[60] M. Payrits, Á. Horváth, T. Biró-Sütő, J. Erostyák, G. Makkai, É. Sághy, et al., Resolvin D1 and D2 inhibit transient receptor potential vanilloid 1 and ankyrin 1 ion channel activation on sensory neurons via lipid raft modification, International Journal of Molecular Sciences 21 (14) (2020) 5019.

[61] L. Cristino, T. Becker, V. di Marzo, Endocannabinoids and energy homeostasis: an update, BioFactors 40 (4) (2014) 389–397.

[62] S. Fujita, Y. Ikegaya, M. Nishikawa, N. Nishiyama, N. Matsuki, Docosahexaenoic acid improves long-term potentiation attenuated by phospholipase A2 inhibitor in rat hippocampal slices, British Journal of Pharmacology 132 (7) (2001) 1417.

[63] M.C. Barbosa-Silva, R.M.P. Campos, I. Del Castilo, J.V. França, P.S. Frost, C. Penido, et al., Mice lacking 5-lipoxygenase display motor deficits associated with cortical and hippocampal synapse abnormalities, Brain, Behavior, and Immunity 100 (2022) 183–193.

[64] H.Y. Kim, A.A. Spector, Z.M. Xiong, A synaptogenic amide N-docosahexaenoylethanolamide promotes hippocampal development, Prostaglandins & Other Lipid Mediators 96 (1–4) (2011) 114–120.

[65] X. Wang, M. Zhu, E. Hjorth, V. Cortés-Toro, H. Eyjolfsdottir, C. Graff, et al., Resolution of inflammation is altered in Alzheimer's disease, Alzheimer's & Dementia 11 (1) (2015) 40–50.

[66] S.M. Shalini, C.F.Y. Ho, Y.K. Ng, J.X. Tong, E.S. Ong, D.R. Herr, et al., Distribution of Alox15 in the rat brain and its role in prefrontal cortical resolvin D1 formation and spatial working memory, Molecular Neurobiology 55 (2018) 1537–1550.

[67] J.M. Gray, H.A. Vecchiarelli, M. Morena, T.T. Lee, D.J. Hermanson, A.B. Kim, et al., Corticotropin-releasing hormone drives anandamide hydrolysis in the amygdala to promote anxiety, Journal of Neuroscience 35 (9) (2015) 3879–3892.

[68] J.M. Gray, H.A. Vecchiarelli, M.N. Hill, Endocannabinoid signaling and synaptic plasticity during stress, in: Synaptic Stress and Pathogenesis of Neuropsychiatric Disorders, Springer, 2014, pp. 99–124.

[69] G. Balsevich, G.N. Petrie, M.N. Hill, Endocannabinoids: Effectors of glucocorticoid signaling, Frontiers in Neuroendocrinology 47 (2017) 86–108.

[70] P. Chameau, Y. Qin, S. Spijker, G. Smit, M. Joëls, Glucocorticoids specifically enhance L-type calcium current amplitude and affect calcium channel subunit expression in the mouse hippocampus, Journal of Neurophysiology 97 (1) (2007) 5–14.

[71] G.M. Kuster, S. Lancel, J. Zhang, C. Communal, M.P. Trucillo, C.C. Lim, et al., Redox-mediated reciprocal regulation of SERCA and Na+–Ca2+ exchanger contributes to sar-

coplasmic reticulum Ca2+ depletion in cardiac myocytes, Free Radical Biology & Medicine 48 (9) (2010) 1182–1187.

[72] Y. Wei, X. Wang, L. Wang, Presence and regulation of cannabinoid receptors in human retinal pigment epithelial cells, Molecular Vision 15 (2009) 1243.

[73] C.A. Sandman, L.M. Glynn, E.P. Davis, Neurobehavioral consequences of fetal exposure to gestational stress, in: Fetal Development: Research on Brain and Behavior, Environmental Influences, and Emerging Technologies, 2016, pp. 229–265.

[74] U. Meyer, Neurodevelopmental resilience and susceptibility to maternal immune activation, Trends in Neurosciences 42 (11) (2019) 793–806.

[75] O. Babenko, I. Kovalchuk, G.A. Metz, Stress-induced perinatal and transgenerational epigenetic programming of brain development and mental health, Neuroscience and Biobehavioral Reviews 48 (2015) 70–91.

[76] A.K. Short, T.Z. Baram, Early-life adversity and neurological disease: age-old questions and novel answers, Nature Reviews Neurology 15 (11) (2019) 657–669.

[77] L. Eiland, R. Romeo, Stress and the developing adolescent brain, Neuroscience 249 (2013) 162–171.

[78] M. Szyf, Nongenetic inheritance and transgenerational epigenetics, Trends in Molecular Medicine 21 (2) (2015) 134–144.

[79] A.L.W. Dick, A. Chen, Stress-Mediated Regulation of the DNA Methylome, in: Stress: Genetics, Epigenetics and Genomics, Elsevier, 2021, pp. 37–47.

[80] S. Goldstein Ferber, V. Trezza, A. Weller, Early life stress and development of the endocannabinoid system: A bidirectional process in programming future coping, Developmental Psychobiology 63 (2) (2021) 143–152.

[81] F. Rusconi, T. Rubino, E. Battaglioli, Endocannabinoid-epigenetic cross-talk: a bridge toward stress coping, International Journal of Molecular Sciences 21 (17) (2020) 6252.

[82] A. Demaili, A. Portugalov, M. Dudai, M. Maroun, I. Akirav, K. Braun, et al., Epigenetic (re) programming of gene expression changes of CB1R and FAAH in the medial prefrontal cortex in response to early life and adolescence stress exposure, Frontiers in Cellular Neuroscience 17 (2023) 1129946.

[83] E.E. Zumbrun, J.M. Sido, P.S. Nagarkatti, M. Nagarkatti, Epigenetic regulation of immunological alterations following prenatal exposure to marijuana cannabinoids and its long term consequences in offspring, Journal of Neuroimmune Pharmacology 10 (2015) 245–254.

[84] T.B. Franklin, H. Russig, I.C. Weiss, J. Gräff, N. Linder, A. Michalon, et al., Epigenetic transmission of the impact of early stress across generations, Biological Psychiatry 68 (5) (2010) 408–415.

[85] S. Hong, G. Zheng, J.W. Wiley, Epigenetic regulation of genes that modulate chronic stress-induced visceral pain in the peripheral nervous system, Gastroenterology 148 (1) (2015) 148–157.

[86] M. Wiedmann, S. Kuitunen-Paul, L.A. Basedow, M. Wolff, N. DiDonato, J. Franzen, et al., DNA methylation changes associated with cannabis use and verbal learning performance in adolescents: an exploratory whole genome methylation study, Translational Psychiatry 12 (1) (2022) 317.

[87] J.P. Hapgood, C. Avenant, J.M. Moliki, Glucocorticoid-independent modulation of GR activity: Implications for immunotherapy, Pharmacology & Therapeutics 165 (2016) 93–113.

[88] J. Hendrik Schmidt, M. Perslev, L. Bukowski, M. Stoklund, F. Herborg, R. Herlo, et al., Constitutive internalization across therapeutically targeted GPCRs correlates with constitutive activity, Basic and Clinical Pharmacology and Toxicology 126 (2020) 116–121.

[89] S.A. Robinson, R.E. Loiacono, A. Christopoulos, P.M. Sexton, D.T. Malone, The effect of social isolation on rat brain expression of genes associated with endocannabinoid signaling, Brain Research 1343 (2010) 153–167.

[90] N. Sciolino, M. Bortolato, S. Eisenstein, J. Fu, F. Oveisi, A. Hohmann, Social isolation and chronic handling alter endocannabinoid signaling and behavioral reactivity to context in adult rats, Neuroscience 168 (2) (2010) 371–386.

[91] E. Zamberletti, F. Piscitelli, T. Rubino, V. Di Marzo, D. Parolaro, Chronic blockade of CB1 receptors reverses startle gating deficits and associated neurochemical alterations in rats reared in isolation, British Journal of Pharmacology 167 (8) (2012) 1652–1664.
[92] E.M. Marco, V. Echeverry-Alzate, J.A. López-Moreno, E. Giné, S. Peñasco, M.P. Viveros, Consequences of early life stress on the expression of endocannabinoid-related genes in the rat brain, Behavioural Pharmacology 25 (5-6) (2014) 547–556.
[93] P. Schneider, L. Bindila, C. Schmahl, M. Bohus, A. Meyer-Lindenberg, B. Lutz, et al., Adverse social experiences in adolescent rats result in enduring effects on social competence pain sensitivity and endocannabinoid signaling, Frontiers in Behavioral Neuroscience 10 (2016) 203.
[94] G. Boero, M.G. Pisu, F. Biggio, L. Muredda, G. Carta, S. Banni, et al., Impaired glucocorticoid-mediated HPA axis negative feedback induced by juvenile social isolation in male rats, Neuropharmacology 133 (2018) 242–253.
[95] T. Uz, Y. Dwivedi, A. Qeli, M. Peters-Golden, G. Pandey, H. Manev, Glucocorticoid receptors are required for up-regulation of neuronal 5-lipoxygenase (5LOX) expression by dexamethasone, The FASEB Journal 15 (10) (2001) 1792–1794.
[96] E. Elliott, C. Hanson, A. Anderson-Berry, T. Nordgren, The role of specialized pro-resolving mediators in maternal-fetal health, Prostaglandins Leukotrienes and Essential Fatty Acids 126 (2017) 98–104.
[97] M. Imbesi, S. Dzitoyeva, L.W. Ng, H. Manev, 5-Lipoxygenase and epigenetic DNA methylation in aging cultures of cerebellar granule cells, Neuroscience 164 (4) (2009) 1531–1537.
[98] W.F. Gattaz, M. Köllisch, T. Thuren, J.A. Virtanen, P.K. Kinnunen, Increased plasma phospholipase-A2 activity in schizophrenic patients: reduction after neuroleptic therapy, Biological Psychiatry 22 (4) (1987) 421–426.
[99] M. Noponen, M. Sanfilipo, K. Samanich, H. Ryer, G. Ko, B. Angrist, et al., Elevated PLA2 activity in schizophrenics and other psychiatric patients, Biological Psychiatry 34 (9) (1993) 641–649.
[100] W.F. Gattaz, A. Schmitt, A. Maras, Increased platelet phospholipase A2 activity in schizophrenia, Schizophrenia Research 16 (1) (1995) 1–6.
[101] B.M. Ross, C. Hudson, J. Erlich, J.J. Warsh, S.J. Kish, Increased phospholipid breakdown in schizophrenia: evidence for the involvement of a calcium-independent phospholipase A2, Archives of General Psychiatry 54 (5) (1997) 487–494.
[102] B.M. Ross, S. Turenne, A. Moszczynska, J.J. Warsh, S.J. Kish, Differential alteration of phospholipase A2 activities in brain of patients with schizophrenia, Brain Research 821 (2) (1999) 407–413.
[103] H. Tavares Jr, J. Yacubian, L.L. Talib, N.R. Barbosa, W.F. Gattaz, Increased phospholipase A2 activity in schizophrenia with absent response to niacin, Schizophrenia Research 61 (1) (2003) 1–6.
[104] S. Smesny, D. Kinder, I. Willhardt, T. Rosburg, J. Lasch, G. Berger, et al., Increased calcium-independent phospholipase A2 activity in first but not in multiepisode chronic schizophrenia, Biological Psychiatry 57 (4) (2005) 399–405.
[105] S. Smesny, B. Milleit, I. Nenadic, C. Preul, D. Kinder, J. Lasch, et al., Phospholipase A2 activity is associated with structural brain changes in schizophrenia, NeuroImage 52 (4) (2010) 1314–1327.
[106] S. Smesny, C. Kunstmann, S. Kunstmann, I. Willhardt, J. Lasch, R.A. Yotter, et al., Phospholipase A2 activity in first episode schizophrenia: associations with symptom severity and outcome at week 12, The World Journal of Biological Psychiatry 12 (8) (2011) 598–607.
[107] C. Xu, X. Yang, L. Sun, T. Yang, C. Cai, P. Wang, et al., An investigation of calcium-independent phospholipase A2 (iPLA2) and cytosolic phospholipase A2 (cPLA2) in schizophrenia, Psychiatry Research 273 (2019) 782–787.
[108] X. Yang, M. Li, J. Jiang, X. Hu, Y. Qing, L. Sun, et al., Dysregulation of phospholipase and cyclooxygenase expression is involved in Schizophrenia, eBioMedicine 64 (2021) 103239.

[109] L.L. Talib, A.C. Costa, H.P. Joaquim, Pereira CA Van de Bilt MT, A.A. Loch, et al., Increased PLA 2 activity in individuals at ultra-high risk for psychosis. European archives of psychiatry and clinical neuroscience:1-7.
[110] M. Li, Y. Gao, D. Wang, X. Hu, J. Jiang, Y. Qing, et al., Impaired Membrane Lipid Homeostasis in Schizophrenia, Schizophrenia Bulletin 48 (5) (2022) 1125–1135.
[111] M. Albers, H. Meurer, F. Märki, J. Klotz, Phospholipase A2 activity in serum of neuroleptic-naive psychiatric inpatients, Pharmacopsychiatry 26 (03) (1993) 94–98.
[112] M.J. Clancy, M.C. Clarke, D.J. Connor, M. Cannon, D.R. Cotter, The prevalence of psychosis in epilepsy a systematic review and meta-analysis, BMC Psychiatry 14 (1) (2014) 1–9.
[113] W.F. Gattaz, K.D. Valente, N.R. Raposo, S. Vincentiis, L.L. Talib, Increased PLA2 activity in the hippocampus of patients with temporal lobe epilepsy and psychosis, Journal of Psychiatric Research 45 (12) (2011) 1617–1620.
[114] B. Elliott, E. Joyce, S. Shorvon, Delusions illusions and hallucinations in epilepsy: 2. Complex phenomena and psychosis, Epilepsy Research 85 (2–3) (2009) 172–186.
[115] G. Onder, F. Pellicciotti, G. Gambassi, R. Bernabei, NSAID-related psychiatric adverse events: who is at risk?, Drugs 64 (2004) 2619–2627.
[116] X.R. Lu, W.Y. Ong, B. Halliwell, L.A. Horrocks, A.A. Farooqui, Differential effects of calcium-dependent and calcium-independent phospholipase A2 inhibitors on kainate-induced neuronal injury in rat hippocampal slices, Free Radical Biology & Medicine 30 (11) (2001) 1263–1273.
[117] F.J. Charlson, A.J. Ferrari, D.F. Santomauro, S. Diminic, E. Stockings, J.G. Scott, et al., Global epidemiology and burden of schizophrenia: findings from the global burden of disease study 2016, Schizophrenia Bulletin 44 (6) (2018) 1195–1203.
[118] M. Peet, J. Laugharne, N. Rangarajan, D. Horrobin, G. Reynolds, Depleted red cell membrane essential fatty acids in drug-treated schizophrenic patients, Journal of Psychiatric Research 29 (3) (1995) 227–232.
[119] J.K. Yao, D.P. van Kammen, J.A. Gurklis, Abnormal incorporation of arachidonic acid into platelets of drug-free patients with schizophrenia, Psychiatry Research 60 (1) (1996) 11–21.
[120] J.K. Yao, S. Leonard, R.D. Reddy, Membrane phospholipid abnormalities in postmortem brains from schizophrenic patients, Schizophrenia Research 42 (1) (2000) 7–17.
[121] M.M. Khan, D.R. Evans, V. Gunna, R.E. Scheffer, V.V. Parikh, S.P. Mahadik, Reduced erythrocyte membrane essential fatty acids and increased lipid peroxides in schizophrenia at the never-medicated first-episode of psychosis and after years of treatment with antipsychotics, Schizophrenia Research 58 (1) (2002) 1–10.
[122] M. Arvindakshan, S. Sitasawad, V. Debsikdar, M. Ghate, D. Evans, D.F. Horrobin, et al., Essential polyunsaturated fatty acid and lipid peroxide levels in never-medicated and medicated schizophrenia patients, Biological Psychiatry 53 (1) (2003) 56–64.
[123] R.D. Reddy, M.S. Keshavan, J.K. Yao, Reduced red blood cell membrane essential polyunsaturated fatty acids in first episode schizophrenia at neuroleptic-naive baseline, Schizophrenia Bulletin 30 (4) (2004) 901–911.
[124] R. Kemperman, M. Veurink, T. van der Wal, H. Knegtering, R. Bruggeman, M. Fokkema, et al., Low essential fatty acid and B-vitamin status in a subgroup of patients with schizophrenia and its response to dietary supplementation, Prostaglandins Leukotrienes and Essential Fatty Acids 74 (2) (2006) 75–85.
[125] R.K. McNamara, R. Jandacek, T. Rider, P. Tso, C.G. Hahn, N.M. Richtand, et al., Abnormalities in the fatty acid composition of the postmortem orbitofrontal cortex of schizophrenic patients: gender differences and partial normalization with antipsychotic medications, Schizophrenia Research 91 (1–3) (2007) 37–50.
[126] M. Sethom, S. Fares, N. Bouaziz, W. Melki, R. Jemaa, M. Feki, et al., Polyunsaturated fatty acids deficits are associated with psychotic state and negative symptoms in patients with schizophrenia, Prostaglandins Leukotrienes and Essential Fatty Acids 83 (3) (2010) 131–136.
[127] S.M. Rice, M.R. Schäfer, C. Klier, N. Mossaheb, N. Vijayakumar, G.P. Amminger, Erythrocyte polyunsaturated fatty acid levels in young people at ultra-high risk for psychotic disorder and healthy adolescent controls, Psychiatry Research 228 (1) (2015) 174–176.

[128] K. Hamazaki, M. Maekawa, T. Toyota, Y. Iwayama, B. Dean, T. Hamazaki, et al., Fatty acid composition and fatty acid binding protein expression in the postmortem frontal cortex of patients with schizophrenia: A case–control study, Schizophrenia Research 171 (1–3) (2016) 225–232.
[129] D. Wang, X. Sun, J. Yan, B. Ren, B. Cao, Q. Lu, et al., Alterations of eicosanoids and related mediators in patients with schizophrenia, Journal of Psychiatric Research 102 (2018) 168–178.
[130] A. Alqarni, T.W. Mitchell, P.D. McGorry, B. Nelson, C. Markulev, H.P. Yuen, et al., Comparison of erythrocyte omega-3 index, fatty acids and molecular phospholipid species in people at ultra-high risk of developing psychosis and healthy people, Schizophrenia Research 226 (2020) 44–51.
[131] X. Zhou, T. Long, G.L. Haas, H. Cai, J.K. Yao, Reduced levels and disrupted biosynthesis pathways of plasma free fatty acids in first-episode antipsychotic-naïve schizophrenia patients, Frontiers in Neuroscience 14 (2020) 784.
[132] N. Li, P. Yang, M. Tang, Y. Liu, W. Guo, B. Lang, et al., Reduced erythrocyte membrane polyunsaturated fatty acid levels indicate diminished treatment response in patients with multi-versus first-episode schizophrenia, Schizophrenia 8 (1) (2022) 7.
[133] Y.H. Yu, H.M. Su, S.H. Lin, P.C. Hsiao, Y.T. Lin, C.M. Liu, et al., Niacin skin flush and membrane polyunsaturated fatty acids in schizophrenia from the acute state to partial remission: a dynamic relationship, Schizophrenia 8 (1) (2022) 38.
[134] I. Das, N. Khan, Increased arachidonic acid induced platelet chemiluminescence indicates cyclooxygenase overactivity in schizophrenic subjects, Prostaglandins Leukotrienes and Essential Fatty Acids 58 (3) (1998) 165–168.
[135] M. Berger, B. Nelson, C. Markulev, H.P. Yuen, M.R. Schäfer, N. Mossaheb, et al., Relationship between polyunsaturated fatty acids and psychopathology in the NEURAPRO clinical trial, Frontiers in Psychiatry 10 (2019) 393.
[136] A. Kale, S. Joshi, N. Naphade, S. Sapkale, M. Raju, A. Pillai, et al., Opposite changes in predominantly docosahexaenoic acid (DHA) in cerebrospinal fluid and red blood cells from never-medicated first-episode psychotic patients, Schizophrenia Research 98 (1–3) (2008) 295–301.
[137] S.P. Mahadik, S. Mukherjee, D.F. Horrobin, K. Jenkins, E.E. Correnti, R.E. Scheffer, Plasma membrane phospholipid fatty acid composition of cultured skin fibroblasts from schizophrenic patients: comparison with bipolar patients and normal subjects, Psychiatry Research 63 (2–3) (1996) 133–142.
[138] A. Frajerman, B. Chaumette, D. Farabos, G. Despres, C. Simonard, A. Lamazière, et al., Membrane Lipids in Ultra-High-Risk Patients: Potential Predictive Biomarkers of Conversion to Psychosis, Nutrients 15 (9) (2023) 2215.
[139] S. Smesny, B. Milleit, U. Hipler, C. Milleit, M. Schäfer, C. Klier, et al., Omega-3 fatty acid supplementation changes intracellular phospholipase A2 activity and membrane fatty acid profiles in individuals at ultra-high risk for psychosis, Molecular Psychiatry 19 (3) (2014) 317–324.
[140] S. Medema, R.J. Mocking, M.W. Koeter, F.M. Vaz, C. Meijer, L. de Haan, et al., Levels of red blood cell fatty acids in patients with psychosis, their unaffected siblings, and healthy controls, Schizophrenia Bulletin 42 (2) (2016) 358–368.
[141] M. Watari, K. Hamazaki, T. Hirata, T. Hamazaki, Y. Okubo, Hostility of drug-free patients with schizophrenia and n-3 polyunsaturated fatty acid levels in red blood cells, Psychiatry Research 177 (1–2) (2010) 22–26.
[142] P.R. Szeszko, R.K. McNamara, J.A. Gallego, A.K. Malhotra, U. Govindarajulu, B.D. Peters, et al., Longitudinal investigation of the relationship between omega-3 polyunsaturated fatty acids and neuropsychological functioning in recent-onset psychosis: a randomized clinical trial, Schizophrenia Research 228 (2021) 180–187.
[143] M.E. Maida, S.D. Hurley, J.A. Daeschner, A.H. Moore, M.K. O'banion, Cytosolic prostaglandin E2 synthase (cPGES) expression is decreased in discrete cortical regions in psychiatric disease, Brain Research 1103 (1) (2006) 164–172.

[144] B. Dean, A. Gibbons, A. Gogos, M. Udawela, E. Thomas, E. Scarr, Studies on prostaglandin-endoperoxide synthase 1: lower levels in schizophrenia and after treatment with antipsychotic drugs in conjunction with aspirin, International Journal of Neuropsychopharmacology 21 (3) (2018) 216–225.
[145] S. Ganzinelli, E. Borda, L. Sterin-Borda, Autoantibodies from schizophrenia patients induce cerebral COX-1/iNOS mRNA expression with NO/PGE2/MMP-3 production, International Journal of Neuropsychopharmacology 13 (3) (2010) 293–303.
[146] Y. Abdulla, K. Hamadah, Effect of ADP on PGE1 formation in blood platelets from patients with depression, mania and schizophrenia, British Journal of Psychiatry 127 (6) (1975) 591–595.
[147] H. Kaiya, Prostaglandin E1 suppression of platelet aggregation response in schizophrenia, Schizophrenia Research 5 (1) (1991) 67–80.
[148] B. Tang, C. Capitao, B. Dean, E.A. Thomas, Differential age- and disease-related effects on the expression of genes related to the arachidonic acid signaling pathway in schizophrenia, Psychiatry Research 196 (2–3) (2012) 201–206.
[149] J. Caso, M. García-Portilla, L. De la Fuente-Tomás, L. González-Blanco, P.S. Martínez, J. Leza, et al., Regulation of inflammatory pathways in schizophrenia: a comparative study with bipolar disorder and healthy controls, European Psychiatry 47 (2018) 50–59.
[150] R.N. Yüksel, A.P. Titiz, E.T. Yaylacı, K. Ünal, T. Turhan, G. Erzin, et al., Serum PGE2, 15d-PGJ, PPARγ and CRP levels in patients with schizophrenia, Asian Journal of Psychiatry 46 (2019) 24–28.
[151] M. Fromer, P. Roussos, S.K. Sieberts, J.S. Johnson, D.H. Kavanagh, T.M. Perumal, et al., Gene expression elucidates functional impact of polygenic risk for schizophrenia, Nature Neuroscience 19 (11) (2016) 1442–1453.
[152] H. Kaiya, M. Uematsu, M. Ofuji, A. Nishida, K. Takeuchi, M. Nozaki, et al., Elevated plasma prostaglandin E2 levels in schizophrenia, Journal of Neural Transmission 77 (1989) 39–46.
[153] I. Martínez-Gras, B.G. Pérez-Nievas, B. García-Bueno, J.L. Madrigal, E. Andrés-Esteban, R. Rodríguez-Jiménez, et al., The anti-inflammatory prostaglandin 15d-PGJ2 and its nuclear receptor PPARgamma are decreased in schizophrenia, Schizophrenia Research 128 (1–3) (2011) 15–22.
[154] B. García-Bueno, M. Bioque, K.S. Mac-Dowell, M.F. Barcones, M. Martínez-Cengotitabengoa, L. Pina-Camacho, et al., Pro-/anti-inflammatory dysregulation in patients with first episode of psychosis: toward an integrative inflammatory hypothesis of schizophrenia, Schizophrenia Bulletin 40 (2) (2014) 376–387.
[155] B. Cabrera, R. Penadés, A. González-Pinto, M. Parellada, J. Bobes, A. Lobo, et al., Cognition and psychopathology in first-episode psychosis: are they related to inflammation?, Psychological Medicine 46 (10) (2016) 2133–2144.
[156] C.A. Pereira, A.C. Costa, H.P. Joaquim, L.L. Talib, M.T. van de Bilt, A.A. Loch, et al., COX-2 pathway is upregulated in ultra-high risk individuals for psychosis, The World Journal of Biological Psychiatry 23 (3) (2022) 236–241.
[157] S. Nadalin, A. Buretić-Tomljanović, G. Rubeša, D. Tomljanović, L. Gudelj, Niacin skin flush test: a research tool for studying schizophrenia, Psychiatria Danubina 22 (1) (2010) 14–27.
[158] L. Dong, H. Zou, C. Yuan, Y.H. Hong, D.V. Kuklev, W.L. Smith, Different fatty acids compete with arachidonic acid for binding to the allosteric or catalytic subunits of cyclooxygenases to regulate prostanoid synthesis, Journal of Biological Chemistry 291 (8) (2016) 4069–4078.
[159] R.S. Lacombe, R. Chouinard-Watkins, R.P. Bazinet, Brain docosahexaenoic acid uptake and metabolism, Molecular Aspects of Medicine 64 (2018) 109–134.
[160] R.K. McNamara, R. Jandacek, T. Rider, P. Tso, Y. Dwivedi, G.N. Pandey, Adult medication-free schizophrenic patients exhibit long-chain omega-3 fatty acid deficiency: implications for cardiovascular disease risk, Cardiovascular Psychiatry and Neurology 2013 (2013) 796462.
[161] J. McEvoy, R.A. Baillie, H. Zhu, P. Buckley, M.S. Keshavan, H.A. Nasrallah, et al., Lipidomics reveals early metabolic changes in subjects with schizophrenia: effects of atypical antipsychotics, PLoS ONE (2013), 8(7):e68717.

[162] J. Assies, R. Lieverse, P. Vreken, R.J. Wanders, P.M. Dingemans, D.H. Linszen, Significantly reduced docosahexaenoic and docosapentaenoic acid concentrations in erythrocyte membranes from schizophrenic patients compared with a carefully matched control group, Biological Psychiatry 49 (6) (2001) 510–522.
[163] P.L. Wood, G. Unfried, W. Whitehead, A. Phillipps, J.A. Wood, Dysfunctional plasmalogen dynamics in the plasma and platelets of patients with schizophrenia, Schizophrenia Research 161 (2–3) (2015) 506–510.
[164] S. Mahadik, R. Scheffer, S. Mukherjee, E. Correnti, Utilization of precursor essential fatty acids in culture by skin fibroblasts from schizophrenic patients and normal controls, Prostaglandins Leukotrienes and Essential Fatty Acids 55 (1–2) (1996) 65–70.
[165] M. Berger, S. Smesny, S. Kim, C. Davey, S. Rice, Z. Sarnyai, et al., Omega-6 to omega-3 polyunsaturated fatty acid ratio and subsequent mood disorders in young people with at-risk mental states: a 7-year longitudinal study, Translational Psychiatry (2017), 7(8):e1220-0.
[166] J.W. Pettegrew, M.S. Keshavan, K. Panchalingam, S. Strychor, D.B. Kaplan, M.G. Tretta, et al., Alterations in brain high-energy phosphate and membrane phospholipid metabolism in first-episode, drug-naive schizophrenics: A pilot study of the dorsal prefrontal cortex by in vivo phosphorus 31 nuclear magnetic resonance spectroscopy, Archives of General Psychiatry 48 (6) (1991) 563–568.
[167] M.S. Keshavan, A.G. Mallinger, J.W. Pettegrew, C. Dippold, Erythrocyte membrane phospholipids in psychotic patients, Psychiatry Research 49 (1) (1993) 89–95.
[168] S.P. Mahadik, S. Mukherjee, E.E. Correnti, H.S. Kelkar, C.G. Wakade, R.M. Costa, et al., Plasma membrane phospholipid and cholesterol distribution of skin fibroblasts from drug-naive patients at the onset of psychosis, Schizophrenia Research 13 (3) (1994) 239–247.
[169] J.A. Stanley, P.C. Williamson, D.J. Drost, T.J. Carr, R.J. Rylett, A. Malla, et al., An in vivo study of the prefrontal cortex of schizophrenic patients at different stages of illness via phosphorus magnetic resonance spectroscopy, Archives of General Psychiatry 52 (5) (1995) 399–406.
[170] A. Schmitt, A. Maras, G. Petroianu, D. Braus, L. Scheuer, Effects of antipsychotic treatment on membrane phospholipid metabolism in schizophrenia, Journal of Neural Transmission 108 (2001) 1081–1091.
[171] A. Ponizovsky, I. Modai, Y. Nechamkin, G. Barshtein, M. Ritsner, S. Yedgar, et al., Phospholipid patterns of erythrocytes in schizophrenia: relationships to symptomatology, Schizophrenia Research 52 (1–2) (2001) 121–126.
[172] N. Ryazantseva, V. Novitsky, N. Vlasova, N. Tokareva, O. Zhukova, S. Mikheev, et al., Changes in the Composition, Structure, and Metabolism of Erythrocyte Membranes in Schizophrenia and Other Psychopathologies, Neurophysiology 34 (2002) 332–341.
[173] A. Schmitt, K. Wilczek, K. Blennow, A. Maras, A. Jatzko, G. Petroianu, et al., Altered thalamic membrane phospholipids in schizophrenia: a postmortem study, Biological Psychiatry 56 (1) (2004) 41–45.
[174] R. Kaddurah-Daouk, J. McEvoy, R. Baillie, H. Zhu, J.K. Yao, V.L. Nimgaonkar, et al., Impaired plasmalogens in patients with schizophrenia, Psychiatry Research 198 (3) (2012) 347–352.
[175] D. Wang, S.L. Cheng, Q. Fei, H. Gu, D. Raftery, B. Cao, et al., Metabolic profiling identifies phospholipids as potential serum biomarkers for schizophrenia, Psychiatry Research 272 (2019) 18–29.
[176] D. Wang, X. Sun, M. Maziade, W. Mao, C. Zhang, J. Wang, et al., Characterising phospholipids and free fatty acids in patients with schizophrenia: A case-control study, The World Journal of Biological Psychiatry 22 (3) (2021) 161–174.
[177] M. Song, Y. Liu, J. Zhou, H. Shi, X. Su, M. Shao, et al., Potential plasma biomarker panels identification for the diagnosis of first-episode schizophrenia and monitoring antipsychotic monotherapy with the use of metabolomics analyses, Psychiatry Research 321 (2023) 115070.

[178] P. Nuss, C. Tessier, F. Ferreri, M. De Hert, J. Peuskens, G. Trugnan, et al., Abnormal transbilayer distribution of phospholipids in red blood cell membranes in schizophrenia, Psychiatry Research 169 (2) (2009) 91–96.
[179] J.R. Atack, J. Levine, R.H. Belmaker, Cerebrospinal fluid inositol monophosphatase: elevated activity in depression and neuroleptic-treated schizophrenia, Biological Psychiatry 44 (6) (1998) 433–437.
[180] H. Shimon, Y. Sobolev, M. Davidson, V. Haroutunian, R.H. Belmaker, G. Agam, Inositol levels are decreased in postmortem brain of schizophrenic patients, Biological Psychiatry 44 (6) (1998) 428–432.
[181] R.S. Jope, L. Song, C.A. Grimes, M.A. Pacheco, G.E. Dilley, X. Li, et al., Selective increases in phosphoinositide signaling activity and G protein levels in postmortem brain from subjects with schizophrenia or alcohol dependence, Journal of Neurochemistry 70 (2) (1998) 763–771.
[182] M.A. Essali, I. Das, J. de Belleroche, S.R. Hirsch, The platelet polyphosphoinositide system in schizophrenia: the effects of neuroleptic treatment, Biological Psychiatry 28 (6) (1990) 475–487.
[183] I. Das, M. Essali, J. De Belleroche, S. Hirsch, Inositol phospholipid turnover in platelets of schizophrenic patients, Prostaglandins Leukotrienes and Essential Fatty Acids 46 (1) (1992) 65–66.
[184] J. Yao, P. Yasaei, D. Van Kammen, Increased turnover of platelet phosphatidylinositol in schizophrenia, Prostaglandins Leukotrienes and Essential Fatty Acids 46 (1) (1992) 39–46.
[185] J. Rybakowski, W. Lehmann, Increased erythrocyte inositol monophosphatase activity in schizophrenia, European Psychiatry 12 (1) (1997) 44–45.
[186] Y. Kunii, J. Matsumoto, R. Izumi, A. Nagaoka, M. Hino, R. Shishido, et al., Evidence for altered phosphoinositide signaling-associated molecules in the postmortem prefrontal cortex of patients with schizophrenia, International Journal of Molecular Sciences 22 (15) (2021) 8280.
[187] P.F. Durrenberger, F.S. Fernando, S.N. Kashefi, T.P. Bonnert, D. Seilhean, B. Nait-Oumesmar, et al., Common mechanisms in neurodegeneration and neuroinflammation: a BrainNet Europe gene expression microarray study, Journal of Neural Transmission 122 (2015) 1055–1068.
[188] I.S. Piras, M. Manchia, M.J. Huentelman, F. Pinna, C.C. Zai, J.L. Kennedy, et al., Peripheral biomarkers in schizophrenia: a meta-analysis of microarray gene expression datasets, International Journal of Neuropsychopharmacology 22 (3) (2019) 186–193.
[189] T. Kim, H.J. Kim, J.K. Park, J.W. Kim, J.H. Chung, Association between polymorphisms of arachidonate 12-lipoxygenase (ALOX12) and schizophrenia in a Korean population, Behavioral and Brain Functions 6 (1) (2010) 1–4.
[190] S. Akiyama, H. Nagai, S. Oike, I. Horikawa, M. Shinohara, Y. Lu, et al., Chronic social defeat stress increases the amounts of 12-lipoxygenase lipid metabolites in the nucleus accumbens of stress-resilient mice, Scientific Reports 12 (1) (2022) 11385.
[191] R. Junqueira, Q. Cordeiro, I. Meira-Lima, W.F. Gattaz, H. Vallada, Allelic association analysis of phospholipase A2 genes with schizophrenia, Psychiatric Genetics 14 (3) (2004) 157–160.
[192] Y. Yu, R. Tao, J. Shi, X. Zhang, C. Kou, Y. Guo, et al., A genetic study of two calcium-independent cytosolic PLA2 genes in schizophrenia, Prostaglandins Leukotrienes and Essential Fatty Acids 73 (5) (2005) 351–354.
[193] R. Tao, Y. Yu, X. Zhang, Y. Guo, J. Shi, X. Zhang, et al., Cytosolic PLA2 genes possibly contribute to the etiology of schizophrenia, American Journal of Medical Genetics. Part B, Neuropsychiatric Genetics 137 (1) (2005) 56–58.
[194] S. Nadalin, A. Buretić-Tomljanović, An association between PLA2G6 and PLA2G4C gene polymorphisms and schizophrenia risk and illness severity in a Croatian population, Prostaglandins Leukotrienes and Essential Fatty Acids 121 (2017) 57–59.

[195] S. Le Hellard, T. Mühleisen, S. Djurovic, J. Fernø, Z. Ouriaghi, M. Mattheisen, et al., Polymorphisms in SREBF1 and SREBF2, two antipsychotic-activated transcription factors controlling cellular lipogenesis, are associated with schizophrenia in German and Scandinavian samples, Molecular Psychiatry 15 (5) (2010) 463–472.
[196] N.R. Barbosa, R.M. Junqueira, H.P. Vallada, W.F. Gattaz, Association between Ban I genotype and increased phospholipase A2 activity in schizophrenia, European Archives of Psychiatry and Clinical Neuroscience 257 (2007) 340–343.
[197] S. Nadalin, G. Rubeša, J. Giacometti, M. Vulin, D. Tomljanović, J. Vraneković, et al., BanI polymorphism of cytosolic phospholipase A2 gene is associated with age at onset in male patients with schizophrenia and schizoaffective disorder, Prostaglandins Leukotrienes and Essential Fatty Acids 78 (6) (2008) 351–360.
[198] D.B. Allison, J.W. Newcomer, A.L. Dunn, J.A. Blumenthal, A.N. Fabricatore, G.L. Daumit, et al., Obesity among those with mental disorders: a National Institute of Mental Health meeting report, American Journal of Preventive Medicine 36 (4) (2009) 341–350.
[199] N. Garrido-Torres, M. Ruiz-Veguilla, L. Alameda, M. Canal-Rivero, M.J. Ruiz, M. Gómez-Revuelta, et al., Prevalence of metabolic syndrome and related factors in a large sample of antipsychotic naïve patients with first-episode psychosis: Baseline results from the PAFIP cohort, Schizophrenia Research 246 (2022) 277–285.
[200] M. Strassnig, J. Brar, R. Ganguli, Dietary intake of patients with schizophrenia, Psychiatry (Edgmont (Pa: Township)) 2 (2) (2005) 31–35.
[201] M. Strassnig, J.S. Brar, R. Ganguli, Dietary fatty acid and antioxidant intake in community-dwelling patients suffering from schizophrenia, Schizophrenia Research 76 (2–3) (2005) 343–351.
[202] S. Dipasquale, C.M. Pariante, P. Dazzan, E. Aguglia, P. McGuire, V. Mondelli, The dietary pattern of patients with schizophrenia: a systematic review, Journal of Psychiatric Research 47 (2) (2013) 197–207.
[203] T. Pawełczyk, E. Trafalska, M. Kotlicka-Antczak, A. Pawełczyk, The association between polyunsaturated fatty acid consumption and the transition to psychosis in ultra-high risk individuals, Prostaglandins Leukotrienes and Essential Fatty Acids 108 (2016) 30–37.
[204] T. Pawełczyk, E. Trafalska, A. Pawełczyk, M. Kotlicka-Antczak, Differences in omega-3 and omega-6 polyunsaturated fatty acid consumption in people at ultra-high risk of psychosis, first-episode schizophrenia, and in healthy controls, Early Intervention in Psychiatry 11 (6) (2017) 498–508.
[205] E.J. Kim, S.Y. Lim, H.J. Lee, J.Y. Lee, S. Choi, S.Y. Kim, et al., Low dietary intake of n-3 fatty acids, niacin, folate, and vitamin C in Korean patients with schizophrenia and the development of dietary guidelines for schizophrenia, Nutrition Research 45 (2017) 10–18.
[206] R. McNamara, Modulation of polyunsaturated fatty acid biosynthesis by antipsychotic medications: Implications for the pathophysiology and treatment of schizophrenia, Clinical Lipidology 4 (6) (2009) 809–820.
[207] P. Bozzatello, P. Rocca, E. Mantelli, S. Bellino, Polyunsaturated fatty acids: what is their role in treatment of psychiatric disorders?, International Journal of Molecular Sciences 20 (21) (2019) 5257.
[208] M.C. Hsu, Y.S. Huang, W.C. Ouyang, Beneficial effects of omega-3 fatty acid supplementation in schizophrenia: Possible mechanisms, Lipids in Health and Disease 19 (2020) 1–17.
[209] J. Kim, Y. Li, B.A. Watkins, Fat to treat fat: emerging relationship between dietary PUFA, endocannabinoids, and obesity, Prostaglandins & Other Lipid Mediators 104 (2013) 32–41.
[210] M. Hedelin, M. Löf, M. Olsson, T. Lewander, B. Nilsson, C.M. Hultman, et al., Dietary intake of fish, omega-3, omega-6 polyunsaturated fatty acids and vitamin D and the prevalence of psychotic-like symptoms in a cohort of 33,000 women from the general population, BMC Psychiatry 10 (1) (2010) 1–13.
[211] Y. Gao, X. Hu, D. Wang, J. Jiang, M. Li, Y. Qing, et al., Association between arachidonic acid and the risk of schizophrenia: a cross-national study and Mendelian randomization analysis, Nutrients 15 (5) (2023) 1195.

[212] A. Fogerty, F. Whitfield, D. Svoronos, G. Ford, The composition of the fatty acids and aldehydes of the ethanolamine and choline phospholipids of various meats, International Journal of Food Science & Technology 26 (4) (1991) 363–371.
[213] M. Trépanier, K. Hopperton, R. Mizrahi, N. Mechawar, R. Bazinet, Postmortem evidence of cerebral inflammation in schizophrenia: a systematic review, Molecular Psychiatry 21 (8) (2016) 1009–1026.
[214] B.J. Miller, P. Buckley, W. Seabolt, A. Mellor, B. Kirkpatrick, Meta-analysis of cytokine alterations in schizophrenia: clinical status and antipsychotic effects, Biological Psychiatry 70 (7) (2011) 663–671.
[215] R. Khoury, H.A. Nasrallah, Inflammatory biomarkers in individuals at clinical high risk for psychosis (CHR-P): State or trait?, Schizophrenia Research 199 (2018) 31–38.
[216] A.E. Cullen, S. Holmes, T.A. Pollak, G. Blackman, D.W. Joyce, M.J. Kempton, et al., Associations between non-neurological autoimmune disorders and psychosis: a meta-analysis, Biological Psychiatry 85 (1) (2019) 35–48.
[217] L.Y. Wang, S.F. Chen, J.H. Chiang, C.Y. Hsu, Y.C. Shen, Autoimmune diseases are associated with an increased risk of schizophrenia: a nationwide population-based cohort study, Schizophrenia Research 202 (2018) 297–302.
[218] Y.H. Chen, H.C. Lee, H.C. Lin, Prevalence and risk of atopic disorders among schizophrenia patients: a nationwide population based study, Schizophrenia Research 108 (1–3) (2009) 191–196.
[219] M.S. Pedersen, M.E. Benros, E. Agerbo, A.D. Børglum, P.B. Mortensen, Schizophrenia in patients with atopic disorders with particular emphasis on asthma: a Danish population-based study, Schizophrenia Research 138 (1) (2012) 58–62.
[220] S. Tiosano, A. Farhi, A. Watad, N. Grysman, R. Stryjer, H. Amital, et al., Schizophrenia among patients with systemic lupus erythematosus: population-based cross-sectional study, Epidemiology and Psychiatric Sciences 26 (4) (2017) 424–429.
[221] R.J. Oken, M. Schulzer, At issue: schizophrenia and rheumatoid arthritis: the negative association revisited, Schizophrenia Bulletin 25 (4) (1999) 625–638.
[222] S. Matthysse, J. Lipinski, Biochemical aspects of schizophrenia, Annual Review of Medicine 26 (1) (1975) 551–565.
[223] E. Heleniak, O'Desky I. Histamine and prostaglandins in schizophrenia: revisited, Medical Hypotheses 52 (1) (1999) 37–42.
[224] J.M. McCoy, J.R. Wicks, L.P. Audoly, et al., The role of prostaglandin E2 receptors in the pathogenesis of rheumatoid arthritis, The Journal of Clinical Investigation 110 (5) (2002) 651–658.
[225] R. Pettipher, The roles of the prostaglandin D2 receptors DP1 and CRTH2 in promoting allergic responses, British Journal of Pharmacology 153 (S1) (2008) S191.
[226] T.S. Hallstrand, W.R. Henderson Jr, An update on the role of leukotrienes in asthma, Current Opinion in Allergy and Clinical Immunology 10 (1) (2010) 60.
[227] T. Ruzicka, T. Simmet, B.A. Peskar, J. Ring, Skin levels of arachidonic acid-derived inflammatory mediators and histamine in atopic dermatitis and psoriasis, Journal of Investigative Dermatology 86 (2) (1986) 105–108.
[228] D. Horrobin, Schizophrenia as a prostaglandin deficiency disease, The Lancet 309 (8018) (1977) 936–937.
[229] G. Engels, A.L. Francke, B. van Meijel, J.G. Douma, H. de Kam, W. Wesselink, et al., Clinical pain in schizophrenia: a systematic review, The Journal of Pain 15 (5) (2014) 457–467.
[230] F.M. Leweke, A. Giuffrida, U. Wurster, H.M. Emrich, D. Piomelli, Elevated endogenous cannabinoids in schizophrenia, NeuroReport 10 (8) (1999) 1665–1669.
[231] N. De Marchi, L. De Petrocellis, P. Orlando, F. Daniele, F. Fezza, V. Di Marzo, Endocannabinoid signalling in the blood of patients with schizophrenia, Lipids in Health and Disease 2 (2003) 1–9.
[232] A. Giuffrida, F.M. Leweke, C.W. Gerth, D. Schreiber, D. Koethe, J. Faulhaber, et al., Cerebrospinal anandamide levels are elevated in acute schizophrenia and are inversely correlated with psychotic symptoms, Neuropsychopharmacology 29 (11) (2004) 2108–2114.

[233] F.M. Leweke, A. Giuffrida, D. Koethe, D. Schreiber, B.M. Nolden, L. Kranaster, et al., Anandamide levels in cerebrospinal fluid of first-episode schizophrenic patients: impact of cannabis use, Schizophrenia Research 94 (1–3) (2007) 29–36.
[234] S. Potvin, É. Kouassi, O. Lipp, R.H. Bouchard, M.A. Roy, M.F. Demers, et al., Endogenous cannabinoids in patients with schizophrenia and substance use disorder during quetiapine therapy, Journal of Psychopharmacology 22 (3) (2008) 262–269.
[235] D. Koethe, A. Giuffrida, D. Schreiber, M. Hellmich, F. Schultze-Lutter, S. Ruhrmann, et al., Anandamide elevation in cerebrospinal fluid in initial prodromal states of psychosis, British Journal of Psychiatry 194 (4) (2009) 371–372.
[236] C. Muguruza, M. Lehtonen, N. Aaltonen, B. Morentin, J.J. Meana, L.F. Callado, Quantification of endocannabinoids in postmortem brain of schizophrenic subjects, Schizophrenia Research 148 (1–3) (2013) 145–150.
[237] D. Koethe, F. Pahlisch, M. Hellmich, C. Rohleder, J.K. Mueller, A. Meyer-Lindenberg, et al., Familial abnormalities of endocannabinoid signaling in schizophrenia, The World Journal of Biological Psychiatry 20 (2) (2019) 117–125.
[238] S. Potvin, L. Mahrouche, R. Assaf, M. Chicoine, C.É. Giguère, A. Furtos, et al., Peripheral endogenous cannabinoid levels are increased in schizophrenia patients evaluated in a psychiatric emergency setting, Frontiers in Psychiatry 11 (2020) 628.
[239] I. Ibarra-Lecue, P. Unzueta-Larrinaga, R. Barrena-Barbadillo, A. Villate, I. Horrillo, B. Mendivil, et al., Cannabis use selectively modulates circulating biomarkers in the blood of schizophrenia patients, Addiction Biology 27 (6) (2022) e13233.
[240] M. Parksepp, L. Haring, K. Kilk, K. Koch, K. Uppin, R. Kangro, et al., The expanded endocannabinoid system contributes to metabolic and body mass shifts in first-episode schizophrenia: a 5-year follow-up study, Biomedicines 10 (2) (2022) 243.
[241] T.B. Rømer, R. Jeppesen, R.H.B. Christensen, M.E. Benros, Biomarkers in the cerebrospinal fluid of patients with psychotic disorders compared to healthy controls: a systematic review and meta-analysis, Molecular Psychiatry (2023) 1–14.
[242] A. Minichino, M. Senior, N. Brondino, S.H. Zhang, B.R. Godlewska, P.W. Burnet, et al., Measuring disturbance of the endocannabinoid system in psychosis: a systematic review and meta-analysis, JAMA Psychiatry 76 (9) (2019) 914–923.
[243] E. Appiah-Kusi, R. Wilson, M. Colizzi, E. Foglia, E. Klamerus, A. Caldwell, et al., Childhood trauma and being at-risk for psychosis are associated with higher peripheral endocannabinoids, Psychological Medicine 50 (11) (2020) 1862–1871.
[244] H.P. Joaquim, A.C. Costa, C.A. Pereira, L.L. Talib, M.M. Bilt, A.A. Loch, et al., Plasmatic endocannabinoids are decreased in subjects with ultra-high risk of psychosis, European Journal of Neuroscience 55 (4) (2022) 1079–1087.
[245] C. Muguruza, B. Morentin, J.J. Meana, S.P. Alexander, L.F. Callado, Endocannabinoid system imbalance in the postmortem prefrontal cortex of subjects with schizophrenia, Journal of Psychopharmacology 33 (9) (2019) 1132–1140.
[246] M. Bioque, B. García-Bueno, K.S. MacDowell, A. Meseguer, P.A. Saiz, M. Parellada, et al., Peripheral endocannabinoid system dysregulation in first-episode psychosis, Neuropsychopharmacology 38 (13) (2013) 2568–2577.
[247] C.J. Morgan, E. Page, C. Schaefer, K. Chatten, A. Manocha, S. Gulati, et al., Cerebrospinal fluid anandamide levels, cannabis use and psychotic-like symptoms, British Journal of Psychiatry 202 (5) (2013) 381–382.
[248] P. Si, S. Liu, D. Tong, M. Cheng, L. Wang, X. Cheng, Association of polymorphisms of NAPE-PLD and FAAH genes with schizophrenia in Chinese Han population, Zhonghua yi xue yi chuan xue za zhi= Zhonghua yixue yichuanxue zazhi= Chinese Journal of Medical Genetics 35 (2) (2018) 215–218.
[249] P.L. Wood, Targeted lipidomics and metabolomics evaluations of cortical neuronal stress in schizophrenia, Schizophrenia Research 212 (2019) 107–112.
[250] R. Bradbury, D. Copolov, Studies on [3H] CP-55940 binding in the human central nervous system: regional specific changes in density of cannabinoid-1 receptors associated with schizophrenia and cannabis use, Neuroscience 103 (1) (2001) 9–15.

[251] K. Zavitsanou, T. Garrick, X.F. Huang, Selective antagonist [3H] SR141716A binding to cannabinoid CB1 receptors is increased in the anterior cingulate cortex in schizophrenia, Progress in Neuro-Psychopharmacology & Biological Psychiatry 28 (2) (2004) 355–360.
[252] K.A. Newell, C. Deng, X.F. Huang, Increased cannabinoid receptor density in the posterior cingulate cortex in schizophrenia, Experimental Brain Research 172 (2006) 556–560.
[253] D.F. Wong, H. Kuwabara, A.G. Horti, V. Raymont, J. Brasic, M. Guevara, et al., Quantification of cerebral cannabinoid receptors subtype 1 (CB1) in healthy subjects and schizophrenia by the novel PET radioligand [11C] OMAR, NeuroImage 52 (4) (2010) 1505–1513.
[254] K.J. Jenko, J. Hirvonen, I.D. Henter, K.B. Anderson, S.S. Zoghbi, T.M. Hyde, et al., Binding of a tritiated inverse agonist to cannabinoid CB1 receptors is increased in patients with schizophrenia, Schizophrenia Research 141 (2–3) (2012) 185–188.
[255] J. Ceccarini, M. De Hert, R. Van Winkel, J. Peuskens, G. Bormans, L. Kranaster, et al., Increased ventral striatal CB1 receptor binding is related to negative symptoms in drug-free patients with schizophrenia, NeuroImage 79 (2013) 304–312.
[256] D.W. Volk, S.M. Eggan, A.G. Horti, D.F. Wong, D.A. Lewis, Reciprocal alterations in cortical cannabinoid receptor 1 binding relative to protein immunoreactivity and transcript levels in schizophrenia, Schizophrenia Research 159 (1) (2014) 124–129.
[257] K.A. Chase, B. Feiner, C. Rosen, D.P. Gavin, R.P. Sharma, Characterization of peripheral cannabinoid receptor expression and clinical correlates in schizophrenia, Psychiatry Research 245 (2016) 346–353.
[258] R. Tao, C. Li, A.E. Jaffe, J.H. Shin, A. Deep-Soboslay, R. Yamin, et al., Cannabinoid receptor CNR1 expression and DNA methylation in human prefrontal cortex hippocampus and caudate in brain development and schizophrenia, Translational Psychiatry 10 (1) (2020) 158.
[259] S. Chou, K.N. Fish, D.A. Lewis, R.A. Sweet, Terminal type-specific cannabinoid CB1 receptor alterations in patients with schizophrenia: a pilot study, bioRxiv 2023 (2023) 04.
[260] V.S. Dalton, L.E. Long, C.S. Weickert, K. Zavitsanou, Paranoid schizophrenia is characterized by increased CB1 receptor binding in the dorsolateral prefrontal cortex, Neuropsychopharmacology 36 (8) (2011) 1620–1630.
[261] S.M. Eggan, T. Hashimoto, D.A. Lewis, Reduced cortical cannabinoid 1 receptor messenger RNA and protein expression in schizophrenia, Archives of General Psychiatry 65 (7) (2008) 772–784.
[262] L. Urigüen, M.J. García-Fuster, L.F. Callado, B. Morentin, R. La Harpe, V. Casadó, et al., Immunodensity and mRNA expression of A2A adenosine, D2 dopamine, and CB1 cannabinoid receptors in postmortem frontal cortex of subjects with schizophrenia: effect of antipsychotic treatment, Psychopharmacology 206 (2009) 313–324.
[263] S.M. Eggan, S.R. Stoyak, C.D. Verrico, D.A. Lewis, Cannabinoid CB1 receptor immunoreactivity in the prefrontal cortex: comparison of schizophrenia and major depressive disorder, Neuropsychopharmacology 35 (10) (2010) 2060–2071.
[264] M. Ranganathan, J. Cortes-Briones, R. Radhakrishnan, H. Thurnauer, B. Planeta, P. Skosnik, et al., Reduced brain cannabinoid receptor availability in schizophrenia, Biological Psychiatry 79 (12) (2016) 997–1005.
[265] F. Borgan, H. Laurikainen, M. Veronese, T.R. Marques, M. Haaparanta-Solin, O. Solin, et al., In vivo availability of cannabinoid 1 receptor levels in patients with first-episode psychosis, JAMA Psychiatry 76 (10) (2019) 1074–1084.
[266] C. Deng, M. Han, X.F. Huang, No changes in densities of cannabinoid receptors in the superior temporal gyrus in schizophrenia, Neuroscience Bulletin 23 (6) (2007) 341.
[267] D. Koethe, I. Llenos, J. Dulay, C. Hoyer, E. Torrey, F. Leweke, et al., Expression of CB1 cannabinoid receptor in the anterior cingulate cortex in schizophrenia, bipolar disorder, and major depression, Journal of Neural Transmission 114 (2007) 1055–1063.
[268] M.A. Wallace, E. Claro, Transmembrane signaling through phospholipase C in human cortical membranes, Neurochemical Research 18 (1993) 139–145.
[269] C. D'Addario, V. Micale, M. Di Bartolomeo, T. Stark, M. Pucci, A. Sulcova, et al., A preliminary study of endocannabinoid system regulation in psychosis: Distinct alterations of

CNR1 promoter DNA methylation in patients with schizophrenia, Schizophrenia Research 188 (2017) 132–140.
[270] D. Navarro, A. Gasparyan, F. Navarrete, A.B. Torregrosa, G. Rubio, M. Marín-Mayor, et al., Molecular alterations of the endocannabinoid system in psychiatric disorders, International Journal of Molecular Sciences 23 (9) (2022) 4764.
[271] D.P. Covey, Y. Mateo, D. Sulzer, J.F. Cheer, D.M. Lovinger, Endocannabinoid modulation of dopamine neurotransmission, Neuropharmacology 124 (2017) 52–61.
[272] A.F. Carvalho, E.J. Van Bockstaele, Cannabinoid modulation of noradrenergic circuits: implications for psychiatric disorders, Progress in Neuro-Psychopharmacology & Biological Psychiatry 38 (1) (2012) 59–67.
[273] S. Haj-Dahmane, R.Y. Shen, Modulation of the serotonin system by endocannabinoid signaling, Neuropharmacology 61 (3) (2011) 414–420.
[274] T.V. Maia, M.J. Frank, An integrative perspective on the role of dopamine in schizophrenia, Biological Psychiatry 81 (1) (2017) 52–66.
[275] G. Juckel, Serotonin: from sensory processing to schizophrenia using an electrophysiological method, Behavioural Brain Research 277 (2015) 121–124.
[276] T. Harkany, W. Härtig, P. Berghuis, M.B. Dobszay, Y. Zilberter, R.H. Edwards, et al., Complementary distribution of type 1 cannabinoid receptors and vesicular glutamate transporter 3 in basal forebrain suggests input-specific retrograde signalling by cholinergic neurons, European Journal of Neuroscience 18 (7) (2003) 1979–1992.
[277] E.T. Tzavara, M. Wade, G.G. Nomikos, Biphasic effects of cannabinoids on acetylcholine release in the hippocampus: site and mechanism of action, The Journal of Neuroscience 23 (28) (2003) 9374–9384.
[278] A. Saunders, A.J. Granger, B.L. Sabatini, Corelease of acetylcholine and GABA from cholinergic forebrain neurons, eLife (2015) 4:e06412.
[279] A. Gibbons, B. Dean, The cholinergic system: an emerging drug target for schizophrenia, Current Pharmaceutical Design 22 (14) (2016) 2124–2133.
[280] L. Robinson, A.V. Goonawardena, R. Pertwee, R.E. Hampson, B. Platt, G. Riedel, WIN55, 212-2 induced deficits in spatial learning are mediated by cholinergic hypofunction, Behavioural Brain Research 208 (2) (2010) 584–592.
[281] S. Navakkode, M. Korte, Pharmacological activation of CB1 receptor modulates long term potentiation by interfering with protein synthesis, Neuropharmacology 79 (2014) 525–533.
[282] L. Gonzalez-Blanco, A.M.D. Greenhalgh, C. Garcia-Rizo, E. Fernandez-Egea, B.J. Miller, B. Kirkpatrick, Prolactin concentrations in antipsychotic-naive patients with schizophrenia and related disorders: a meta-analysis, Schizophrenia Research 174 (1–3) (2016) 156–160.
[283] J. Labad, A. Stojanovic-Pérez, I. Montalvo, M. Solé, Á. Cabezas, L. Ortega, et al., Stress biomarkers as predictors of transition to psychosis in at-risk mental states: roles for cortisol, prolactin and albumin, Journal of Psychiatric Research 60 (2015) 163–169.
[284] L. Grandison, Stimulation of anterior pituitary prolactin release by melittin, an activator of phospholipase A2, Endocrinology 114 (1) (1984) 1–7.
[285] P.C. Ross, A.M. Judd, R.M. Macleod, The dynamics of arachidonic acid liberation and prolactin release: a comparison of thyrotropin-releasing hormone, angiotensin II, and neurotensin stimulation in perifused rat anterior pituitary cells, Endocrinology 123 (5) (1988) 2445–2453.
[286] M. Pruessner, A.E. Cullen, M. Aas, E.F. Walker, The neural diathesis-stress model of schizophrenia revisited: an update on recent findings considering illness stage and neurobiological and methodological complexities, Neuroscience and Biobehavioral Reviews 73 (2017) 191–218.
[287] T. Unger, J. Maldonado-Aviles, H. Morris, D. Volk, K. Mirnics, D. Lewis, Alterations in GABA-related transcriptome in the dorsolateral prefrontal cortex of subjects with schizophrenia, Molecular Psychiatry 13 (2) (2008) 147–161.
[288] J. Hammond, D. Shan, J. Meador-Woodruff, R. McCullumsmith, Evidence of glutamatergic dysfunction in the pathophysiology of schizophrenia, Synaptic Stress and Pathogenesis of Neuropsychiatric Disorders (2014) 265–294.

[289] K. Friston, H.R. Brown, J. Siemerkus, K.E. Stephan, The dysconnection hypothesis (2016), Schizophrenia Research 176 (2–3) (2016) 83–94.
[290] V. Peralta, M.S. Campos, E.G. de Jalon, M.J. Cuesta, DSM-IV catatonia signs and criteria in first-episode, drug-naive, psychotic patients: psychometric validity and response to antipsychotic medication, Schizophrenia Research 118 (1–3) (2010) 168–175.
[291] M.J. Cuesta, Campos MS de Jalón EG, L. Moreno-Izco, R. Lorente-Omeñaca, A.M. Sánchez-Torres, et al., Motor abnormalities in first-episode psychosis patients and long-term psychosocial functioning, Schizophrenia Research 200 (2018) 97–103.
[292] A.E. Pinkham, P. Liu, H. Lu, M. Kriegsman, C. Simpson, C. Tamminga, Amygdala hyperactivity at rest in paranoid individuals with schizophrenia, The American Journal of Psychiatry 172 (8) (2015) 784–792.
[293] S.F. Taylor, K. Luan Phan, J.C. Britton, I. Liberzon, Neural response to emotional salience in schizophrenia, Neuropsychopharmacology 30 (5) (2005) 984–995.
[294] S. Potvin, A. Tikàsz, A. Mendrek, Emotionally neutral stimuli are not neutral in schizophrenia: a mini review of functional neuroimaging studies, Frontiers in Psychiatry 7 (2016) 115.
[295] N.L. Matthews, K.P. Collins, K.N. Thakkar, S. Park, Visuospatial imagery and working memory in schizophrenia, Cognitive Neuropsychiatry 19 (1) (2014) 17–35.
[296] M. Bodatsch, A. Brockhaus-Dumke, J. Klosterkötter, S. Ruhrmann, Forecasting psychosis by event-related potentials–systematic review and specific meta-analysis, Biological Psychiatry 77 (11) (2015) 951–958.
[297] L. Berkovitch, A. Del Cul, M. Maheu, S. Dehaene, Impaired conscious access and abnormal attentional amplification in schizophrenia, NeuroImage Clinical 18 (2018) 835–848.
[298] J.K. Wynn, W.P. Horan, A.M. Kring, R.F. Simons, M.F. Green, Impaired anticipatory event-related potentials in schizophrenia, International Journal of Psychophysiology 77 (2) (2010) 141–149.
[299] P.D. Skosnik, J.A. Cortes-Briones, M. Hajós, It's all in the rhythm: the role of cannabinoids in neural oscillations and psychosis, Biological Psychiatry 79 (7) (2016) 568–577.
[300] P.J. Uhlhaas, W. Singer, Oscillations and neuronal dynamics in schizophrenia: the search for basic symptoms and translational opportunities, Biological Psychiatry 77 (12) (2015) 1001–1009.
[301] R. Lopes, R. Soares, R. Coelho, M. Figueiredo-Braga, Angiogenesis in the pathophysiology of schizophrenia–a comprehensive review and a conceptual hypothesis, Life Sciences 128 (2015) 79–93.
[302] E. Mısır, G.G. Akay, Synaptic dysfunction in schizophrenia, Synapse:e22276.
[303] V.D. Mouchlis, D. Limnios, M.G. Kokotou, E. Barbayianni, G. Kokotos, J.A. McCammon, et al., Development of potent and selective inhibitors for group VIA calcium-independent phospholipase A2 guided by molecular dynamics and structure–activity relationships, Journal of Medicinal Chemistry 59 (9) (2016) 4403–4414.
[304] C. Dedaki, M.G. Kokotou, V.D. Mouchlis, D. Limnios, X. Lei, C.T. Mu, et al., β-Lactones: A novel class of Ca2+-independent phospholipase A2 (group VIA iPLA2) inhibitors with the ability to inhibit β-cell apoptosis, Journal of Medicinal Chemistry 62 (6) (2019) 2916–2927.
[305] A. Smyrniotou, M.G. Kokotou, V.D. Mouchlis, E. Barbayianni, G. Kokotos, E.A. Dennis, et al., 2-Oxoamides based on dipeptides as selective calcium-independent phospholipase A2 inhibitors, Bioorganic & Medicinal Chemistry 25 (3) (2017) 926–940.
[306] N.H. Dubin, D.A. Blake, M.C. DiBlasi, T.H. Parmley, T.M. King, Pharmacokinetic studies on quinacrine following intrauterine administration to cynomolgus monkeys, Fertility and Sterility 38 (6) (1982) 735–740.
[307] R.L. Nevin, A.M. Croft, Psychiatric effects of malaria and anti-malarial drugs: historical and modern perspectives, Malaria Journal 15 (1) (2016) 1–13.
[308] K.A. O'Donnell, A.C. Howlett, Muscarinic receptor binding is inhibited by quinacrine, Neuroscience Letters 127 (1) (1991) 46–48.
[309] S. Tamamizu, A.P. Todd, M.G. McNamee, Mutations in the M1 region of the nicotinic acetylcholine receptor alter the sensitivity to inhibition by quinacrine, Cellular and Molecular Neurobiology 15 (1995) 427–438.

[310] T. Lidz, R.L. Kahn, Toxicity of quinacrine (atabrine) for the central nervous system: III. An experimental study on human subjects, Archives of Neurology and Psychiatry 56 (3) (1946) 284–299.

[311] H.W. Newell, T. Lidz, The toxicity of atabrine to the central nervous system, The American Journal of Psychiatry 102 (6) (1946) 805–818.

[312] T. Kitagawa, A. Matsumoto, I. Terashima, Y. Uesono, Antimalarial quinacrine and chloroquine lose their activity by decreasing cationic amphiphilic structure with a slight decrease in pH, Journal of Medicinal Chemistry 64 (7) (2021) 3885–3896.

[313] P. Vadas, E. Stefanski, W. Pruzanski, Potential therapeutic efficacy of inhibitors of human phospholipase A2 in septic shock, Agents and Actions 19 (3–4) (1986) 194–202.

[314] R. Christensen, P.K. Kristensen, E.M. Bartels, H. Bliddal, A. Astrup, Efficacy and safety of the weight-loss drug rimonabant: a meta-analysis of randomised trials, The Lancet 370 (9600) (2007) 1706–1713.

[315] D.L. Kelly, D.A. Gorelick, R.R. Conley, D.L. Boggs, J. Linthicum, F. Liu, et al., Effects of the cannabinoid-1 receptor antagonist rimonabant on psychiatric symptoms in overweight people with schizophrenia: a randomized, double-blind, pilot study, Journal of Clinical Psychopharmacology 31 (1) (2011) 86.

[316] H.Y. Meltzer, L. Arvanitis, D. Bauer, W. Rein, M.T.S. Group, Placebo-controlled evaluation of four novel compounds for the treatment of schizophrenia and schizoaffective disorder, The American Journal of Psychiatry 161 (6) (2004) 975–984.

[317] Sanofi, Efficacy and Safety of AVE1625 as a Co-treatment With Antipsychotic Therapy in Schizophrenia, http://ClinicalTrials.gov/show/NCT00439634, 2009. (Accessed 28 June 2023).

[318] T.A. Iseger, M.G. Bossong, A systematic review of the antipsychotic properties of cannabidiol in humans, Schizophrenia Research 162 (1–3) (2015) 153–161.

[319] X. Xu, G. Shao, X. Zhang, Y. Hu, J. Huang, Y. Su, et al., The efficacy of nutritional supplements for the adjunctive treatment of schizophrenia in adults: a systematic review and network meta-analysis, Psychiatry Research 311 (2022) 114500.

[320] X. Chen, A. Gresham, A. Morrison, A.P. Pentland, Oxidative stress mediates synthesis of cytosolic phospholipase A2 after UVB injury, Biochimica et Biophysica Acta (BBA)-Lipids and Lipid Metabolism 1299 (1) (1996) 23–33.

[321] C. Quintana, J.M. Beaulieu, A fresh look at cortical dopamine D2 receptor expressing neurons, Pharmacological Research 139 (2019) 440–445.

[322] A. De La Mora MP Gallegos-Cari, M. Crespo-Ramirez, D. Marcellino, A. Hansson, K. Fuxe, Distribution of dopamine D2-like receptors in the rat amygdala and their role in the modulation of unconditioned fear and anxiety, Neuroscience 201 (2012) 252–266.

[323] A. Giuffrida, L. Parsons, T. Kerr, F.R. De Fonseca, M. Navarro, D. Piomelli, Dopamine activation of endogenous cannabinoid signaling in dorsal striatum, Nature Neuroscience 2 (4) (1999) 358–563.

[324] S. Patel, D.J. Rademacher, C.J. Hillard, Differential regulation of the endocannabinoids anandamide and 2-arachidonylglycerol within the limbic forebrain by dopamine receptor activity, The Journal of Pharmacology and Experimental Therapeutics 306 (3) (2003) 880–888.

[325] D. Centonze, N. Battista, S. Rossi, N.B. Mercuri, A. Finazzi-Agro, G. Bernardi, et al., A critical interaction between dopamine D2 receptors and endocannabinoids mediates the effects of cocaine on striatal GABAergic transmission, Neuropsychopharmacology 29 (8) (2004) 1488–1497.

[326] D.S. Kerr, L.L. Talib, V.J. Yamamoto, A.S. Ferreira, M.V. Zanetti, M.H. Serpa, et al., Antipsychotic drugs decrease iPLA2 gene expression in schizophrenia, Schizophrenia Research 147 (1) (2013) 203–204.

[327] Y. Yuhas, S. Ashkenazi, E. Berent, A. Weizman, Clozapine Suppresses the Gene Expression and the Production of Cytokines and Up-Regulates Cyclooxygenase 2 mRNA in Human Astroglial Cells, Brain Sciences 12 (12) (2022) 1703.

[328] H.R. Modi, A.Y. Taha, H.W. Kim, L. Chang, S.I. Rapoport, Y. Cheon, Chronic clozapine reduces rat brain arachidonic acid metabolism by reducing plasma arachidonic acid availability, Journal of Neurochemistry 124 (3) (2013) 376–387.
[329] C. Felder, H. Williams, J. Axelrod, A transduction pathway associated with receptors coupled to the inhibitory guanine nucleotide binding protein Gi that amplifies ATP-mediated arachidonic acid release, Proceedings of the National Academy of Sciences 88 (15) (1991) 6477–6480.
[330] D. Piomelli, C. Pilon, B. Giros, P. Sokolofff, M.P. Martres, J.C. Schwartz, Dopamine activation of the arachidonic acid cascade as a basis for D1/D2 receptor synergism, Nature 353 (6340) (1991) 164–167.
[331] C. Felder, R. Kanterman, A. Ma, J. Axelrod, Serotonin stimulates phospholipase A2 and the release of arachidonic acid in hippocampal neurons by a type 2 serotonin receptor that is independent of inositolphospholipid hydrolysis, Proceedings of the National Academy of Sciences 87 (6) (1990) 2187–2191.
[332] S. Dzitoyeva, H. Chen, H. Manev, et al., 5-lipoxygenase-activating protein as a modulator of olanzapine-induced lipid accumulation in adipocyte, Journal of Lipids (2013).
[333] M.B. Raeder, J. Fernø, A.O. Vik-Mo, V.M. Steen, SREBP activation by antipsychotic- and antidepressant-drugs in cultured human liver cells: relevance for metabolic side-effects?, Molecular and Cellular Biochemistry 289 (2006) 167–173.
[334] M.H. Polymeropoulos, L. Licamele, S. Volpi, K. Mack, S.N. Mitkus, E.D. Carstea, et al., Common effect of antipsychotics on the biosynthesis and regulation of fatty acids and cholesterol supports a key role of lipid homeostasis in schizophrenia, Schizophrenia Research 108 (1–3) (2009) 134–142.
[335] R.K. McNamara, R. Jandacek, T. Rider, P. Tso, A. Cole-Strauss, J.W. Lipton, Differential effects of antipsychotic medications on polyunsaturated fatty acid biosynthesis in rats: Relationship with liver delta6-desaturase expression, Schizophrenia Research 129 (1) (2011) 57–65.
[336] H.W. Kim, Y. Cheon, H.R. Modi, S.I. Rapoport, J.S. Rao, Effects of chronic clozapine administration on markers of arachidonic acid cascade and synaptic integrity in rat brain, Psychopharmacology 222 (2012) 663–674.
[337] Y. Cheon, J.Y. Park, H.R. Modi, H.W. Kim, H.J. Lee, L. Chang, et al., Chronic olanzapine treatment decreases arachidonic acid turnover and prostaglandin E2 concentration in rat brain, Journal of Neurochemistry 119 (2) (2011) 364–376.
[338] C.S. Wu, S.C. Wang, I.J. Yeh, S.K. Liu, Comparative risk of seizure with use of first- and second-generation antipsychotics in patients with schizophrenia and mood disorders, The Journal of Clinical Psychiatry 77 (5) (2016) 3433.
[339] C.S. Kearn, K. Blake-Palmer, E. Daniel, K. Mackie, M. Glass, Concurrent stimulation of cannabinoid CB1 and dopamine D2 receptors enhances heterodimer formation: a mechanism for receptor cross-talk?, Molecular Pharmacology 67 (5) (2005) 1697–1704.
[340] A.M. Bagher, R.B. Laprairie, M.E. Kelly, E.M. Denovan-Wright, Antagonism of dopamine receptor 2 long affects cannabinoid receptor 1 signaling in a cell culture model of striatal medium spiny projection neurons, Molecular Pharmacology 89 (6) (2016) 652–666.
[341] D. Guinart, E. Moreno, L. Galindo, A. Cuenca-Royo, M. Barrera-Conde, E.J. Pérez, et al., Altered signaling in CB1R-5-HT2AR heteromers in olfactory neuroepithelium cells of schizophrenia patients is modulated by cannabis use, Schizophrenia Bulletin 46 (6) (2020) 1547–1557.
[342] R. Carhart-Harris, D. Nutt, Serotonin and brain function: a tale of two receptors, Journal of Psychopharmacology 31 (9) (2017) 1091–1120.
[343] M.L. Chew, B.H. Mulsant, B.G. Pollock, M.E. Lehman, A. Greenspan, R.A. Mahmoud, et al., Anticholinergic activity of 107 medications commonly used by older adults, Journal of the American Geriatrics Society 56 (7) (2008) 1333–1341.
[344] T. Bordia, D. Zhang, X.A. Perez, M. Quik, Striatal cholinergic interneurons and D2 receptor-expressing GABAergic medium spiny neurons regulate tardive dyskinesia, Experimental Neurology 286 (2016) 32–39.

[345] G. Kharkwal, K. Brami-Cherrier, J.E. Lizardi-Ortiz, A.B. Nelson, M. Ramos, D. Del Barrio, et al., Parkinsonism driven by antipsychotics originates from dopaminergic control of striatal cholinergic interneurons, Neuron 91 (1) (2016) 67–78.
[346] M. Harrow, T.H. Jobe, L. Tong, Twenty-year effects of antipsychotics in schizophrenia and affective psychotic disorders, Psychological Medicine 52 (13) (2022) 2681–2691.
[347] J. Moncrieff, N. Crellin, J. Stansfeld, R. Cooper, L. Marston, N. Freemantle, et al., Antipsychotic dose reduction and discontinuation versus maintenance treatment in people with schizophrenia and other recurrent psychotic disorders in England (the RADAR trial): an open, parallel-group, randomised controlled trial, Lancet Psychiatry (2023) S2215-0366.
[348] H. Cai, C. Zeng, X. Zhang, Y. Liu, R. Wu, W. Guo, et al., Diminished treatment response in relapsed versus first-episode schizophrenia as revealed by a panel of blood-based biomarkers: A combined cross-sectional and longitudinal study, Psychiatry Research 316 (2022) 114762.
[349] S.M. Francey, B. O'Donoghue, B. Nelson, J. Graham, L. Baldwin, H.P. Yuen, et al., Psychosocial intervention with or without antipsychotic medication for first-episode psychosis: a randomized noninferiority clinical trial, Schizophrenia Bulletin Open 1 (1) (2020) sgaa015.
[350] J. Desfossés, E. Stip, L.A. Bentaleb, S. Potvin, Endocannabinoids schizophrenia, Pharmaceuticals 3 (10) (2010) 3101–3126.
[351] A.S. Cohen, K.S. Minor, Emotional experience in patients with schizophrenia revisited: meta-analysis of laboratory studies, Schizophrenia Bulletin 36 (1) (2010) 143–150.
[352] A.M. Kring, J.M. Caponigro, Emotion in schizophrenia: where feeling meets thinking, Current Directions in Psychological Science 19 (4) (2010) 255–259.
[353] C. Yan, S.S. Lui, Zou Lq, Wang Cy, Zhou Fc, E.F. Cheung, et al., Anticipatory pleasure for future rewards is attenuated in patients with schizophrenia but not in individuals with schizotypal traits, Schizophrenia Research 206 (2019) 118–126.
[354] D.I. Driver, N. Gogtay, J.L. Rapoport, Childhood onset schizophrenia and early onset schizophrenia spectrum disorders, Child and Adolescent Psychiatric Clinics 22 (4) (2013) 539–555.
[355] D. Sinclair, M. Webster, J. Wong, C. Weickert, Dynamic molecular and anatomical changes in the glucocorticoid receptor in human cortical development, Molecular Psychiatry 16 (5) (2011) 504–516.
[356] J.A. Markham, Sex steroids and schizophrenia, Reviews in Endocrine and Metabolic Disorders 13 (2012) 187–207.
[357] B.B. Gorzalka, S.S. Dang, Minireview: Endocannabinoids and gonadal hormones: bidirectional interactions in physiology and behavior, Endocrinology 153 (3) (2012) 1016–1024.
[358] E. Engler-Chiurazzi, C. Brown, J. Povroznik, J. Simpkins, Estrogens as neuroprotectants: estrogenic actions in the context of cognitive aging and brain injury, Progress in Neurobiology 157 (2017) 188–211.

Chapter 4

A dynorphin theory of depression and bipolar disorder

4.1 Introduction

Major depressive disorder (MDD) affects hundreds of millions of people worldwide, and is one of the leading causes of years lost to disability, with increasing prevalence over the last decades [1]. The efficacy of current pharmaceutical treatment is moderate at best, with substantial negative side effects [2,3]. MDD is closely linked to bipolar disorder (BP), the distinction depending on the presence of manic episodes. At present, there is no theory that explains MDD or BP [2,3], despite major research activity (over 700K/2M papers in pubmed/Google scholar).

Here I present a theory (T*MDD) that explains the etiology, symptoms, pathology and treatment of MDD and bipolar disorder. The theory is supported by strong preclinical and clinical evidence, and points to novel treatment directions.

Theory overview. MDD is triggered by stress-inducing life events that the person does not manage to resolve. In such situations, animals execute one of the innate survival responses ('fight or flight'). MDD occurs when the 'disengage' (withdraw, give up) response is impaired and chronically executed.

To explain the biological mechanisms involved, I present a novel theory of opioids and survival responses, in which each opioid supports one of the survival responses. The opioid supporting the disengage response is dynorphin (DYN), which acts via the kappa opioid receptor (KOR). KOR mediates disengage by suppressing the phasic responses of neurons releasing dopamine (DA), corticotropin-releasing hormone (CRH), norepinephrine (NEP), and serotonin (SER).

In MDD, KOR signaling is impaired, leading to its chronic activation. The resulting dysregulation of DA, CRH, NEP and SER reduces goal-directed behaviors, dysregulates appetite and sleep, and induces motor agitation or retardation, difficulties in concentration, and fatigue. In humans, this state is associated with dysphoria and reduced positive emotions, and promotes suicidal thoughts (the ultimate 'withdraw' response). Thus, T*MDD explains the defining symptoms of MDD [4]. Females are more vulnerable than males because their expression of CRH1 is higher and their KOR signaling is more prolonged.

The Science of the Brain. https://doi.org/10.1016/B978-0-44-345008-2.00010-2

In addition to MDD, T*MDD explains bipolar disorder. Manic episodes occur when chronic KOR activation leads to its complete desensitization, allowing the dysregulated NEP and DA systems to reach a hyperactivated state. This leads to reduced sleep, increased goal-directed activities, excessively elevated mood, a feeling of omnipotence, and other mania symptoms [3].

The leading treatment of MDD at present is via drugs that increase brain SER levels. Moderate and high SER levels oppose DYN and provide energy, explaining why these drugs suppress most MDD symptoms. However, SER also opposes CRH and NEP, with general suppression of novelty-induced responses, including positive ones. This can result in an unpleasant emotional state. In addition, high SER levels can induce motor and mental agitation. T*MDD points to the KOR pathway as a promising treatment direction.

4.2 Stress responses and MDD

Organisms can be in a state of **satiety** with no needs or threats, or in a **stress** state where these are present. Stressful events trigger internal body responses collectively known as **stress responses**, whose goal is to recruit resources (e.g., glucose, oxygen) that allow the organism to deal with the event. Stressful events can involve both threats (e.g., predators) and need-satisfying opportunities (e.g., food, sex).

There are two major stress response systems, the **sympathetic nervous system (SNS)** and the **hypothalamus-pituitary-adrenal (HPA) axis**. At stress onset, external surprises trigger an alert conveyed by high frequency neural firing in sensory input paths. This alert recruits the SNS, which provides immediate energy via glycogenolysis and elevated blood glucose and heart rate. It also enhances sensory inputs (e.g., by increasing pupil diameter). In parallel, sensory input induces the release of CRH, mainly from neurons in the central nucleus of the amygdala (CeA) and the paraventricular hypothalamus (PVH). CRH stimulates the HPA axis, acting on CRH1 receptors in the pituitary to induce the release of ACTH, which in turn induces the secretion of glucocorticoids (cortisol in humans) from the adrenal gland [5]. Within minutes, cortisol increases blood glucose and promotes food intake. CRH also sustains the recruitment of the SNS, and recruits its brain counterpart, NEP from the locus coeruleus (LC).

MDD is known to be triggered by life events involving strong stress [6]. In some people, MDD can be triggered by mild stress. However, this type of susceptibility is usually associated with early life or parental stress, and can be attributed to stress-induced epigenetic or genetic adaptations [6,7]. Thus, stress is the underlying cause of MDD in virtually all cases.

In accordance with chronic stress, MDD patients show chronically dysregulated (mainly elevated) SNS and HPA axis activity [8–17]. However, stress is involved in many, probably most, psychiatric disorders [18]. Thus, although depression is triggered by stress, stress responses alone do not explain the unique characteristics of MDD.

4.3 A theory of opioids and survival responses

A central thesis of T*MDD is that the occurrence of MDD is related to the concrete actions that the person takes to deal with stress, rather than to general stress responses. Specifically, T*MDD posits that MDD is due to the chronic execution of the 'disengage' survival response.

A major contribution of the present chapter is a theory of opioids (T*OPS) that connects survival responses with opioids (OPs), allowing a mechanistic understanding of MDD. In principle, T*MDD only requires a theory of DYN function. However, presenting the full theory of OPs strengthens the case for both DYN function and its effect in MDD.

Survival responses. Animals have a repertoire of innate survival responses, the main ones being **charge** (prey or sex), **fight, flight, chase**, and **disengage (withdraw, give up)**. These responses promote survival of the individual or the species. Stress responses are body internal, and their main function is metabolic, while survival responses involve external actions. Note that both stress and survival responses respond to both rewarding and aversive stimuli [19].

The disengage response is crucial for survival in confrontations with a strong adversary. Some animals have a 'faint' response, which is a variant of disengage. Another variant is freezing without muscle flexing and with reduced heart rate. Freezing with muscle flexing and increased heart rate accompanies the SNS response to an initial surprise, and is not one of the survival responses strategies.

Opioid signaling. Survival responses are crucial to the animal and to its species, so it is reasonable to expect that there would be molecular agents that have evolved to support each specific survival response. According to T*OPS, **opioids are the major agents mediating survival responses.**

There are four well-known OPs, beta-endorphin (BEND), enkephalin (ENK), nociceptin (NOCP), and dynorphin (DYN). These signal via the G protein-coupled receptors (GPCRs) mu opioid receptor (MOR), delta opioid receptor (DOR), NOCP receptor (NOCPR, also known as nociceptin/orphanin FQ receptor and opioid receptor like 1, ORL1), and kappa opioid receptor (KOR), respectively [20].

Endomorphin1 (EM1) and endomorphin2 (EM2) have received less research attention than the other OPs, but are probably just as important (see below). Like BEND, they are MOR ligands, but may act on different alternatively spliced MOR subtypes [21,22].

The opioid receptors (OPRs) are usually described as coupled to Gi/o proteins, with inhibitory actions on their cells via suppression of cAMP production, and activation of G protein-coupled inwardly-rectifying potassium channels (GIRKs) [20]. A lesser-known fact is that OPRs also couple to Gs, which has opposite effect on cells, exciting them by decreasing potassium currents and activating adenylate cyclase (AC) isoforms [20,23,24]. Low (nanomolar) and high (micromolar) agonist concentrations activate Gs and Gi/o binding, respectively [23,25].

Once bound to their ligand, OPRs undergo phosphorylation (mainly by G protein receptor kinases (GRKs)), which allows binding by beta-arrestin and endocytosis. Endocytosed receptors can be degraded or recycled to the plasma membrane. Importantly, they can also yield prolonged signaling in intracellular compartments (mainly endosomes) [26].

In light of these data, T*OPS uses the following description of OPR signaling, which is more accurate than labeling it as 'inhibitory'. **OPRs suppress phasic cellular responses to novel extracellular inputs, while allowing continuation of, and quickly suppressing, responses that have already started.** For the first part of this description, new extracellular responses are suppressed by suppressing AC and thus cAMP production and PKA. OPR binding to Gs can activate AC isoforms, but these isoforms are linked to PKC [27], which is associated with the release of calcium from intracellular stores, less with responses to acute extracellular inputs. For the second part of this description, OPRs oppose (via Gs) or slow down (via Gi/o) outward potassium currents. This does not rapidly hyperpolarize the cell, but keeps it depolarized (i.e., allows on-going activity). Thus, OPRs disconnect neurons from new acute inputs, but increase their on-going activity and intrinsic excitability. Eventually, the response is terminated.

Opioid release and signaling. According to T*OPS, each opioid agent is expressed in cells that act as sensors for the execution of the agent's survival response. When this condition is detected, the cell releases the OP in large quantities. Release in smaller quantities can occur prior to the execution of the survival response, due to brain plasticity. Past events in which the survival response has been executed enhance synaptic connections from neurons activated by the sensory context to the OP releasing neurons. As a result, OP-releasing neurons are excited when the animal is in similar contexts. Thus, past experience teaches the brain to anticipate survival responses in certain situations, which can lead to low-grade OP release before survival response execution.

The OPR activated by the OP agent is expressed in neurons involved in response execution (we refer to these neurons as the OP's **path**). Small ligand concentrations indicate anticipation of imminent execution, and activate Gs to enhance the path's excitation and accelerate the response. Once execution successfully commences, opioid ligand concentrations are increased, switching the OPR to Gi/o to ensure response completion. This strongly prevents the path from being activated by new inputs, while still allowing its on-going activity. This architecture minimizes interference with the execution of survival responses, which are crucial to the animal and the species.

This is why all OPs have a strong anti-pain effect. Pain is conveyed by sensory neurons to indicate states that may harm cells, and thus stimulates responses. However, survival responses, by their very definition, enjoy precedence over other responses. Once they start executing, they suppress any interference generated by new inputs. Hence, in T*OPS, pain suppression is part of OP-mediated potentiation of survival responses, not the main physiological role of OPs.

Opioid function. According to T*OPS, each opioid mediates one of the basic survival responses. Specifically, **MOR, DOR, NOCPR, and KOR mediate charge, chase/flight, fight, and disengage, respectively**. As to ligands, BEND may be specific to charge for food (i.e., preying), while EM1 and EM2 may be specific to charge for sex.

Since the focus of the present paper is MDD, the description of DYN/KOR below is more detailed than that of the other OPs.

BEND, endomorphins, MOR. The role of MOR in T*OPS is to support charge survival responses, for food or for sex. Successful charge for food involves a rapid increase in blood food metabolites. Indeed, POMC neurons in the arcuate nucleus of the hypothalamus, which are known sensors of food metabolites in blood, release BEND and increase its CSF concentrations during fat eating [28]. MORs in the basolateral amygdala (BLA) promote vigorous food approach to predictive cues [29]. Stimulation of nucleus accumbens (NAc) MORs induces appetite for high-fat food, while their antagonism decreases intake of food items containing fat and sugar [30,31].

MOR is also clearly involved in sexual behavior. MOR agonists produce sensations similar to orgasm in people [32], and orgasm in men is accompanied by significant release of an endogenous MOR ligand at the hippocampus [33]. MOR can trigger ejaculation without sensory stimulation [34], and sexual behavior induces MOR-dependent conditioned place preference (CPP) [32]. The precise mechanisms through which OP-releasing cells sense successful sexual climax are not known, but include a rapid increase in estrogen [35].

A major way in which MOR achieves its function is by promoting the action of dopamine. MOR agonists disinhibit DA neurons, and can also directly induce DA release, in both the ventral tegmental area (VTA) and the A11 DA group, which innervates the spinal cord and promotes vigorous movements [36,37].

T*OPS hypothesizes that BEND's main role is charge for food (prey), while endomorphins promote charge for sex. There is some evidence supporting this idea (see also DYN below), but more research is needed to validate it.

ENK, DOR. The role of ENK and DOR in T*OPS is to support fast locomotion, in the flight or chase (predation) survival responses. ENK is widely expressed in non-neuronal tissue, including the heart, skeletal muscle, and glia, and is released in response to exercise and hypoxia [38,39]. DOR is expressed in the spinal ventral horn, where neurons supporting motor movements are located. It is expressed in inhibitory interneurons (IINs) [40], so its activation disinhibits excitatory neurons (motor neurons and interneurons) that drive movement. DOR agonists promote locomotion and suppress MOR-induced feeding [41,42]. ENK controls the cortical release of acetylcholine (ACh) [43]. Since ACh is the agent that drives muscle contraction and locomotion, this shows that ENK supports locomotion. ENK specifically enhances horizontal locomotion (running), with no effect of even a negative effect on vertical movements (rearing) [44–46]. In the spinal cord dorsal horn, DOR controls mechanical but not thermal pain, supporting involvement in external movement [47].

It can be argued that although chase and flight responses involve the same motor movements, they are made in completely different survival contexts and should hence involve different OPs. This may be the reason why there are two dominant ENK isoforms. However, their specific support in chase vs flight is not known. ENK is also a MOR agonist, supporting involvement in chase for food.

NOCP, NOCPR. In T*OPS, the role of NOCP is to support the fight survival response. BNST NOCP neurons are stimulated by aversive odor [48]. Aversive social confrontations increase NOCPR mRNA in the amygdala and hypothalamus [49], while NOCP mRNA is decreased in suicide [50]. NOCP agonists increase aggression [51], and induce scratching and biting movements [52–54]. NOCP achieves its function at least partly via substance P [52,53], which is known to be involved in aggression [55].

DYN, KOR. DYN is mainly expressed in the central amygdala (CeA), hypothalamus, prefrontal cortex (PFC), basal ganglia (striatum), hippocampus, and the spinal cord dorsal horn [56]. It is strongly expressed in neurons whose activity indicates acute needs and effort, including CeA CRH neurons [57], hypothalamus and pituitary arginine vasopressin (AVP) and oxytocin (OXT) neurons [58–60], hypothalamus orexin neurons [61], and striatum principal neurons expressing the dopamine D1 receptor [56]. Its release is stimulated by sustained intense neural activity [62], indicating that prolonged efforts have already been made to address the external challenge and maybe it is time to give up. Importantly, it has been explicitly shown that DYN (the A isoform) yields persistent signaling (AC suppression) when most KORs are in late endosomes and lysosomes [63].

Unlike MOR and DOR, which are mainly expressed in IINs (except in the spinal cord), KOR has substantial expression in principal neurons, including excitatory projections from CeA to the locus coeruleus [57,64], amygdala, thalamus, and contralateral cortical projections to mPFC [65], and BLA projections to the BNST [66] and the striatum [67]. KOR exerts an especially strong control over CRH [68], VTA DA [69,70], and brain NEP [64] neurons, and regulates dorsal raphe SER neurons [71,72]. It also controls adrenal medulla epinephrine release [73], SNS responses [74], and the HPA axis [75].

Amygdala DYN neurons are activated during fear memory [76], supporting the T*OPS model. DYN is released in virtually all animal models of chronic or repeated stress, including social defeat stress, forced swim test, and restraint stress. In these models, the effect of KOR is clearly that of 'give up', manifested as immobility, defeated posture, and decreased social interaction, heart rate, and blood pressure [74,77–83]. The aversive effects of KOR are learned and remain present after the event, as shown by KOR promotion of conditioned place aversion (CPA) [68,80,84–86]. KOR effects on midbrain DA are central in its aversive effects [70,87], including social avoidance [88]. KOR reduces intracranial self-stimulation, usually interpreted as reduced motivation, goal-directed behavior, and pleasure [78,89,90]. These effects are generally blocked by KOR antagonist given before the event [81,82] (see [91] for a highly detailed review).

It is well-known that infralimbic mPFC (ILmPFC) mediates fear extinction, mainly via amygdala projections [92]. Fear extinction is successful when the animal stops executing survival responses that involve movements, learning to disengage instead. ILmPFC KORs decrease restraint stress-induced SNS responses [74], supporting KOR's involvement in extinction.

DYN use is not limited to negative experience, also participating in positive social survival responses, namely birth and sex. DYN regulates AVP and OXT, which control stress-induced fluid management. AVP indicates a need for water, while OXT stimulates fluid secretion during birth, sex, and maternal behavior [93]. DYN assists reproduction also by cooperating with MOR. EM2 binds a MOR isoform that induces DYN release [21], and induces conditioned place aversion [94]. This may be the mechanism behind post-sex aversion to sexual touch.

There are some reports where low KOR agonist doses induce a positive response (CPP, self-administration) rather than a negative one [95]. Recall that in T*OPS, DYN suppresses new inputs to DA neurons, but increases their intrinsic excitability [36]. Low dose DYN can thus induce DA release and positive DA-mediated responses.

In summary, the role of opioids is to mediate the basic survival responses. DYN is released in situations of high stress, and mediates the disengage (withdraw, give up) survival response. Mechanistically, it does this by acting on DA, CRH, NEP, and SER neurons, amygdala-PFC connections, the SNS, and the HPA axis. KOR initially excites neurons, and quickly suppresses their phasic responses while increasing their intrinsic excitability.

4.4 A theory of depression and bipolar disorder

Now that we understand the role of DYN in survival responses, it is possible to formulate a theory of MDD. The same theory also explains bipolar disorder and some major aspects of drug addiction.

Depression. MDD is triggered by stress, mainly due to external social challenges. Stress stimulates effortful responses. If these responses do not manage to solve the problem, the person needs to disengage, which is normally mediated by the DYN/KOR pathway. DYN allows people to stop treating stressful challenges as requiring action, and lets them go on with their lives.

In some people, the DYN path is weaker than in other people, in the following sense. Generally, healthy biological responses are of high amplitude and short duration, and non-healthy ones have a blunted amplitude and a prolonged duration. We refer to such responses as **chronic**. The two aspects of chronicity enhance each other in a positive feedback loop. Specifically with GPCRs, prolonged agonist-induced activation leads to endocytosis and reduced cell surface receptor expression, decreasing the amplitude of future responses. Reduced response amplitude diminishes the probability of resolving the problem, leading to prolonged signaling. In the case of MDD, a weaker DYN path leads to an impaired disengage response.

In people with a tendency towards chronic DYN signaling, unresolved stress and an impaired disengage response cause persistent thoughts about the problem (rumination), and chronic activation of the systems and agents regulated by DYN, including the SNS, NEP, the HPA axis, DA, SER, AVP and OXT. Since these systems are crucial for recruiting energy and engaging in goal-directed and pleasurable behavior, these capacities are reduced. In addition, since the SNS and HPA axis control sleep and food intake, these are dysregulated. This can manifest as both increased or decreased sleep and appetite, because chronic states involve both increased excitability and decreased activation amplitude. The subjective experience of this state is what we call 'sad' or 'depressed'. Since the person keeps viewing the problem as highly stressful (i.e., requiring action), and since they cannot find a conventional way to resolve the situation, they tend to suicidal thoughts and attempts. Thus, chronic DYN signaling and the resulting impaired disengage response can explain all of the symptoms that define MDD [4].

Why are some people predisposed to MDD? MDD risk is greatly increased by stress during sensitive developmental periods (pregnancy, perinatal, early life, and adolescence) [96–98], via epigenetic modifications and/or mutations, which can be heritable [18]. Predisposition to MDD can involve a very large number of genes. These genes do not have to be directly linked to DYN or KOR, because chronic DYN signaling can result from anything that diminishes the person's capacity of resolving external problems in a reasonable amount of time. Thus, a weakness in any of the pathways described above (CRH, SNS, HPA, DA, SER, the other OPs, etc) can increase MDD risk. This explains why depression is so common. However, it is still exhibited by a minority of humans, because impaired disengage can be seriously harmful to the survival of the species. Animals in which such a predisposition is very common would perish during evolution.

Women are about twice as likely to have MDD than men [2]. This can be explained by higher female sensitivity of stress responses to CRH [99], and by estrogen's stimulation of KOR signaling (at least in hypothalamus sex-related neurons) [100]. Estrogen increases KOR endocytosis and its intracellular signaling [101], thereby instigating a more chronic-like KOR profile.

Bipolar disorder (BP). BP is characterized by the occurrence of both manic and depressive episodes [4]. Mania involves abnormally increased goal-directed activity, energy, and self-confidence, decreased sleep, distractibility, psychomotor agitation, and abnormal risk taking. All of these symptoms can be explained by excessive NEP and/or DA signaling. In T*MDD, depressive episodes involve chronic KOR activity, which leads to chronic NEP and DA activity. However, chronic KOR activity can lead to its complete desensitization. When this happens, KOR no longer restrains the phasic activation of NEP and DA. Since KOR mediates one of the fundamental survival responses, it is a major factor in restraining NEP and DA, and the disappearance of this factor allows them to signal strongly and persistently.

This account holds when mania is specifically accompanied by depressive episodes, and does not purport to explain mania in general. Mania can stem from other causes. For example, mania-like behavior is not uncommon in ADHD [102]. ADHD has a strong comorbidity with MDD, so it can be argued that all three disorders share a common cause. However, the episodic nature and age of onset of MDD and BP, as opposed to the continuous manifestation and very early onset in ADHD, point to different diagnoses [102].

Drug addiction. Any condition that induces chronic DA, NEP and/or CRH can induce DYN release and trigger MDD, especially in predisposed people. In particular, all addictive drugs increase the release of these agents, and are indeed associated with higher rates of depression [103].

Different substances of abuse have different properties, and there are aspects of addiction that are not directly related to MDD (e.g., their rewarding properties and the plasticity changes that they induce). However, T*MDD can naturally explain two major aspects of addiction.

First, the dysphoria associated with drugs appears during drug withdrawal, not during drug use. T*MDD explains this by noting that during withdrawal, cues associated with drug use excite DA, CRH and NEP neurons, and these release DYN that acts on KORs to yield dysphoria as in MDD. Drug use opposes this process (at least as long as the drug-activated reward system is not desensitized), and this may be a major factor in craving and relapse. Second, chronic KOR signaling induces chronic SNS activity, which explains the somatic symptoms of drug withdrawal (sweating, increased heart and blood pressure, pupil dilation, stomach cramps) [104].

4.5 Evidence

Overwhelming preclinical evidence for the involvement of DYN/KOR in aversion, immobility, decreased social interaction, and dysregulated DA, CRH, and NEP has been presented above. Here we provide evidence from MDD and bipolar patients that KOR signaling is chronic in MDD, and is associated with symptoms. This includes direct evidence, via DYN release, KOR expression and activation, and the effects of KOR agonists on mood in healthy humans and patients, and indirect evidence, via chronic activation of the systems regulated by DYN.

DYN/KOR data in patients. A major route through which KOR achieves its MDD effects are amygdala projections. There is direct evidence for both chronic amygdala DYN and chronic amygdala excitability. Amygdaloid complex pDYN mRNA is significantly decreased in MDD and bipolar patients (41-68% and 37-38% respectively) [105]. pDYN mRNA in the amygdala nucleus of the periamygdaloid cortex is decreased in MDD [106]. Using PET rCBF data subtraction, significantly increased left amygdala (and left dlPFC-mPFC) activity was shown in active MDD patients, with a trend in remitted patients [107]. MDD patients have an increased early (300 ms) amygdala response to sad faces, showing higher excitability of the negative paths [108]. The same paper reported a decreased late (600 ms) response to happy faces, with increased PFC-amygdala connectivity. One paper using PET reported no amygdala KOR binding differences, but it did not have sufficient power to detect effects that are not very large [109].

Another major route of KOR effects is PFC, mainly ILmPFC (subgenual cingulate cortex (SgCC) in humans), which mediates extinction and hence disengage. KOR expression in right ACC, dorsomedial PFC, and insula negatively correlates with symptoms in unmedicated patients in a depressive episode, indicating chronic KOR activation in threat and stress areas [110].

Blood KOR levels have been reported to be both lower [111] and higher [112] than control levels. Lower levels may indicate lower brain levels, and the higher levels were accompanied by higher serum DYN levels. Both pieces of data support chronic signaling. Gene linkage association, expression profiling, and network analysis in MDD patients point to KOR [113].

There is high comorbidity of MDD and drug addiction, and strong clinical and preclinical evidence link DYN to addiction (reviewed in [56,114]). For example, a significant association between depression severity and two DYN gene mutations has been found in heroin addicts [115].

KOR agonists and mood in healthy humans and patients. KOR agonists readily induce dysphoria in healthy humans [116–118]. They can also cause perceptual distortions, nervousness, anxiety, depersonalization, confusion, and abnormal thinking [119–121]. DYN is the only agent discovered so far that is consistently associated with dysphoria. CRH can induce anxiety, a sense of needing to be prepared for negative future events, but does not induce depression.

Based on the strong preclinical data, KOR antagonists have been proposed as MDD treatment. Their potential as treatment is not clear (see below), but their beneficial effects in initial clinical trials with MDD patients provide strong support for T*MDD. A combination of the KOR antagonist and partial MOR agonist buprenorphine, and the MOR antagonist samidorphan (to offset the MOR action of buprenorphine) helped treatment-resistant patients [122]. Buprenorphine was found to provide a small benefit for depressive symptoms in a systematic review and meta-analysis [123]. The selective KOR antagonist aticaprant significantly increased ventral striatum activity during reward anticipation and decreased some anhedonia measures [124]. In a phase II RCT, aticaprant (as adjunctive treatment) significantly decreased depressive symptoms, more so in patients with higher anhedonia [125]. Another selective antagonist, navicaprant, has also shown benefits in a phase II trial [126]. However, at present (March 2025) all KOR-based drugs have failed phase III trials, possibly due to experimental protocols and continues intracellular signaling.

Adenylate cyclase (AC). The main effect of prolonged Gi/o signaling is suppression of cellular AC. Indeed, decreased AC activity and cAMP have been repeatedly shown in MDD and bipolar patients, both in brain [127,128] and platelets [129]. Depressed suicide victims show decreased brain AC activity [130] and increased Gi2 and decreased Gi3 protein in platelets [131]. This result may provide direct evidence for increased KOR activity. KOR is expressed in platelets [132], KOR equally binds Gi2 and Gi3 (in transfected CHO cells) [133], and the only other significant GPCRs that couple to Gi in platelets are P2Y12, which binds Gi2, and the alpha2 adrenergic receptor, which binds Gz [134].

There is also some genetic data pointing to AC. MDD-associated genes include various AC isoforms (as well as CRH1 and CRH2) [135], and DNA hypo-methylation of AC9, associated with decreased expression and increased CRH, has been found in suicide victims [136]. Importantly, AC9 signals from endosomes [137], supporting sustained intracellular signaling of a Gi/o-bound GPCR.

Relatedly, BDNF, which cooperates with cAMP in early plasticity, is also decreased in MDD, in brain and serum [138], and is highlighted by genetic analysis [113].

Prefrontal cortex. KOR has a strong effect in PFC, especially SgCC. Increased functional connectivity between the SgCC and the default-mode network (the brain network engaged in thinking when not doing anything special) was reported in patients [139]. Moreover, there was a positive correlation of the effect with the length of the current depressive episode. Increased functional connectivity between the SgCC and the insula and amygdala was reported in depressed adolescents [140]. These results imply chronic SgCC activity (including with the amygdala) that does not manage to mediate disengage. Using data subtraction with PET regional cerebral blood flow, increased activity was shown in left mPFC and amygdala in active patients, with a trend in patients in remission [107]. MDD and bipolar patients showed increased amplitude of low-freq fluctuations in resting state fMRI, mainly in the insula and mPFC, indicating higher spontaneous activity [141]. Remitted MDD patients showed decreased PFC responses to both pleasant and aversive stimuli [142]. A highly thorough review of fMRI and PET imaging in MDD concluded that patients show increased activity and decreased volume in ventral PFC and hippocampus [143]. This review also found hypometabolism in dorsal PFC, indicating reduced actions.

SNS, brain norepinephrine. As mentioned above, MDD patients show chronic dysregulation of the SNS [8,12,14–16,144] and brain NEP [11–13,15,145], mostly involving higher excitability.

HPA axis, cortisol. MDD patients show higher CRH release, CSF CRH, blunted stimulation of ACTH by CRH, higher plasma cortisol and ACTH, lower morning cortisol, and decreased GR receptor (the cortisol receptor) function [9–13,17,145]. These data clearly point to chronically higher HPA axis activity, with desensitized function.

Dopamine, reward. DA supports vigorous goal-directed movements and reward motivation [146]. DA function can be assessed via an animal's DA and/or behavioral response to positive and negative stimuli. There is strong evidence for decreased phasic DA release and reward-related learning signals in MDD [142,147,148]. A recent systematic review and meta-analysis found higher DA release in the basal ganglia without synthesis capacity differences, indicating chronic activity [149].

Serotonin. The role of SER in MDD seems paradoxical. On one hand, drugs that elevate brain SER levels oppose many MDD symptoms, at least in the short term [150] (but see [151]). On the other hand, despite many research efforts, and reports of dysregulation of various components of the SER system, no serious impairment in brain SER has been consistently identified [152]. Here I explain why this indirectly supports T*MDD.

In T*MDD, SER-based drugs help because medium SER levels generally oppose DYN, NEP, and CRH [153–158]. Moreover, since DYN regulates SER, we can expect SER signaling to be impaired in MDD. However, DYN's regulation of SER is weaker than its regulation of other agents (see below), so the impairment is not large. In addition, since chronic effects involve both increased tonic release and decreased signaling, the effects of a small-scale chronic impairment are difficult to identify. Moreover, SER is much more abundant than DYN, so the effect of DYN should be limited to specific neural paths. Thus, the profile of the reported state of SER in MDD fits a DYN-induced problem.

To better understand the mutual effects of SER, DYN, and other agents, we need to examine the physiological role of SER, which has been the subject of much debate [159]. In my view, the main relevant observation is that the vast majority of body SER is present in the gut, where SER release is stimulated by excessive glucose [160]. In addition, release is stimulated by high temperature [161]. In turn, SER signaling promotes glucose uptake, and suppresses thermogenesis [162]. In other words, SER signaling is activated in situations of excess, and its role is excess disposal. This stands in sharp contrast to the stress systems relevant to MDD, which are activated in situations of deficiency (glucose, oxygen, cold). Indeed, SER suppresses fight and flight survival responses, thereby promoting 'do nothing' (i.e., healthy disengage, covering for impaired DYN signaling) [163]. In fact, DYN has been reported to decrease the SER transporter [164], implying that DYN may use SER's 'do nothing' function as part of DYN's disengage. Thus, SER has a fundamental opposition to deficiency-induced stress, explaining why SER drugs are beneficial in MDD. However, deficiency-induced stress is more common in nature than excess-induced stress, and DYN may use SER, explaining why the SER system is only weakly regulated by DYN and why only weak SER impairment (if at all) is identified MDD.

Oxytocin. OXT is strongly regulated by KOR. As with other such agents, OXT levels are mainly reported to be decreased in MDD, with some reports of increased levels with high variability [165,166]. One paper reported higher plasma AVP in MDD, probably reflecting its recruitment by stress responses [166].

Immunity. Cytokines and inflammation are leading recurrent themes in MDD theories [2,167,168]. Chronic inflammation should be expected in MDD, since chronic stress yields chronic immune activation [169]. However, immunity also has a tight connection to DYN, which is synthesized by immune cells (macrophages, T cells, other cells) following stimulation by CRH [170]. Indeed, unmedicated MDD patients show significantly higher serum DYN and KOR than controls, and these are strongly associated with increased levels of the cytokines IL-6 and IL-10 [112].

4.6 Treatment

Behavioral treatment. MDD involves an impaired behavioral response, occurring when the disengage survival response is impaired. Thus, the basic treatment for MDD would be to enhance the disengage response via behavioral techniques. Cognitive behavioral therapy techniques such as relaxed breathing normalize SNS activity, and emulate the effect of a successful disengage response. Engaging in actions that are unrelated to the stressful challenge would make it easier for the brain to disengage, while talking or thinking about the challenge, which increase chronic DYN signaling, are generally not recommended unless they can lead to concrete ways of solving the problem.

Serotonin. As discussed above, T*MDD explains the beneficial effects of SER-based drugs on MDD symptoms via SER's inherent opposition to deficiency-induced stress responses. These beneficial effects come with a painful price, however. SER is associated with a state of satiety, so its suppresses goal-directed actions (DA) and energy recruitment (NEP, SNS). This is fine for a few hours after a meal, but chronically elevated SER continuously suppresses motivated responses to all challenges, including challenges of a positive nature. Thus, it is not surprising that SSRIs reduce excitement and sex drive and are associated with apathy, emotional blunting, and a 'zombie-like' feeling [171]. In addition, to compensate for its opposition to NEP, high doses of SER excite muscles and the SNS, yielding SER syndrome symptoms such as motor agitation and mental confusion [172].

It takes weeks for SSRIs to start producing an effect. This is because initially, SSRIs induce the activation of SER1 receptors, whose affinity to SER is high and which act as autoreceptors on SER axons to reduce SER release [173]. After weeks of SSRI treatment, SER1a receptors are desensitized, and

SER levels begin to increase. During the few initial weeks, SER levels are actually decreased [173], which might explain the higher risk of suicide at this time period [174]. Indeed, SER depletion significantly decreases pDYN mRNA in several brain areas, indicating increased DYN usage [154]. In many cases, SSRIs stop suppressing MDD symptoms after a few months. This is probably due to desensitization of the lower affinity SER2 receptors [175].

A highly controversial aspect of antidepressants is their long-term effect. There are reports that usage of antidepressants (not only SSRIs) is associated with worse long-term prognosis [176], leading to a 'chronification' of the disorder and higher risk of switching to bipolar disorder [177]. This may be due to a long-term desensitization of the SER system. In addition, because GPCR antagonists increase receptor expression [178], chronic SSRI usage probably induces supersensitivity of the stress systems suppressed by SER, making the person more vulnerable to future stressful events.

Mania. Lithium is highly effective for preventing and treating manic episodes [179], yet it is not clear how it achieves this effect. The parsimonious T*MDD account is that lithium suppresses adenylate cyclase, even at very low doses [180]. This effectively opposes NEP (and CRH1) signaling, and thus mania.

Quetiapine is effective in treating BP, both mania and depression [179]. It is usually described as an atypical antipsychotic drug, a drug class associated with SER receptor antagonism. However, quetiapine is also a NEP receptor antagonist. In fact, its affinity to the alpha1 adrenergic receptor is almost 4 times higher than to the SER2a receptor [181]. Thus, as for lithium, the T*MDD assumption is that its efficacy in BP stems from its effect on the NEP system.

KOR antagonism. As mentioned above, selective KOR antagonists have shown promising results in initial RCTs. Such drugs relieve chronic KOR signaling, which should be beneficial in MDD. However, these drugs also weaken acute KOR signaling by reducing response amplitude. Since strong KOR signaling is crucial for mediating disengage, and since impaired disengage is the fundamental issue in MDD, KOR antagonists may also have a detrimental effect. Moreover, strong KOR blockade might induce mania. Nonetheless, in the longer term, GPCR antagonists increase cell surface receptor expression, which should improve resilience to future stress. Thus, it seems that KOR antagonists would be best used during depressive episodes and for a short time after episode termination, but not later. Naturally, the optimal usage guidelines would depend on the precise characteristics of each drug.

GRK3 inhibition. An interesting direction is to inhibit GRK3, which is the kinase promoting KOR (and CRH1) endocytosis and intracellular signaling. This would preserve response amplitude while decreasing its chronic activation. The design of GRK inhibitors (especially brain-penetrating ones) is challenging, but they might work better than KOR antagonists.

NEP-based drugs. Along with SSRIs, NEP reuptake inhibitors that are also SER or DA reuptake inhibitors are used as first line of treatment for MDD [2]. Considering that NEP and DA have a more direct effect on MDD symptoms than SER, we can expect NEP- and DA-based drugs to be effective. Indeed, a recent systematic review and meta-analysis found that stimulants help depressive and fatigue symptoms, and methylphenidate (ritalin) also decreased symptom severity and increased response rate [182].

4.7 Discussion

This chapter presented a complete theory of depression and bipolar disorder. The theory is complete in the sense that it explains the etiology, symptoms, pathology and treatment of the disorders, and addresses all of the salient existing evidence. I am not aware of any other complete theory of MDD or BP.

Besides explaining the desired phenomena and addressing the salient existing evidence, a good biological theory needs to show biological logic, a property that's hard to define but easy to recognize. Biological systems are extremely complicated, involving a very large number of components. A good theory positions itself inside existing bodies of biological knowledge that are related to the explained phenomenon. In the current case, T*MDD makes use of a novel complete theory of opioids. Strictly speaking, T*MDD does not need to explain the roles of opioids besides DYN. However, the presentation of T*OPS strengthens the case for the fundamental role of DYN in stress, its mediation of the disengage survival response, and the precise mechanisms of its signaling. Thus, T*OPS provides a strong biological logic for T*MDD.

T*MDD includes a complete theory of emotions, which would have positioned it even more firmly in the wider biological context. I have opted to discuss emotions elsewhere, because the subject requires much more space than is available here, and is contentious and would unnecessarily complicate the presentation.

The main current theories of MDD involve monoamines (SER, NEP, DA), the HPA stress axis, and cytokines (inflammation) [2,168]. None of these directions can explain the defining symptoms of MDD or the salient evidence. Given that people have already taken active steps for treating MDD using KOR antagonists, an interesting question is why a DYN-based theory has not been formulated already. This may be due to the dominance of the serotonin direction, and to the lack of a theory of opioids that positions DYN in the wider biological context. In any case, this paper makes the case that T*MDD should be the default theory of MDD until some other better theory emerges, or until the evidence supporting it is so large that it can be viewed as correct.

T*MDD also explains some of the central aspects of drug addiction. Since other central aspects are basically understood, the distance to a complete theory of drug addiction is in my opinion very small. This will be detailed elsewhere.

The evidence supporting T*MDD is overall strong, but more evidence pertaining to the behavior of DYN and KOR in MDD patients is called for. Compared to the overwhelming preclinical evidence about DYN and KOR, and to the indirect evidence supporting DYN involvement in MDD, the direct evidence is smaller.

As discussed in the treatment section, KOR antagonists constitute a promising treatment direction, but their success is far from assured. GRK3 inhibitors may have higher chances of success, but are more difficult to design. Discussing this direction in depth is beyond the scope of this chapter. As mentioned above, platelet Gi3 might be a biomarker, but this need to be verified.

Finally, T*MDD makes a very strong theory prediction: that normalizing DYN secretion and KOR signaling to be strong and non-chronic would completely resolve the mood symptoms of MDD, and would improve its somatic symptoms. This would dramatically improve the quality of life of hundreds of millions of people.

List of abbreviations

AC: adenylate cyclase.

ACh: acetylcholine. ACTH: adrenocorticotropic hormone.

ADHD: attention deficit hyperactivity disorder.

BEND: beta-endorphin.

BLA: basolateral amygdala.

BNST: bed nucleus of the stria terminalis.

BP: bipolar disorder.

cAMP: cyclic adenosine monophosphate. CeA: central nucleus of the amygdala.

CRH (CRH1): corticotropin-releasing hormone (receptor type 1).

CPP: conditioned place preference.

CSF: cerebrospinal fluid. DA: dopamine.

DOR: delta opioid receptor.

DYN: dynorphin.

ENK: enkephalin.

Gi/o: a G protein alpha subunit.

GIRK: G protein-coupled inwardly rectifying potassium channel.

GPCR: G protein-coupled receptor.

Gs: a G protein alpha subunit that stimulates PKA.

HPA: hypothalamus pituitary adrenal (axis).

IIN: inhibitory interneuron.

ILmPFC: infralimbic medial prefrontal cortex.

KOR: kappa opioid receptor.

LC: locus coeruleus.

MDD: major depressive disorder.

MOR: mu opioid receptor.
mPFC: medial prefrontal cortex.
NAc: nucleus accumbens.
NEP: norepinephrine.
NOCP (NOCPR): nociceptin opioid (receptor).
OP (OPR): opioid (receptor).
PFC: prefrontal cortex. PKA: protein kinase A.
PKC: protein kinase C.
POMC: pro-opiomelanocortin.
RCT: randomized controlled trial.
SER: serotonin.
SgCC: subgenual cingulate cortex.
SNS: sympathetic nervous system.
SSRI: selective serotonin reuptake inhibitor.
T*MDD: the theory of depression presented in this paper.
T*OPS: the theory of opioids presented in this paper.
VTA: ventral tegmental area.

References

[1] S.L. James, D. Abate, K.H. Abate, S.M. Abay, C. Abbafati, N. Abbasi, et al., Global, regional, and national incidence, prevalence, and years lived with disability for 354 diseases and injuries for 195 countries and territories, 1990–2017: a systematic analysis for the Global Burden of Disease Study 2017, The Lancet 392 (10159) (2018) 1789–1858.

[2] G. Malhi, J. Mann, Depression, The Lancet 392 (2018) 2299–2312.

[3] C. Otte, S.M. Gold, B.W. Penninx, C.M. Pariante, A. Etkin, M. Fava, et al., Major depressive disorder, Nature Reviews Disease Primers 2 (1) (2016) 1–20.

[4] A.P.A. American, Psychiatric Association: Diagnostic and Statistical Manual of Mental Disorders, Fifth Edition (DSM-5), American Psychiatric Association, Arlington, VA, 2013.

[5] T.L. Bale, W.W. Vale, CRF and CRF receptors: role in stress responsivity and other behaviors, Annual Review of Pharmacology and Toxicology 44 (2004) 525–557.

[6] P. Willner, J. Scheel-Krüger, C. Belzung, The neurobiology of depression and antidepressant action, Neuroscience and Biobehavioral Reviews 37 (10) (2013) 2331–2371.

[7] A.G. Bertollo, A.C.L. Galvan, C. Dallagnol, A.D. Cortez, Z.M. Ignácio, Early life stress and major depressive disorder–an update on molecular mechanisms and synaptic impairments, Molecular Neurobiology (2024).

[8] R.C. Veith, N. Lewis, O.A. Linares, R.F. Barnes, M.A. Raskind, E.C. Villacres, et al., Sympathetic nervous system activity in major depression: basal and desipramine-induced alterations in plasma norepinephrine kinetics, Archives of General Psychiatry 51 (5) (1994) 411–422.

[9] M. Owens, P. Plotsky, The role of corticotropin-releasing factor in depression and anxiety disorders, Journal of Endocrinology 160 (1) (1999) 1–12.

[10] F. Holsboer, The corticosteroid receptor hypothesis of depression, Neuropsychopharmacology 23 (5) (2000) 477–501.

[11] M.L. Wong, M.A. Kling, P.J. Munson, S. Listwak, J. Licinio, P. Prolo, et al., Pronounced and sustained central hypernoradrenergic function in major depression with melancholic features: relation to hypercortisolism and corticotropin-releasing hormone, Proceedings of the National Academy of Sciences 97 (1) (2000) 325–330.

[12] P.W. Gold, M.L. Wong, D.S. Goldstein, H.K. Gold, D.S. Ronsaville, M. Esler, et al., Cardiac implications of increased arterial entry and reversible 24-h central and peripheral norepinephrine levels in melancholia, Proceedings of the National Academy of Sciences 102 (23) (2005) 8303–8308.

[13] T. Rein, O. Ambrée, G.R. Fries, V. Rappeneau, U. Schmidt, C. Touma, The hypothalamic-pituitary-adrenal axis in depression: molecular regulation, pathophysiological role, and translational implications, in: Neurobiology of Depression, Elsevier, 2019, pp. 89–96.
[14] M. Xie, Y. Huang, W. Cai, B. Zhang, H. Huang, Q. Li, et al., Neurobiological underpinnings of hyperarousal in depression: a comprehensive review, Brain Sciences 14 (1) (2024) 50.
[15] C. Cottingham, Q. Wang, $\alpha 2$ adrenergic receptor dysregulation in depressive disorders: implications for the neurobiology of depression and antidepressant therapy, Neuroscience and Biobehavioral Reviews 36 (10) (2012) 2214–2225.
[16] W.J. Cubała, J. Landowski, B. Wielgomas, W. Czarnowski, Low baseline salivary 3-methoxy-4-hydroxyphenylglycol (MHPG) in drug-naïve patients with short-illness-duration first episode major depressive disorder, Journal of Affective Disorders 161 (2014) 4–7.
[17] L. Izakova, N. Hlavacova, V. Segeda, D. Kapsdorfer, E. Morovicsova, D. Jezova, Salivary aldosterone, cortisol, and their morning to evening slopes in patients with depressive disorder and healthy subjects: acute episode and follow-up 6 months after reaching remission, Neuroendocrinology 110 (11–12) (2020) 1001–1009.
[18] O. Babenko, I. Kovalchuk, G.A. Metz, Stress-induced perinatal and transgenerational epigenetic programming of brain development and mental health, Neuroscience and Biobehavioral Reviews 48 (2015) 70–91.
[19] J. Koolhaas, A. Bartolomucci, B. Buwalda, S. de Boer, G. Flügge, S. Korte, et al., Stress revisited: a critical evaluation of the stress concept, Neuroscience and Biobehavioral Reviews 35 (5) (2011) 1291–1301.
[20] J.M. Bian, N. Wu, R.B. Su, J. Li, Opioid receptor trafficking and signaling: what happens after opioid receptor activation?, Cellular and Molecular Neurobiology 32 (2012) 167–184.
[21] S. Sakurada, T. Sawai, H. Mizoguchi, H. Watanabe, C. Watanabe, A. Yonezawa, et al., Possible involvement of dynorphin a release via $\mu 1$-opioid receptor on supraspinal antinociception of endomorphin-2, Peptides 29 (9) (2008) 1554–1560.
[22] S. Liu, W.J. Kang, A. Abrimian, J. Xu, L. Cartegni, S. Majumdar, et al., Alternative pre-mRNA splicing of the mu opioid receptor gene, OPRM1: insight into complex mu opioid actions, Biomolecules 11 (10) (2021) 1525.
[23] Fan Sf, S.M. Crain, Dual regulation by μ, δ and κ opioid receptor agonists of K+ conductance of DRG neurons and neuroblastoma$\times$ DRG neuron hybrid F11 cells, Brain Research 696 (1–2) (1995) 97–105.
[24] M. Szucs, K. Boda, A.R. Gintzler, Dual effects of Tyr-D-Ala-Gly-(NMe) Phe-Gly-ol (DAMGO) and D-Phe-Cys-Tyr-D-Trp-Arg-Thr-Pen-Thr-NH2 (CTAP) on adenylyl cyclase activity, implications for μ-opioid receptor Gs coupling, The Journal of Pharmacology and Experimental Therapeutics 389 (2) (2004).
[25] A. Kuzmin, J. Sandin, L. Terenius, S.O. Ögren, Dose- and time-dependent bimodal effects of κ-opioid agonists on locomotor activity in mice, The Journal of Pharmacology and Experimental Therapeutics 295 (3) (2000) 1031–1042.
[26] S.E. Crilly, M.A. Puthenveedu, Compartmentalized GPCR signaling from intracellular membranes, The Journal of Membrane Biology 254 (2021) 259–271.
[27] M.L. Halls, D.M. Cooper, Regulation by Ca2+-signaling pathways of adenylyl cyclases, Cold Spring Harbor Perspectives in Biology (2011), 3(1):a004143.
[28] T. Mizushige, K. Saitoh, Y. Manabe, T. Nishizuka, Y. Taka, A. Eguchi, et al., Preference for dietary fat induced by release of beta-endorphin in rats, Life Sciences 84 (21) (2009) 760–765.
[29] N.T. Lichtenberg, K.M. Wassum, Amygdala mu-opioid receptors mediate the motivating influence of cue-triggered reward expectations, European Journal of Neuroscience 121 (3) (2017) 381–387.
[30] A. Kelley, V. Bakshi, S. Haber, T. Steininger, M. Will, M. Zhang, Opioid modulation of taste hedonics within the ventral striatum, Physiology & Behavior 76 (3) (2002) 365–377.
[31] A.C. Shin, P.J. Pistell, C.B. Phifer, H.R. Berthoud, Reversible suppression of food reward behavior by chronic mu-opioid receptor antagonism in the nucleus accumbens, Neuroscience 170 (2) (2010) 580–588.

[32] R. Paredes, Opioids and sexual reward, Pharmacology, Biochemistry and Behavior 121 (2014) 124–131.
[33] P. Jern, J. Chen, J. Tuisku, T. Saanijoki, J. Hirvonen, L. Lukkarinen, et al., Endogenous opioid release after orgasm in man: a combined PET/functional MRI study, Journal of Nuclear Medicine 64 (8) (2023) 1310–1313.
[34] N. Kozyrev, L.M. Coolen, Activation of mu or delta opioid receptors in the lumbosacral spinal cord is essential for ejaculatory reflexes in male rats, PLoS ONE (2015), 10(3):e0121130.
[35] G. Corona, E.A. Jannini, L. Vignozzi, G. Rastrelli, M. Maggi, The hormonal control of ejaculation, Nature Reviews Neurology 9 (9) (2012) 508–519.
[36] H.L. Fields, E.B. Margolis, Understanding opioid reward, Trends Neuroscis 38 (4) (2015) 217–225.
[37] S.S. Pappas, T. Kennedy, J.L. Goudreau, K.J. Lookingland, Opioid-mediated regulation of A11 diencephalospinal dopamine neurons: pharmacological evidence of activation by morphine, Neuropharmacology 61 (4) (2011) 614–621.
[38] W.M. Armstead, Nitric oxide contributes to opioid release from glia during hypoxia, Brain Research 813 (2) (1998) 398–401.
[39] G.M. Denning, L.W. Ackermann, T.J. Barna, J.G. Armstrong, L.L. Stoll, N.L. Weintraub, et al., Proenkephalin expression and enkephalin release are widely observed in non-neuronal tissues, Peptides 29 (1) (2008) 83–92.
[40] D. Wang, V.L. Tawfik, G. Corder, S.A. Low, A. François, A.I. Basbaum, et al., Functional divergence of delta and mu opioid receptor organization in CNS pain circuits, Neuron 98 (1) (2018) 90–108.
[41] E. Wei, L. Tseng, H. Loh, C.H. Li, Comparison of the behavioral effects of β-endorphin and enkephalin analogs, Life Sciences 21 (3) (1977) 321–327.
[42] Y. Katsuura, S.A. Taha, Modulation of feeding and locomotion through mu and delta opioid receptor signaling in the nucleus accumbens, Neuropeptides 44 (3) (2010) 225–232.
[43] K. Jhamandas, M. Sutak, Action of enkephalin analogues and morphine on brain acetylcholine release: differential reversal by naloxone and an opiate pentapeptide, British Journal of Pharmacology 71 (1) (1980) 201–210.
[44] G. Andrew Mickley, M.A. Mulvihill, M.A. Postler, Brain μ and δ opioid receptors mediate different locomotor hyperactivity responses of the C57BL/6J mouse, Psychopharmacology 101 (1990) 332–337.
[45] P.D. Mendella, R.M. Zacharko, Variations of motor activity following intraventricular (D-Pen2, D-Pen5)-enkephalin administration: interaction with acute uncontrollable foot-shock in mice, Pharmacology, Biochemistry and Behavior 53 (4) (1996) 877–883.
[46] A.L. Hebb, R.M. Zacharko, Central d-Ala2-Met5-enkephalinamide μ/δ-opioid receptor activation reverses the anxiogenic-like properties of cholecystokinin on locomotor and rearing activity in CD-1 mice, Brain Research 970 (1–2) (2003) 9–19.
[47] A.I. Basbaum, D.M. Bautista, G. Scherrer, D. Julius, Cellular and molecular mechanisms of pain, Cell 139 (2) (2009) 267–284.
[48] R.L. Ung, M.M. Ortiz-Juza, V.R. Curtis, R.A. Alghorazi, G. Velazquez-Hernandez, A. Ring, et al., Prepronociceptin-expressing neurons in the extended amygdala signal darting away from an aversive odor, bioRxiv (2022).
[49] M.K. Green, D.P. Devine, Nociceptin/orphanin FQ and NOP receptor gene regulation after acute or repeated social defeat stress, Neuropeptides 43 (6) (2009) 507–514.
[50] P.E. Lutz, Y. Zhou, A. Labbe, N. Mechawar, G. Turecki, Decreased expression of nociceptin/orphanin FQ in the dorsal anterior cingulate cortex of suicides, European Neuropsychopharmacology 25 (11) (2015) 2008–2014.
[51] E.F. Silva, A.I. Silva, L. Asth, L.S. Souza, N.T. Zaveri, R. Guerrini, et al., Nociceptin/orphanin FQ receptor agonists increase aggressiveness in the mouse resident-intruder test, Behavioural Brain Research 356 (2019) 120–126.

[52] M. Inoue, I. Shimohira, A. Yoshida, A. Zimmer, H. Takeshima, T. Sakurada, et al., Dose-related opposite modulation by nociceptin/orphanin FQ of substance P nociception in the nociceptors and spinal cord, The Journal of Pharmacology and Experimental Therapeutics 291 (1) (1999) 308–313.
[53] T. Sakurada, S. Katsuyama, S. Sakurada, M. Inoue, K. Tan-No, K. Kisara, et al., Nociceptin-induced scratching, biting and licking in mice: involvement of spinal NK1 receptors, British Journal of Pharmacology 127 (7) (1999) 1712–1718.
[54] K. Duvan Aydemir, O. Gunduz, A. Ulugol, Effects of a nociceptin receptor antagonist on experimentally induced scratching behavior in mice, Neurophysiology 49 (2017) 130–134.
[55] J. Halasz, D. Zelena, M. Toth, A. Tulogdi, E. Mikics, J. Haller, Substance P neurotransmission and violent aggression: the role of tachykinin NK 1 receptors in the hypothalamic attack area, European Journal of Pharmacology 611 (1) (2009) 35–43.
[56] H. Tejeda, T. Shippenberg, R. Henriksson, The dynorphin/κ-opioid receptor system and its role in psychiatric disorders, Cellular and Molecular Life Sciences 69 (6) (2012) 857–896.
[57] B. Reyes, A. Carvalho, K. Vakharia, E. Van Bockstaele, Amygdalar peptidergic circuits regulating noradrenergic locus coeruleus neurons: linking limbic and arousal centers, Experimental Neurology 230 (1) (2011) 96–105.
[58] M. Dumont, S. Lemaire, Opioid and nonopioid cardiovascular effects of dynorphins, Advances in Pharmacology 37 (1996) 1–33.
[59] K.J. Iremonger, J.S. Bains, Retrograde opioid signaling regulates glutamatergic transmission in the hypothalamus, The Journal of Neuroscience 29 (22) (2009) 7349–7358.
[60] J.A. Russell, G. Leng, A.J. Douglas, The magnocellular oxytocin system the fount of maternity: adaptations in pregnancy, Frontiers in Neuroendocrinology 24 (1) (2003) 27–61.
[61] J.W. Muschamp, J.A. Hollander, J.L. Thompson, G. Voren, L.C. Hassinger, S. Onvani, et al., Hypocretin (orexin) facilitates reward by attenuating the antireward effects of its cotransmitter dynorphin in ventral tegmental area, Proceedings of the National Academy of Sciences 111 (16) (2014) E1648–E1655.
[62] C. Drake, G. Terman, M. Simmons, T. Milner, D. Kunkel, P. Schwartzkroin, et al., Dynorphin opioids present in dentate granule cells may function as retrograde inhibitory neurotransmitters, The Journal of Neuroscience 14 (6) (1994) 3736–3750.
[63] J.M. Kunselman, A. Gupta, I. Gomes, L.A. Devi, M.A. Puthenveedu, Compartment-specific opioid receptor signaling is selectively modulated by different dynorphin peptides, eLife 10 (2021) e60270.
[64] A. Kreibich, B.A. Reyes, A.L. Curtis, L. Ecke, C. Chavkin, E.J. Van Bockstaele, et al., Presynaptic inhibition of diverse afferents to the locus ceruleus by κ-opiate receptors: a novel mechanism for regulating the central norepinephrine system, Journal of Neuroscience 28 (25) (2008) 6516–6525.
[65] H.E. Yarur, S.M. Casello, V.S. Tsai, J. Enriquez-Traba, R. Kore, H. Wang, et al., Dynorphin/kappa-opioid receptor regulation of excitation-inhibition balance toggles afferent control of prefrontal cortical circuits in a pathway-specific manner, Molecular Psychiatry (2023) 1–13.
[66] N.A. Crowley, D.W. Bloodgood, J.A. Hardaway, A.M. Kendra, J.G. McCall, R. Al-Hasani, et al., Dynorphin controls the gain of an amygdalar anxiety circuit, Cell Reports 14 (12) (2016) 2774–2783.
[67] H.A. Tejeda, J. Wu, A.R. Kornspun, M. Pignatelli, V. Kashtelyan, M.J. Krashes, et al., Pathway- and cell-specific kappa-opioid receptor modulation of excitation-inhibition balance differentially gates D1 and D2 accumbens neuron activity, Neuron 93 (1) (2017) 147–163.
[68] M. Hein, G. Ji, D. Tidwell, P. D'Souza, T. Kiritoshi, V. Yakhnitsa, et al., Kappa opioid receptor activation in the amygdala disinhibits CRF neurons to generate pain-like behaviors, Neuropharmacology 185 (2021) 108456.
[69] E.B. Margolis, H. Lock, V.I. Chefer, T.S. Shippenberg, G.O. Hjelmstad, H.L. Fields, κ opioids selectively control dopaminergic neurons projecting to the prefrontal cortex, Proceedings of the National Academy of Sciences 103 (8) (2006) 2938–2942.

[70] V.I. Chefer, C.M. Bäckman, E.D. Gigante, T.S. Shippenberg, Kappa opioid receptors on dopaminergic neurons are necessary for kappa-mediated place aversion, Neuropsychopharmacology 38 (13) (2013) 2623–2631.
[71] J.C. Lemos, C.A. Roth, D.I. Messinger, H.K. Gill, P.E. Phillips, C. Chavkin, Repeated stress dysregulates κ-opioid receptor signaling in the dorsal raphe through a p38α MAPK-dependent mechanism, Journal of Neuroscience 32 (36) (2012) 12325–12336.
[72] R. Tao, S.B. Auerbach, μ-Opioids disinhibit and κ-opioids inhibit serotonin efflux in the dorsal raphe nucleus, Brain Research 1049 (1) (2005) 70–79.
[73] Langley Aunis, Physiological aspects of exocytosis in chromaffin cells of the adrenal medulla, Acta Physiologica Scandinavica 167 (2) (1999) 89–97.
[74] A. Fassini, A.A. Scopinho, L.B. Resstel, F.M. Corrêa, κ-Opioid receptors in the infralimbic cortex modulate the cardiovascular responses to acute stress, Experimental Physiology 100 (4) (2015) 377–387.
[75] B. Varastehmoradi, K.L. Smith, H.K. Müller, B. Elfving, C. Sanchez, G. Wegener, Kappa opioid activation changes protein profiles in different regions of the brain relevant to depression, European Neuropsychopharmacology 72 (2023) 9–17.
[76] K. Jüngling, M.D. Lange, H.J. Szkudlarek, J. Lesting, F.S. Erdmann, M. Doengi, et al., Increased gabaergic efficacy of central amygdala projections to neuropeptide S neurons in the brainstem during fear memory retrieval, Neuropsychopharmacology 40 (12) (2015) 2753–2763.
[77] J.P. McLaughlin, S. Li, J. Valdez, T.A. Chavkin, C. Chavkin, Social defeat stress-induced behavioral responses are mediated by the endogenous kappa opioid system, Neuropsychopharmacology 31 (6) (2006) 1241–1248.
[78] W.A. Carlezon, C. Béguin, J.A. DiNieri, M.H. Baumann, M.R. Richards, M.S. Todtenkopf, et al., Depressive-like effects of the κ-opioid receptor agonist salvinorin A on behavior and neurochemistry in rats, The Journal of Pharmacology and Experimental Therapeutics 316 (1) (2006) 440–447.
[79] R.J. Donahue, S.M. Landino, S.A. Golden, F.I. Carroll, S.J. Russo, W.A. Carlezon Jr, Effects of acute and chronic social defeat stress are differentially mediated by the dynorphin/kappa-opioid receptor system, Behavioural Pharmacology 26 (7) (2015) 654.
[80] A.R. Laman-Maharg, T. Copeland, E.O. Sanchez, K.L. Campi, B.C. Trainor, The long-term effects of stress and kappa opioid receptor activation on conditioned place aversion in male and female California mice, Behavioural Brain Research 332 (2017) 299–307.
[81] A.V. Williams, A. Laman-Maharg, C.V. Armstrong, S. Ramos-Maciel, V.A. Minie, B.C. Trainor, Acute inhibition of kappa opioid receptors before stress blocks depression-like behaviors in California mice, Progress in Neuro-Psychopharmacology & Biological Psychiatry 86 (2018) 166–174.
[82] C.A. Browne, E. Falcon, S.A. Robinson, O. Berton, I. Lucki, Reversal of stress-induced social interaction deficits by buprenorphine, International Journal of Neuropsychopharmacology 21 (2) (2018) 164–174.
[83] G.y. Zan, X. Sun, Y.j. Wang, R. Liu, C.y. Wang, W.j. Du, et al., Amygdala dynorphin/κ opioid receptor system modulates depressive-like behavior in mice following chronic social defeat stress, Acta Pharmacologica Sinica 43 (3) (2022) 577–587.
[84] S. Ghozland, H.W. Matthes, F. Simonin, D. Filliol, B.L. Kieffer, R. Maldonado, Motivational effects of cannabinoids are mediated by μ-opioid and κ-opioid receptors, The Journal of Neuroscience 22 (3) (2002) 1146–1154.
[85] B.B. Land, M.R. Bruchas, J.C. Lemos, M. Xu, E.J. Melief, C. Chavkin, The dysphoric component of stress is encoded by activation of the dynorphin κ-opioid system, Journal of Neuroscience 28 (2) (2008) 407–414.
[86] C.F. Robles, M.Z. McMackin, K.L. Campi, I.E. Doig, E.Y. Takahashi, M.C. Pride, et al., Effects of kappa opioid receptors on conditioned place aversion and social interaction in males and females, Behavioural Brain Research 262 (2014) 84–93.

[87] M.A. Robble, M.E. Bozsik, D.S. Wheeler, R.A. Wheeler, Learned avoidance requires VTA KOR-mediated reductions in dopamine, Neuropharmacology 167 (2020) 107996.
[88] S.L. Resendez, P.C. Keyes, J.J. Day, C. Hambro, C.J. Austin, F.K. Maina, et al., Dopamine and opioid systems interact within the nucleus accumbens to maintain monogamous pair bonds, eLife 5 (2016) e15325.
[89] M.S. Todtenkopf, J.F. Marcus, P.S. Portoghese, W.A. Carlezon, Effects of κ-opioid receptor ligands on intracranial self-stimulation in rats, Psychopharmacology 172 (2004) 463–470.
[90] S.S. Negus, E.M. Morrissey, M. Rosenberg, K. Cheng, K.C. Rice, Effects of kappa opioids in an assay of pain-depressed intracranial self-stimulation in rats, Psychopharmacology 210 (2010) 149–159.
[91] C.A. Browne, H. Wulf, I. Lucki, Kappa opioid receptors in the pathology and treatment of major depressive disorder, The Kappa Opioid Receptor (2021) 493–524.
[92] F. Sotres-Bayon, G.J. Quirk, Prefrontal control of fear: more than just extinction, Current Opinion in Neurobiology 20 (2) (2010) 231–235.
[93] R. Stoop, Neuromodulation by oxytocin and vasopressin, Neuron 76 (1) (2012) 142–159.
[94] Wu He, R.S. MacDougall, A.D. Clithero, R.J. Leitermann, M. Terashvili, L.F. Tseng, Opposite conditioned place preference responses to endomorphin-1 and endomorphin-2 in the mouse, Neuroscience Letters 365 (3) (2004) 157–161.
[95] D. Braida, V. Limonta, V. Capurro, P. Fadda, T. Rubino, P. Mascia, et al., Involvement of κ-opioid and endocannabinoid system on Salvinorin A-induced reward, Biological Psychiatry 63 (3) (2008) 286–292.
[96] C.A. Sandman, L.M. Glynn, E.P. Davis, Neurobehavioral consequences of fetal exposure to gestational stress, Fetal development: Research on brain and behavior, environmental influences, and emerging technologies (2016) 229–265.
[97] A.K. Short, T.Z. Baram, Early-life adversity and neurological disease: age-old questions and novel answers, Nature Reviews Neurology 15 (11) (2019) 657–669.
[98] L. Eiland, R. Romeo, Stress and the developing adolescent brain, Neuroscience 249 (2013) 162–171.
[99] A.L. Curtis, T. Bethea, R.J. Valentino, Sexually dimorphic responses of the brain norepinephrine system to stress and corticotropin-releasing factor, Neuropsychopharmacology 31 (3) (2006) 544–554.
[100] M.P. Mostari, N. Ieda, C. Deura, S. Minabe, S. Yamada, Y. Uenoyama, et al., Dynorphin-kappa opioid receptor signaling partly mediates estrogen negative feedback effect on LH pulses in female rats, Journal of Reproduction and Development 59 (3) (2013) 266–272.
[101] A.D. Abraham, S.S. Schattauer, K.L. Reichard, J.H. Cohen, H.M. Fontaine, A.J. Song, et al., Estrogen regulation of GRK2 inactivates kappa opioid receptor signaling mediating analgesia, but not aversion, The Journal of Neuroscience 38 (37) (2018) 8031–8043.
[102] B. Birmaher, Bipolar disorder in children and adolescents, Child and Adolescent Mental Health 18 (3) (2013) 140–148.
[103] N.D. Volkow, M. Michaelides, R. Baler, The neuroscience of drug reward and addiction, Physiological Reviews 99 (4) (2019) 2115–2140.
[104] W.B. Solecki, N. Kus, K. Gralec, A. Klasa, K. Pradel, R. Przewłocki, Noradrenergic and corticosteroid receptors regulate somatic and motivational symptoms of morphine withdrawal, Behavioural Brain Research 360 (2019) 146–157.
[105] Y. Hurd, Subjects with major depression or bipolar disorder show reduction of prodynorphin mRNA expression in discrete nuclei of the amygdaloid complex, Molecular Psychiatry 7 (1) (2002) 75–81.
[106] S.A.R. Anderson, M. Michaelides, P. Zarnegar, Y. Ren, P. Fagergren, P.K. Thanos, et al., Impaired periamygdaloid-cortex prodynorphin is characteristic of opiate addiction and depression, The Journal of Clinical Investigation 123 (12) (2013) 5334–5341.
[107] W. Drevets, T. Videen, J. Price, S. Preskorn, S. Carmichael, M. Rarchle, A functional anatomical study of unipolar depression, The Journal of Neuroscience 12 (9) (1992) 3628–3641.

[108] X. Fan, M. Mocchi, B. Pascuzzi, J. Xiao, B.A. Metzger, R.K. Mathura, et al., Brain mechanisms underlying the emotion processing bias in treatment-resistant depression, Nature Mental Health (2024).

[109] J.M. Miller, F. Zanderigo, P.D. Purushothaman, C. DeLorenzo, H. Rubin-Falcone, R.T. Ogden, et al., Kappa opioid receptor binding in major depression: a pilot study, Synapse (2018), 72(9):e22042.

[110] K. Smart, A. Yttredahl, M.A. Oquendo, J.J. Mann, A.T. Hillmer, R.E. Carson, et al., Data-driven analysis of kappa opioid receptor binding in major depressive disorder measured by positron emission tomography, Translational Psychiatry 11 (1) (2021) 602.

[111] B. Quintanilla, G.C. Medeiros, D. Greenstein, P. Yuan, J.N. Johnston, L.T. Park, et al., κ-opioid receptor plasma levels are associated with sex and diagnosis of major depressive disorder but not response to ketamine, Journal of Clinical Psychopharmacology 43 (2) (2023) 89–96.

[112] H.K. Al-Hakeim, S.Z. Al-Fadhel, A.H. Al-Dujaili, M. Maes, In major depression, increased kappa and mu opioid receptor levels are associated with immune activation, Acta Neuropsychiatrica 32 (2) (2020) 99–108.

[113] A.J. Deo, Huang Yy, C.A. Hodgkinson, Y. Xin, M.A. Oquendo, A.J. Dwork, et al., A large-scale candidate gene analysis of mood disorders: evidence of neurotrophic tyrosine kinase receptor and opioid receptor signaling dysfunction, Psychiatric Genetics 23 (2) (2013) 47–55.

[114] C. Chavkin, G.F. Koob, Dynorphin, dysphoria, and dependence: the stress of addiction, Neuropsychopharmacology 41 (1) (2016) 373.

[115] D. Kaya-Akyüzlü, S. Özkan-Kotiloğlu, Ş Ayaz N. Yalçın-Şahiner, Effect of PDYN rs2281285, rs2235749 and rs910080 gene polymorphisms on the intensity of depression symptoms and negative craving in heroin addicts, Archives of Biological Sciences 73 (4) (2021).

[116] K. Kumor, C. Haertzen, R. Johnson, T. Kocher, D. Jasinski, Human psychopharmacology of ketocyclazocine as compared with cyclazocine, morphine and placebo, The Journal of Pharmacology and Experimental Therapeutics 238 (3) (1986) 960–968.

[117] A. Pfeiffer, V. Brantl, A. Herz, H.M. Emrich, Psychotomimesis mediated by κ opiate receptors, Science 233 (4765) (1986) 774–776.

[118] G. Rimoy, D. Wright, N. Bhaskar, P. Rubin, The cardiovascular and central nervous system effects in the human of U-62066E: a selective opioid receptor agonist, European Journal of Clinical Pharmacology 46 (1994) 203–207.

[119] A.C. Pande, R.E. Pyke, M. Greiner, G.L. Wideman, R. Benjamin, M.W. Pierce, Analgesic efficacy of enadoline versus placebo or morphine in postsurgical pain, Clinical Neuropharmacology 19 (5) (1996) 451–456.

[120] S.L. Walsh, E.C. Strain, M.E. Abreu, G.E. Bigelow, Enadoline, a selective kappa opioid agonist: comparison with butorphanol and hydromorphone in humans, Psychopharmacology 157 (2001) 151–162.

[121] M. Ranganathan, A. Schmakenberg, P.D. Skosnik, B.M. Cohen, B. Pittman, R.A. Sewell, et al., Dose-related behavioral, subjective, endocrine, and psychophysiological effects of the κ opioid agonist Salvinorin A in humans, Biological Psychiatry 72 (10) (2012) 871–879.

[122] E. Ehrich, R. Turncliff, Y. Du, R. Leigh-Pemberton, E. Fernandez, R. Jones, et al., Evaluation of opioid modulation in major depressive disorder, Neuropsychopharmacology 40 (6) (2015) 1448–1455.

[123] N.B. Riblet, Y. Young-Xu, B. Shiner, P.P. Schnurr, B.V. Watts, The efficacy and safety of buprenorphine for the treatment of depression: a systematic review and meta-analysis, Journal of Psychiatric Research 161 (2023) 393–401.

[124] A.D. Krystal, D.A. Pizzagalli, M. Smoski, S.J. Mathew, J. Nurnberger Jr., S.H. Lisanby, et al., A randomized proof-of-mechanism trial applying the 'fast-fail' approach to evaluating κ-opioid antagonism as a treatment for anhedonia, Nature Medicine 26 (5) (2020) 760–768.

[125] M.E. Schmidt, I. Kezic, V. Popova, R. Melkote, P. Van Der Ark, D.J. Pemberton, et al., Efficacy and safety of aticaprant, a kappa receptor antagonist, adjunctive to oral SSRI/SNRI

antidepressant in major depressive disorder: results of a phase 2 randomized, double-blind, placebo-controlled study, Neuropsychopharmacology (2024) 1–11.
[126] E. Hampsey, L. Jelen, A.H. Young, Aticaprant: (a κ-opioid receptor antagonist) for major depressive disorder, Expert Opinion on Emerging Drugs 29 (3) (2024) 193–204.
[127] L.T. Young, D. Dowlatshahi, G.M. MacQueen, J.F. Wang, Increased temporal cortex CREB concentrations and antidepressant treatment in major depression, The Lancet 352 (9142) (1998) 1754–1755.
[128] M. Fujita, C.S. Hines, S.S. Zoghbi, A.G. Mallinger, L.P. Dickstein, J.S. Liow, et al., Downregulation of brain phosphodiesterase type IV measured with 11C-(R)-rolipram positron emission tomography in major depressive disorder, Biological Psychiatry 72 (7) (2012) 548–554.
[129] L.M. Hines, B. Tabakoff, et al., Platelet adenylyl cyclase activity: a biological marker for major depression and recent drug use, Biological Psychiatry 58 (12) (2005) 955–962.
[130] Y. Dwivedi, H.S. Rizavi, P.K. Shukla, J. Lyons, G. Faludi, M. Palkovits, et al., Protein kinase A in postmortem brain of depressed suicide victims: altered expression of specific regulatory and catalytic subunits, Biological Psychiatry 55 (3) (2004) 234–243.
[131] J.A. García-Sevilla, C. Walzer, X. Busquets, P.V. Escribá, L. Balant, J. Guimón, Density of guanine nucleotide-binding proteins in platelets of patients with major depression: increased abundance of the Gαi2 subunit and down-regulation by antidepressant drug treatment, Biological Psychiatry 42 (8) (1997) 704–712.
[132] S.M. Gruba, D.H. Francis, A.F. Meyer, E. Spanolios, J. He, B.M. Meyer, et al., Characterization of the presence and function of platelet opioid receptors, ACS Measurement Science Au 2 (1) (2022) 4–13.
[133] P. Prather, T. McGinn, P. Claude, L. Liu-Chen, Properties of a κ-opioid receptor expressed in CHO cells: interaction with multiple G-proteins is not specific for any individual Gα subunit and is similar to that of other opioid receptors, Molecular Brain Research 29 (2) (1995) 336–346.
[134] S. Offermanns, Activation of platelet function through G protein–coupled receptors, Circulation Research 99 (12) (2006) 1293–1304.
[135] T. Fan, Y. Hu, J. Xin, M. Zhao, J. Wang, Analyzing the genes and pathways related to major depressive disorder via a systems biology approach, Brain and Behavior (2020), 10(2):e01502.
[136] A.L. Romero-Pimentel, D. Almeida, S. Muñoz-Montero, C. Rangel, R. Mendoza-Morales, E.E. Gonzalez-Saenz, et al., Integrative DNA methylation and gene expression analysis in the prefrontal cortex of Mexicans who died by suicide, International Journal of Neuropsychopharmacology 24 (12) (2021) 935–947.
[137] A.M. Lazar, R. Irannejad, T.A. Baldwin, A.B. Sundaram, J.S. Gutkind, A. Inoue, et al., G protein-regulated endocytic trafficking of adenylyl cyclase type 9, eLife 9 (2020) e58039.
[138] E. Castrén, M. Kojima, Brain-derived neurotrophic factor in mood disorders and antidepressant treatments, Neurobiology of Disease 97 (2017) 119–126.
[139] M.D. Greicius, B.H. Flores, V. Menon, G.H. Glover, H.B. Solvason, H. Kenna, et al., Resting-state functional connectivity in major depression: abnormally increased contributions from subgenual cingulate cortex and thalamus, Biological Psychiatry 62 (5) (2007) 429–437.
[140] C.G. Connolly, J. Wu, T.C. Ho, F. Hoeft, O. Wolkowitz, S. Eisendrath, et al., Resting-state functional connectivity of subgenual anterior cingulate cortex in depressed adolescents, Biological Psychiatry 74 (12) (2013) 898–907.
[141] J. Gong, J. Wang, S. Qiu, P. Chen, Z. Luo, J. Wang, et al., Common and distinct patterns of intrinsic brain activity alterations in major depression and bipolar disorder: voxel-based meta-analysis, Translational Psychiatry 10 (1) (2020) 353.
[142] C. McCabe, P.J. Cowen, C.J. Harmer, Neural representation of reward in recovered depressed patients, Psychopharmacology 205 (2009) 667–677.
[143] J. Savitz, W.C. Drevets, Bipolar and major depressive disorder: neuroimaging the developmental-degenerative divide, Neuroscience and Biobehavioral Reviews 33 (5) (2009) 699–771.

[144] J.H. Meyer, N. Ginovart, A. Boovariwala, S. Sagrati, D. Hussey, A. Garcia, et al., Elevated monoamine oxidase a levels in the brain: an explanation for the monoamine imbalance of major depression, Archives of General Psychiatry 63 (11) (2006) 1209–1216.
[145] J. Zhao, X.R. Qi, S.F. Gao, J. Lu, D. van Wamelen, W. Kamphuis, et al., Different stress-related gene expression in depression and suicide, Journal of Psychiatric Research 68 (2015) 176–185.
[146] M.O. Klein, D.S. Battagello, A.R. Cardoso, D.N. Hauser, J.C. Bittencourt, R.G. Correa, Dopamine: functions, signaling, and association with neurological diseases, Cellular and Molecular Neurobiology 39 (1) (2019) 31–59.
[147] M. Stoy, F. Schlagenhauf, P. Sterzer, F. Bermpohl, C. Hägele, K. Suchotzki, et al., Hyporeactivity of ventral striatum towards incentive stimuli in unmedicated depressed patients normalizes after treatment with escitalopram, Journal of Psychopharmacology 26 (5) (2012) 677–688.
[148] H. Geugies, R.J. Mocking, C.A. Figueroa, P.F. Groot, J.B.C. Marsman, M.N. Servaas, et al., Impaired reward-related learning signals in remitted unmedicated patients with recurrent depression, Brain 142 (8) (2019) 2510–2522.
[149] Y. Mizuno, A.H. Ashok, B.B. Bhat, S. Jauhar, O.D. Howes, Dopamine in major depressive disorder: a systematic review and meta-analysis of in vivo imaging studies, Journal of Psychopharmacology 37 (11) (2023) 1058–1069.
[150] F. Hieronymus, J. Emilsson, S. Nilsson, E. Eriksson, Consistent superiority of selective serotonin reuptake inhibitors over placebo in reducing depressed mood in patients with major depression, Molecular Psychiatry 21 (4) (2016) 523–530.
[151] J.C. Jakobsen, C. Gluud, I. Kirsch, Should antidepressants be used for major depressive disorder?, BMJ Evidence-Based Medicine 25 (4) (2020) 130.
[152] J. Moncrieff, R.E. Cooper, T. Stockmann, S. Amendola, M.P. Hengartner, M.A. Horowitz, The serotonin theory of depression: a systematic umbrella review of the evidence, Molecular Psychiatry 28 (8) (2023) 3243–3256.
[153] M.J. Mijnster, Y. Galis-de Graaf, P. Voorn, Serotonergic regulation of neuropeptide and glutamic acid decarboxylase mRNA levels in the rat striatum and globus pallidus: studies with fluoxetine and DOI, Molecular Brain Research 54 (1) (1998) 64–73.
[154] S. Izenwasser, Role of serotonin in the regulation of the dynorphinergic system by a κ-opioid agonist and cocaine treatment in rat CNS, Neuroscience 144 (1) (2007) 157–164.
[155] B.P. Guiard, M. El Mansari, Z. Merali, P. Blier, Functional interactions between dopamine, serotonin and norepinephrine neurons: an in-vivo electrophysiological study in rats with monoaminergic lesions, International Journal of Neuropsychopharmacology 11 (5) (2008) 625–639.
[156] J.P. Tassin, Uncoupling between noradrenergic and serotonergic neurons as a molecular basis of stable changes in behavior induced by repeated drugs of abuse, Biochemical Pharmacology 75 (1) (2008) 85–97.
[157] R. Zhang, T. Tachibana, T. Takagi, T. Koutoku, D.M. Denbow, M. Furuse, Serotonin modifies corticotropin-releasing factor-induced behaviors of chicks, Behavioural Brain Research 151 (1–2) (2004) 47–52.
[158] E.I. Flandreau, C.H. Bourke, K.J. Ressler, W.W. Vale, C.B. Nemeroff, M.J. Owens, Escitalopram alters gene expression and HPA axis reactivity in rats following chronic overexpression of corticotropin-releasing factor from the central amygdala, Psychoneuroendocrinology 38 (8) (2013) 1349–1361.
[159] R. Carhart-Harris, D. Nutt, Serotonin and brain function: a tale of two receptors, Journal of Psychopharmacology 31 (9) (2017) 1091–1120.
[160] T. Babic, A. Troy, S. Fortna, K. Browning, Glucose-dependent trafficking of 5-HT3 receptors in rat gastrointestinal vagal afferent neurons, Neurogastroenterology and Motility 24 (10) (2012) e476–e488.
[161] I.P. Voronova, 5-HT receptors and temperature homeostasis, Biomolecules 11 (12) (2021) 1914.

[162] J.M. Yabut, J.D. Crane, A.E. Green, D.J. Keating, W.I. Khan, G.R. Steinberg, Emerging roles for serotonin in regulating metabolism: new implications for an ancient molecule, Endocrine Reviews 40 (4) (2019) 1092–1107.
[163] E.D. Paul, C.A. Lowry, Functional topography of serotonergic systems supports the Deakin/Graeff hypothesis of anxiety and affective disorders, Journal of Psychopharmacology 27 (12) (2013) 1090–1106.
[164] B. Kivell, Z. Uzelac, S. Sundaramurthy, J. Rajamanickam, A. Ewald, V. Chefer, et al., Salvinorin A regulates dopamine transporter function via a kappa opioid receptor and ERK1/2-dependent mechanism, Neuropharmacology 86 (2014) 228–240.
[165] R.J. McQuaid, O.A. McInnis, A. Abizaid, H. Anisman, Making room for oxytocin in understanding depression, Neuroscience and Biobehavioral Reviews 45 (2014) 305–322.
[166] L. Van Londen, J.G. Goekoop, G.M. Van Kempen, A.C. Frankhuijzen-Sierevogel, V.M. Wiegant, E.A. van der Velde, et al., Plasma levels of arginine vasopressin elevated in patients with major depression, Neuropsychopharmacology 17 (4) (1997) 284–292.
[167] A.H. Miller, V. Maletic, C.L. Raison, Inflammation and its discontents: the role of cytokines in the pathophysiology of major depression, Biological Psychiatry 65 (9) (2009) 732–741.
[168] H. Alawie, J.C. Hu, A. McLeod, What are the recurring theories regarding the pathogenesis of major depressive disorder?, Undergraduate Research in Natural and Clinical Science and Technology Journal 5 (2021) 1–8.
[169] D.A. Padgett, R. Glaser, How stress influences the immune response, Trends in Immunology 24 (8) (2003) 444–448.
[170] S. Gein, Dynorphins in Regulation of Immune System Functions, vol. 79, Biochemistry, Moscow, 2014, pp. 397–405.
[171] V.G. Masdrakis, M. Markianos, D.S. Baldwin, Apathy associated with antidepressant drugs: a systematic review, Acta Neuropsychiatrica 35 (4) (2023) 189–204.
[172] N.A. Buckley, A.H. Dawson, G.K. Isbister, Serotonin syndrome, BMJ. British Medical Journal 348 (2014) g1626.
[173] P. Blier, G. Pineyro, M. El Mansari, R. Bergeron, Montigny Cd, Role of somatodendritic 5-HT autoreceptors in modulating 5-HT neurotransmission, Annals of the New York Academy of Sciences 861 (1) (1998) 204–216.
[174] J. Forsman, T. Masterman, J. Ahlner, G. Isacsson, A.K. Hedström, Selective serotonin reuptake inhibitors and the risk of violent suicide: a nationwide postmortem study, European Journal of Clinical Pharmacology 75 (2019) 393–400.
[175] E. Sanders-Bush, M. Breeding, K. Knoth, M. Tsutsumi, Sertraline-induced desensitization of the serotonin 5HT-2 receptor transmembrane signaling system, Psychopharmacology 99 (1989) 64–69.
[176] M.P. Hengartner, J. Angst, W. Rössler, Antidepressant use prospectively relates to a poorer long-term outcome of depression: results from a prospective community cohort study over 30 years, Psychotherapy and Psychosomatics 87 (3) (2018) 181–183.
[177] G.A. Fava, May antidepressant drugs worsen the conditions they are supposed to treat? The clinical foundations of the oppositional model of tolerance, Therapeutic Advances in Psychopharmacology 10 (2020) 2045125320970325.
[178] E.M. Unterwald, Upregulating G protein-coupled receptors with receptor antagonists, Methods for the Discovery and Characterization of G Protein-Coupled Receptors (2011) 403–419.
[179] I. Grande, M. Berk, B. Birmaher, E. Vieta, Bipolar disorder, The Lancet 387 (10027) (2016) 1561–1572.
[180] J. Forn, F. Valdecasas, Effects of lithium on brain adenyl cyclase activity, Biochemical Pharmacology 20 (10) (1971) 2773–2779.
[181] C.B. Nemeroff, B. Kinkead, J. Goldstein, Quetiapine: preclinical studies, pharmacokinetics, drug interactions, and dosing, The Journal of Clinical Psychiatry 63 (13) (2002) 5–11.
[182] A. Bahji, L. Mesbah-Oskui, Comparative efficacy and safety of stimulant-type medications for depression: a systematic review and network meta-analysis, Journal of Affective Disorders 292 (2021) 416–423.

Chapter 5

A CRH-HCN theory of obsessive-compulsive disorder (OCD)

5.1 Theory

I present a **CRH-HCN theory of obsessive-compulsive disorder (OCD) (T*OCD).** T*OCD is the first complete theory of OCD, explaining its etiology, symptoms, pathophysiology, and treatment.

The core cause of OCD is chronically increased release of corticotropin-releasing hormone (CRH), coupled with chronic activation of hyperpolarization-activated cyclic nucleotide-gated (HCN) channels. HCN channels explain the mechanisms behind OCD symptoms, while CRH excites HCN channels and also explains the association with stress.

CRH is the major brain agent released following deviations from homeostasis (i.e., stress), conveying the need for restoration responses. It acts on two receptors, CRH1 and CRH2, with higher affinity for CRH1. Both receptors are G protein-coupled receptors that mainly bind Gs to induce cAMP, but also Gi/o and Gq.

Strong or chronic stress during sensitive developmental periods can induce persistent alterations to the stress response system. Such alterations commonly involve chronically increased release of stress-related agents, and can be heritable (e.g., via epigenetics).

According to T*OCD, **OCD occurs when chronically released CRH induces excessive activation of CRH1 and possibly CRH2**. This yields excessive cAMP, which induces chronic HCN channel activity as explained below. Alternatively, OCD can occur due to **CRH-independent chronic activation of HCN channels**.

HCN channels are activated by small hyperpolarization and inactivated by small polarization. They are permeable to Na^{+} and K^{+}, and when open yield an excitatory current (Ih) that increases polarization close to the action potential threshold. Thus, their opening facilitates **intrinsic slow cellular oscillations**. HCN channels are crucial to heart rhythmic activity, and are strongly expressed in the brain, including in stress-related areas, cortical response neurons (layer 5 pyramidal neurons that project outside of cortex), the basal ganglia (BG), and the thalamus.

The Science of the Brain. https://doi.org/10.1016/B978-0-44-345008-2.00011-4

cAMP is a major stimulator of HCN channel opening. Thus, chronic CRH signaling induces chronic activation of HCN channels, which promotes repeated neural firing in stress-related areas (i.e., areas with CRHR expression).

Activation of CRH1 by CRH normally leads to its endocytosis and desensitization. However, in the presence of chronic CRH, this does not prevent chronic cAMP synthesis, because (i) if CRH does not bind CRH1, it accumulates and binds the lower affinity CRH2, which also stimulates cAMP, (ii) endocytosed CRH1 and CRH2 continue producing cAMP via lysosomes, and (iii) chronic CRH activates CRH1 receptors again when they are retransported to the plasma membrane.

According to T*OCD, **the obsessions exhibited by OCD patients are due to chronic neural firing driven by cAMP and HCNs**. Due to the increased push for HCN activation, it is very difficult for the brain to suppress repeated activations in paths that express CRHR-HCN. Thus, stress-related thoughts and actions are continuously reactivated without control.

OCD is strongly associated with a phenomenon called **'not just right'**, a feeling of **incompleteness** commonly manifesting as confirmation questions. This phenomenon results from the same chronic CRH-HCN process that drives obsessions. The need to answer a question/challenge (even simple questions), which is normally conveyed by CRH, continues reverberating due to HCN-induced oscillations, even after a response has been reached. **This also explains continuous rechecking behavior in OCD**.

Many OCD patients exhibit **strong binary views** and **rigid personality**. These occur because response neurons are sometimes not re-activated, making the person very confident in these responses (since patients are used to uncertainty). A lack of re-activation often results from inputs from valence areas (e.g., the amygdala), which provide strong excitation of cortical response neurons, especially to frontal layer 2 pyramidal cells, which are also the ones where CRH-HCN expression is highest. **This explains why the rigid personality in OCD is often related to moral issues**.

OCD **compulsions** are a form of self-treatment in which patients voluntarily activate neurons. They do this because **neural activation induces moderate Ca^{2+} influx, which temporarily inhibits cAMP and relieves obsessions and the feeling of uncertainty**. With repeated execution, compulsions get desensitized, gradually losing their ability to stimulate Ca^{2+} influx and prompting patients to increase compulsion complexity and/or number of repeats.

OCD behaviors related to **cleanliness** (e.g., hand washing) are very common. This occurs due to two reasons. First, CRH activates mast cells, and induces the release of histamine (both directly and via mast cells). Mast cells are innate immune cells activated by various pathogens. Histamine induces a feeling of itch, and a large variety of agents released by mast cells report the presence of pathogens and/or inflammation to the brain. Second, CRH yields ACTH release in skin. This can induce the production of beta-endorphin, which is known to induce itch via mu-opioid receptors. **The chronic CRH in OCD yields chronic**

activation of circuits conveying skin-related pathogen threats, and an uncomfortable feeling. Hand-washing can temporarily relieve the problem as in other compulsions, and via the activation and desensitization of TRPV1 channels.

A similar account also explains **trichotillomania** and **excoriation**, OCD sub-types that involve hair pulling and skin picking, respectively, and nail picking in OCD. CRH1, mast cells and histamine are involved in hair growth. **Hoarding** is another OCD subtype. It is explained by the feeling of incompleteness applied to object use ('Am I finished with this object?' 'I'm not sure. I may need it in the future, so I won't throw it away').

From the patient perspective, OCD behavior is a rational response to the inputs that their brain receives. The problem in OCD is that these inputs are not connected to the real state of the organism, but result from erroneous release of a molecule. However, patients experience such inputs exactly as they experience real ones. This explains the (small) subset of patients who do not show **'insight'** as to their symptoms.

Beyond the biological logic related to the known effects of CRH and HCN channels, there is **empirical evidence** supporting T*OCD. CRH1 recruits the sympathetic nervous system (SNS) and the hypothalamus-pituitary-adrenal (HPA) stress axis (resulting in the release of the human glucocorticoid, cortisol). OCD patients show increased CRH, ACTH, and cortisol (indicating chronic CRH), reduced sensitivity to CRH challenge (showing chronic release), reduced cortisol-induced negative feedback (which is partly done via CRH1), reduced prepulse inhibition of the startle reflex (indicating primed CRH), and chronically higher activity in brain areas expressing HCN ('CSTC loops'). In addition, OCD is associated with genetic mutations in HCN and PDE (cAMP suppressor) genes, with increased allergies (indicating mast cell, histamine), and with trauma (supporting stress-related etiology). There is no contradictory evidence.

OCD patients have **trouble falling asleep**. This provides additional evidence for T*OCD, since CRH1 stimulates the SNS and cortical norepinephrine (NEP), both of which oppose sleep.

T*OCD is also supported by known OCD comorbidities. There is high comorbidity with **anxiety**, which is known to be linked to CRH.

OCD shows high comorbidity with **panic disorder**. T*OCD explains this by noting that the enhanced HCN channel and SNS activity in OCD are expected to increase the likelihood of panic attacks, due to their effects on the heart.

Supporting SNS dysregulation, OCD patients show higher rates of **cardiovascular disease**.

Traumatic brain injury (TBI) can induce a variety of psychiatric conditions, including OCD. TBI increases CRH and affects HCN channels.

In summary, OCD involves both stress (CRH) and HCN channels. Most of the features that are unique to OCD stem from chronically active HCN channels rather than directly from CRH, but in many or most cases, chronic CRH is what produces the excessive cAMP that drives HCN channels.

5.2 Treatment

Cognitive behavioral therapy (CBT) is helpful in OCD, especially when combined with medication treatment. CBT teaches patients to reduce the attention given to OCD paths, thereby reducing their excitability and enhancing non-OCD paths.

The best drug treatment for OCD would be to **reduce CRH release**. Unfortunately, at present there is no selective drug that directly has this effect.

Selective serotonin reuptake inhibitors (SSRIs) increase brain serotonin (SER) levels. In high doses, SER opposes the low CRH mode and CRH1 signaling. Moreover, SER reduces HCN currents via PKC. Thus, SSRIs can significantly help OCD. However, in lower doses, SER cooperates with the high CRH mode and CRH2 signaling. Thus, SSRIs only help when provided at the right doses (especially when coupled with antagonists of the CRH2-related SER2 receptors, such as atypical antipsychotics). In practice, this only works in a subset of patients, because it is very difficult to continuously calibrate the doses required, and because the effect of SSRIs is non-selective and indirect.

Alpha2 adrenergic (NEPa2) receptor agonists cross the blood-brain barrier and oppose brain HCN channel activation, and hence might be beneficial in OCD. **NEPa2 agonists such as guanfacine and clonidine** are routinely used to treat ADHD, a disorder with substantial comorbidity with OCD. There are some indications from a small number of case reports that these drugs are helpful in OCD. **Usage of these drugs to treat OCD, alone or with SSRIs, should be seriously explored.**

Guanfacine is preferable over clonidine, because it is more selective to the NEPa2a subtype, which has a higher expression in stress-related areas such as the prefrontal cortex, amygdala, hypothalamus, and locus coeruleus.

When used for ADHD, NEPa2 agonists commonly induce sleepiness and sedation due to suppression of NEP (and possibly epinephrine (EPI)) release. **In OCD, reducing NEP and EPI may actually be desirable**, because the chronic CRH problem in OCD induces chronic NEP and EPI release (see above).

SSRIs and guanfacine can be used alone or in combination. **For patients with minimal anxiety symptoms (i.e., with relatively 'pure' OCD symptoms), guanfacine may suffice**, due to its direct suppression of HCN channels. SSRIs may be essential for addressing patients with higher anxiety symptoms.

In summary, I believe that guanfacine can provide substantial help to OCD patients, and that it might be better than SSRIs for a large subset. Guanfacine is approved for treating ADHD, and since there is some symptom overlap between OCD and ADHD, physicians are allowed to start treating OCD patients with guanfacine.

5.3 Key references

General OCD background. OCD symptoms, epidemiology, pathology and treatment have been the subject of several large reviews [1,2]. A 'not just right' feeling and confirmation questions have been increasingly recognized to be core to the disorder, with components that are not directly explained by stress. Area-wise, OCD involves areas beyond the classical ones of orbital frontal cortex, cortico-striatal-thalamo-cortical loops, ACC, and amygdala (note that these are valence/stress areas) [3].

General HCN channels & cAMP background. HCNs have been extensively reviewed [4,5]. At rest, they counter both hyperpolarization and depolarization, and dampen amplitude and duration of EPSPs and IPSPs. They promote non-burst oscillations (heart, thalamus). Crucially, they can be activated with cAMP, which facilitates their activation by shifting activation voltage to more positive values [5]. Both CRH receptors dramatically increase cAMP [6]. The HCN current Ih increases neural excitability [7].

HCNs are expressed in PFC dendritic spines, colocated with the a2a-adrenergic receptor (NEPa2a) [8]. NEPa2a closes HCN channels and suppresses cAMP [8], which will be important for our proposal of guanfacine treatment. In the ventral tegmental area, NEPa2 agonists (possibly NEPa2c) decrease HCN currents and slow their activation rate [9].

CRH can induce OCD symptoms. OCD is associated with the propensity to move (a large part of the compulsions are physical). CRH induces defensive burying, grooming, mounting, and locomotion. Increased CRH1 yields non-coping and aggression [10]. A thorough review summarized how CRH increases locomotion [11]. CRH increases self-biting and grooming, (self licking and scratching) much higher in novelty (i.e., under stress) [12].

Early life stress (sexual abuse and harsh punishment in early life) are associated with more OCD symptoms in adults [13]. Adult nonhuman primates exposed to early life stress show persistent CSF CRH [14].

There is a very large literature on CRH and early life stress that I assume is well-known and does not need to be cited here.

CRH in OCD. OCD symptoms worsen following childbirth in most women w OCD, and in almost half of men. This we explain by the fact that CRH dramatically rises just before childbirth in women [15]. A genetic association has been found in OCD with the CRH2 receptor (as well as with some others) [16].

There is a large body of evidence showing dysregulation of the hypothalamus-pituitary-adrenal (HPA) axis in OCD, which can be explained via chronically increased CRH release that triggers increased cortisol, followed by increased negative feedback on CRH, optionally now followed by decreased cortisol [17–25].

HCN channels in OCD and stress. Chronic social defeat increases VTA DA spontaneous firing rates, bursts, Ih (in resilient animals too), and avoidance behavior. This behavior can be reversed by Ih inhibitors [26]. HCN inhibitors induced ketamine-like rapid and sustained antidepressant effect in a chronic social defeat stress model [27].

Panic disorder is very common in OCD [28]. Note that panic disorder involves repeated heart beats that are driven by heart HCN channels. In the same direction, OCD involves increased risk of metabolic and cardiovascular disease in a large Sweden cohort [29].

Interoceptive heart inputs reach the insula. Supporting overactivity of HCN channels, OCD involves increased insula activity to unpleasant but also pleasant odors. This is correlated with disgust sensitivity and symptoms [30].

Three HCN4 SNPs are associated with OCD and depression [31]. A PDE4D (cAMP suppressor) SNP is associated with female late-onset (>18y) OCD [32].

CRH, OCD, and allergy. OCD patients show very high (>50%) allergy disorders [33,34], and there is high incidence of OCD among people with systemic autoimmune diseases [35]. Importantly, the skin expresses the full HPA axis, including CRH and cortisol [36], and skin-related CRH promotes stress-enhanced nasal allergy and mast cell proliferation [37]. Mast cells are central in conveying the feeling of itch to the brain [38].

In one report, a 1st generation anti-histamine (diphenhydramine (benadryl)) unexpectedly helped OCD (it was used as control in another experiment) [39].

Traumatic brain injury (TBI). TBI can induce OCD, depression, anxeity, panic, and PTSD [40,41]. The parsimonious account of how this happens is that it induces a large stress response involving CRH and HCN. Indeed, blast-induced mild TBI increases anxiety and spontaneous firing frequency of CRH neurons in the paraventricular hypothalamus [42]. Moreover, TBI is specifically known to drive HCN channels [7], and CRH1 mediates stress-induced high-frequency oscillations in TBI [43].

Guanfacine and clonidine. Guanfacine is a NEPa2a agonist, and clonidine is a general NEPa2 agonist. Clonidine rapidly decreased compulsions in one woman [44], and significantly decreased symptoms in others [45]. More recently, clonidine rapidly and significantly improved OCD following SSRI sertraline failure in a 16yo female [46]. Clonidine augmentation to SSRIs or clomipramine significantly helped vs. baseline, but with only a trend vs. placebo, in an RCT with $n = 57$ [47].

8 weeks guanfacine significantly decreased repetitive behavior (CYBOCS-ASD) in autistic patients with ADHD [48]. There is also a negative result [39].

OCD patients showed a blunted growth hormone response to clonidine, with higher basal plasma NEP and MHPG. This was interpreted as increased presynaptic NEP with decreased receptor responsiveness, according with desensitization of NEP (the SNS) [49]. We add that this can be due to chronic CRH.

Not specific to OCD, chronic guanfacine protects rodent PLmPFC L2/3 pyramidal dendritic spines and working memory from chronic stress [50]. Guanfacine extended release helped symptoms related to traumatic stress [51].

Guanfacine has been used to treat TBI-induced cognitive deficits [52], including working memory [53].

An additional possible treatment direction is via **retigabine**. This opener of potassium channel Kv7 decreased the long term effect of repetitive blast TBI [54].

SSRI. SSRIs decrease hippocampus CRH and increase weight gain [55]. High dose SSRI is safe for treating OCD, but with side effects including sexual dysfunction, weight gain, sedation, sweating, and tremor [56]. Thus, SSRIs help some patients oppose the stress driving the disorder. There is even one report in which fluoxetine downregulated HCN2 in the hippocampus (but not the prefrontal cortex, where OCD matters) [57]. Nonetheless, due to the side effects, the lack of efficacy on about 50% of patients, and the highly indirect action on the core OCD problem (HCNs), there is strong motivation to search for other drugs.

References

[1] J. Zohar, Obsessive Compulsive Disorder: Current Science and Clinical Practice, Wiley, 2012.

[2] H. Szechtman, B.H. Harvey, E.Z. Woody, K.L. Hoffman, The psychopharmacology of obsessive-compulsive disorder: a preclinical roadmap, Pharmacological Reviews 72 (1) (2020) 80–151.

[3] M.R. Milad, S.L. Rauch, Obsessive-compulsive disorder: beyond segregated cortico-striatal pathways, Trends in Cognitive Sciences 16 (1) (2012) 43–51.

[4] C. He, F. Chen, B. Li, Z. Hu, Neurophysiology of HCN channels: from cellular functions to multiple regulations, Progress in Neurobiology 112 (2014) 1–23.

[5] E.E. Benarroch, HCN channels: function and clinical implications, Neurology 80 (3) (2013) 304–310.

[6] C. Inda, N.G. Armando, P.A. dos Santos Claro, S. Silberstein, Endocrinology and the brain: corticotropin-releasing hormone signaling, Endocrine Connections 6 (6) (2017) R99–R120.

[7] P. Deng, Z.C. Xu, Contribution of Ih to neuronal damage in the hippocampus after traumatic brain injury in rats, Journal of Neurotrauma 28 (7) (2011) 1173–1183.

[8] M. Wang, B.P. Ramos, C.D. Paspalas, Y. Shu, A. Simen, A. Duque, et al., α2A-adrenoceptors strengthen working memory networks by inhibiting cAMP-HCN channel signaling in prefrontal cortex, Cell 129 (2) (2007) 397–410.

[9] Alpha-2 noradrenergic receptor activation inhibits the hyperpolarization-activated cation current (Ih) in neurons of the ventral tegmental area, Neuroscience 167 (2) (2010) 287–297.

[10] E. Fekete, Subtype-selective corticotropin-releasing factor receptor agonists exert contrasting, but not opposite, effects on anxiety-related behavior in rats, The Journal of Pharmacology and Experimental Therapeutics 323 (3) (2007) 846–854.

[11] C.A. Lowry, F.L. Moore, Regulation of behavioral responses by corticotropin-releasing factor, General and Comparative Endocrinology 146 (1) (2006) 19–27.

[12] J.E. Sherman, N.H. Kalin, ICV-CRH potently affects behavior without altering antinociceptive responding, Life Sciences 39 (5) (1986) 433–441.

[13] M. Król, Y. Cao, E. Kirkham, Sexual abuse and harsh punishment in early life are associated with more obsessive-compulsive symptoms in adulthood: An online survey, medRxiv (2022) 2022-11.

[14] J. Coplan, M. Andrews, L. Rosenblum, M. Owens, S. Friedman, J. Gorman, et al., Persistent elevations of cerebrospinal fluid concentrations of corticotropin-releasing factor in adult nonhuman primates exposed to early-life stressors: implications for the pathophysiology of mood and anxiety disorders, Proceedings of the National Academy of Sciences 93 (4) (1996) 1619–1623.

[15] J.C. Ramirez, V.L. Buissonnière-Ariza, E. McIngvale, K.A. Rufino, L.J. Puryear, C.A. Treece, et al., Perceived worsening of obsessive-compulsive disorder symptoms after childbirth in women and men: an understudied phenomenon, Bulletin of the Menninger Clinic 88 (1) (2024) 48–60.
[16] X. Wang, P. Zhou, S. Buggs, S. Teng, Genetic biomarker selection for obsessive-compulsive disorder by sparse representation based variable selection method, Journal of Psychiatry and Brain Science 1 (4) (2016).
[17] E.K. Malisiova, I. Mourikis, T. Chalimourdas, N. Nianiakas, M. Michou, A. Mantzou, et al., Low hair cortisol concentrations in obsessive compulsive disorder: a cross-sectional study, Journal of Psychiatric Research 131 (2020) 187–193.
[18] F. Catapano, P. Monteleone, M. Maj, D. Kemali, Dexamethasone suppression test in patients with primary obsessive-compulsive disorder and in healthy controls, Neuropsychobiology 23 (2) (1990) 53–56.
[19] J.A. Cottraux, M. Bouvard, B. Claustrat, C. Juenet, Abnormal dexamethasone suppression test in primary obsessive-compulsive patients: a confirmatory report, Psychiatry Research 13 (2) (1984) 157–165.
[20] F. Catapano, P. Monteleone, A. Fuschino, M. Maj, D. Kemali, Melatonin and cortisol secretion in patients with primary obsessive-compulsive disorder, Psychiatry Research 44 (3) (1992) 217–225.
[21] J. Sousa-Lima, P.S. Moreira, C. Raposo-Lima, N. Sousa, P. Morgado, Relationship between obsessive compulsive disorder and cortisol: systematic review and meta-analysis, European Neuropsychopharmacology 29 (11) (2019) 1185–1198.
[22] M. Altemus, T. Pigott, K.T. Kalogeras, M. Demitrack, B. Dubbert, D.L. Murphy, et al., Abnormalities in the regulation of vasopressin and corticotropin releasing factor secretion in obsessive-compulsive disorder, Archives of General Psychiatry 49 (1) (1992) 9–20.
[23] A. Bilgiç, M. Sertdemir, İ Kılınç, ÖF. Akça, Increased serum brain-derived neurotrophic factor and adrenocorticotropic hormone levels are associated with obsessive compulsive disorder in medication-free children, European Child & Adolescent Psychiatry (2022) 1–11.
[24] D. Bailly, D. Servant, D. Dewailly, R. Beuscart, A. Racadot, P. Fossati, et al., Corticotropin releasing factor stimulation test in obsessive compulsive disorder, Biological Psychiatry 35 (2) (1994) 143–146.
[25] M. Kluge, P. Schüssler, H.E. Künzel, M. Dresler, A. Yassouridis, A. Steiger, Increased nocturnal secretion of ACTH and cortisol in obsessive compulsive disorder, Journal of Psychiatric Research 41 (11) (2007) 928–933.
[26] J.L. Cao, H.E. Covington, A.K. Friedman, M.B. Wilkinson, J.J. Walsh, D.C. Cooper, et al., Mesolimbic dopamine neurons in the brain reward circuit mediate susceptibility to social defeat and antidepressant action, The Journal of Neuroscience 30 (49) (2010) 16453–16458.
[27] M. Cai, Y. Zhu, M.R. Shanley, C. Morel, S.M. Ku, H. Zhang, et al., HCN channel inhibitor induces ketamine-like rapid and sustained antidepressant effects in chronic social defeat stress model, Neurobiology of Stress 26 (2023) 100565.
[28] A.R. Torres, Y.A. Ferrão, R.G. Shavitt, J.B. Diniz, D.L. Costa, M.C. Do Rosário, et al., Panic disorder and agoraphobia in OCD patients: clinical profile and possible treatment implications, Comprehensive Psychiatry 55 (3) (2014) 588–597.
[29] K. Isomura, G. Brander, Z. Chang, R. Kuja-Halkola, C. Rück, C. Hellner, et al., Metabolic and cardiovascular complications in obsessive-compulsive disorder: a total population sibling comparison study with long-term follow-up, Biological Psychiatry 84 (5) (2018) 324–331.
[30] H.A. Berlin, E.R. Stern, J. Ng, S. Zhang, D. Rosenthal, R. Turetzky, et al., Altered olfactory processing and increased insula activity in patients with obsessive-compulsive disorder: an fMRI study, Psychiatry Research. Neuroimaging 262 (2017) 15–24.
[31] B. Kelmendi, M. Holsbach-Beltrame, A.M. McIntosh, L. Hilt, E.D. George, R.R. Kitchen, et al., Association of polymorphisms in HCN4 with mood disorders and obsessive compulsive disorder, Neuroscience Letters 496 (3) (2011) 195–199.

[32] X. Huang, J. Zhang, J. Liu, X. Zhang, Association study of the PDE4D gene and obsessive-compulsive disorder in a Chinese Han population, Psychiatric Genetics 29 (6) (2019) 226–231.
[33] M. Yuce, S. Guner, K. Karabekiroglu, S. Baykal, M. Kilic, R. Sancak, et al., Association of Tourette syndrome and obsessive-compulsive disorder with allergic diseases in children and adolescents: a preliminary study, European Review for Medical and Pharmacological Sciences 18 (3) (2014).
[34] C. Westwell-Roper, K.A. Williams, J. Samuels, O.J. Bienvenu, B. Cullen, F.S. Goes, et al., Immune-related comorbidities in childhood-onset obsessive compulsive disorder: lifetime prevalence in the obsessive compulsive disorder collaborative genetics association study, Journal of Child and Adolescent Psychopharmacology 29 (8) (2019) 615–624.
[35] L.Y. Wang, S.F. Chen, J.H. Chiang, C.Y. Hsu, Y.C. Shen, Systemic autoimmune diseases are associated with an increased risk of obsessive–compulsive disorder: a nationwide population-based cohort study, Social Psychiatry and Psychiatric Epidemiology 54 (2019) 507–516.
[36] A.T. Slominski, M.A. Zmijewski, B. Zbytek, D.J. Tobin, T.C. Theoharides, J. Rivier, Key role of CRF in the skin stress response system, Endocrine Reviews 34 (6) (2013) 827–884.
[37] M. Yamanaka-Takaichi, Y. Mizukami, K. Sugawara, K. Sunami, Y. Teranishi, Y. Kira, et al., Stress and nasal allergy: corticotropin-releasing hormone stimulates mast cell degranulation and proliferation in human nasal mucosa, International Journal of Molecular Sciences 22 (5) (2021) 2773.
[38] F. Wang, A.M. Trier, F. Li, S. Kim, Z. Chen, J.N. Chai, et al., A basophil-neuronal axis promotes itch, Cell 184 (2) (2021) 422–440.
[39] W. Hewlett, S. Vinogradov, W. Agras, Clomipramine, clonazepam, and clonidine treatment of obsessive-compulsive disorder, Journal of Clinical Psychopharmacology 12 (6) (1992) 420–430.
[40] M.A. Grados, Obsessive-compulsive disorder after traumatic brain injury, International Review of Psychiatry 15 (4) (2003) 350–358.
[41] L.M. Li, A. Carson, K. Dams-O'Connor, Psychiatric sequelae of traumatic brain injury-future directions in research, Nature Reviews Neurology 19 (9) (2023) 556–571.
[42] S. Simmons, L.D. Langlois, M.G. Oyola, S. Gouty, T.J. Wu, F.S. Nugent, Blast-induced mild traumatic brain injury alterations of corticotropin-releasing factor neuronal activity in the mouse hypothalamic paraventricular nucleus, Frontiers in Synaptic Neuroscience 13 (2022) 804898.
[43] C. Narla, P.S. Jung, F.B. Cruz, M. Everest, J. Martinez-Trujillo, M.O. Poulter, CRF mediates stress-induced pathophysiological high-frequency oscillations in traumatic brain injury, eNeuro 6 (2) (2019).
[44] J.W. Knesevich, Successful treatment of obsessive-compulsive disorder with clonidine hydrochloride, The American Journal of Psychiatry 139 (1982) 364.
[45] E. Hollander, C. DeCaria, A. Nitescu, T. Cooper, B. Stover, R. Gully, et al., Noradrenergic function in obsessive-compulsive disorder: behavioral and neuroendocrine responses to clonidine and comparison to healthy controls, Psychiatry Research 37 (2) (1991) 161–177.
[46] A. Sarangi, D. Payberah, T. McMahon, The use of clonidine in the treatment of debilitating obsessive-compulsive behaviors comorbid with depression and post-traumatic stress disorder: a case report, Cureus 13 (5) (2021).
[47] S. Akouchakian, M.J. Tarrahi, E. Mohebati, Evaluation of clonidine augmentation therapy for obsessive-compulsive disorder treatment, a randomized clinical trial, Iranian Journal of Psychiatry and Behavioral Sciences 15 (3) (2021).
[48] L.C. Politte, L. Scahill, J. Figueroa, J.T. McCracken, B. King, C.J. McDougle, A randomized, placebo-controlled trial of extended-release guanfacine in children with autism spectrum disorder and ADHD symptoms: an analysis of secondary outcome measures, Neuropsychopharmacology 43 (8) (2018) 1772–1778.
[49] L.J. Siever, T.R. Insel, D.C. Jimerson, C.R. Lake, T.W. Uhde, J. Aloi, et al., Growth hormone response to clonidine in obsessive-compulsive patients, The British Journal of Psychiatry 142 (2) (1983) 184–187.

[50] A.B. Hains, Y. Yabe, A.F. Arnsten, Chronic stimulation of alpha-2A-adrenoceptors with guanfacine protects rodent prefrontal cortex dendritic spines and cognition from the effects of chronic stress, Neurobiology of Stress 2 (2015) 1–9.
[51] D.F. Connor, D.J. Grasso, M.D. Slivinsky, G.S. Pearson, A. Banga, An open-label study of guanfacine extended release for traumatic stress related symptoms in children and adolescents, Journal of Child and Adolescent Psychopharmacology 23 (4) (2013) 244–251.
[52] S. Khasnavis, T. Belliveau, A. Arnsten, A. Fesharaki-Zadeh, Combined use of guanfacine and N-acetylcysteine for the treatment of cognitive deficits after traumatic brain injury, Neurotrauma Reports 5 (1) (2024) 226–231.
[53] T.W. McAllister, B.C. McDonald, L.A. Flashman, R.B. Ferrell, T.D. Tosteson, N.N. Yanofsky, et al., Alpha-2 adrenergic challenge with guanfacine one month after mild traumatic brain injury: altered working memory and BOLD response, International Journal of Psychophysiology 82 (1) (2011) 107–114.
[54] F.A. Vigil, H. Belchior, V. Bugay, I.I. Bazaldua, A. Stoja, D.C. Dantas, et al., Acute treatment with the M-channel (Kv7 KCNQ) opener retigabine reduces the long-term effects of repetitive blast traumatic brain injuries, Neurotherapeutics 20 (3) (2023) 853–869.
[55] E.I. Flandreau, C.H. Bourke, K.J. Ressler, W.W. Vale, C.B. Nemeroff, M.J. Owens, Escitalopram alters gene expression and HPA axis reactivity in rats following chronic overexpression of corticotropin-releasing factor from the central amygdala, Psychoneuroendocrinology 38 (8) (2013) 1349–1361.
[56] D.M. Levy, O.B. Arush, L. Carmi, A.J. Wetzler, J. Zohar, Off-label higher doses of serotonin reuptake inhibitors in the treatment of obsessive-compulsive disorder: safety and tolerability, Comprehensive Psychiatry 133 (2024) 152486.
[57] P. Luo, X. Zhang, Y. Lu, C. Chen, C. Li, M. Zhou, et al., Fluoxetine ameliorates cognitive impairments induced by chronic cerebral hypoperfusion via down-regulation of HCN2 surface expression in the hippocampal CA1 area in rats, Pharmacology, Biochemistry and Behavior 140 (2016) 1–7.

Chapter 6

A KATP channel theory of attention-deficit hyperactivity disorder

6.1 Theory

I present a **KATP channel theory of ADHD (K*ADHD)**. K*ADHD is the first complete theory of ADHD, explaining its etiology, symptoms, pathophysiology, and treatment. The theory is strongly supported by the evidence, and points to **a novel, immediately available, and inexpensive optimal treatment, by a non-stimulant drug**.

According to K*ADHD, **the core cause of ADHD is chronic activation of ATP-inactivated potassium channels (KATPCs)**.

KATPCs are inwardly-rectifying channels, and their chronic opening increases intracellular potassium. High K^+ directly excites the cell, and opposes the activation of the membrane sodium-potassium pump (Na^+/K^+-ATPase), leading to high intracellular sodium as well. The end result is chronic intrinsic cellular hyperexcitability. Thus, **cells tend to spontaneously fire without reason.**

KATPCs are comprised of pore opening Kir6.1 or Kir6.2 subunits, and regulatory SUR1, SUR2A or SUR2B subunits. **The combination most relevant to ADHD is Kir6.2/SUR1**, which is the one expressed in fast twitch skeletal muscle, hypothalamic glucose sensing neurons, pancreas beta cells, adrenal epinephrine (EPI) and norepinephrine (NEP) neurons, heart atria, and various brain areas. The main culprit in ADHD is SUR1, which controls channel opening.

High spontaneous firing directly explains the ADHD symptoms. **In the motor system, it manifests as hyperactivity. In cognition circuits, it manifests as inattention** (a lack of ability to sustain attention, reduced concentration), since any neural activation outside the attended paths can interfere with attention. In both types of circuits, spontaneous activation can manifest as **impulsivity**.

There could be several reasons behind the KATP impairment. A common case is high glucose levels experienced during sensitive developmental periods, by patients or their ancestors. This can lead to persistent protein expression changes to maintain such levels, and these changes **can be heritable (e.g., via epigenetics)**. The relevant mechanisms are explained right below.

The Science of the Brain. https://doi.org/10.1016/B978-0-44-345008-2.00012-6

The brain manages hypoglycemia (hypog) via **counterregulatory responses (CRRs)**. After reduced glucose levels suppress insulin secretion, CRRs include the release of pancreas glucagon, adrenal EPI, cortisol (the human glucocorticoid), and NEP, and pituitary growth hormone (GRH), which increase liver glycogenolysis and gluconeogenesis (GNG) and adipose tissue lipolyis (to produce raw materials for GNG). **CRRs (mostly their EPI part) desensitize** very quickly following repeated activation.

KATP channels are activated by ATP deficiency, and as such are **hypog sensors**. Their opening is a major mechanism participating in the activation and execution of CRRs.

High glucose levels during sensitive periods stimulate adaptation to a high glucose state. When this happens, the brain attempts to maintain glucose levels that are higher than normal (i.e., glucose thresholds that trigger CRRs are higher). Faster opening of KATPCs is one way of elevating CRR thresholds. Thus, adaptation to higher glucose levels can result in faster opening of KATPCs. **This is why high glucose during sensitive periods (pre- or postnatal) is associated with ADHD**.

When CRR thresholds are higher, CRRs are activated more frequently than normal, which can lead to their desensitization. With desensitized CRRs, there is nothing that counters hypog, so **the person is more likely to experience a hypog episode**. Hypog causes ATP deficiency, impairing the activity of the plasma membrane sodium-potassium pump even more. This further exacerbates ADHD symptoms.

The glucose thresholds for the CRR EPI response are higher than those for the cortisol, GRH and NEP ones (i.e., EPI is triggered earlier), and the latter responses are not desensitized as strongly as the EPI one. Thus, cortisol, GRH and NEP protect from severe hypog, and **the patient experiences only mild hypog**. Hence, although ADHD patients experience hypog episodes, they normally do not show the more serious symptoms associated with hypog.

In medical settings, blood glucose levels are normally measured in the morning after a nightly fast. At this time, circadian cortisol secretion is at its peak, and NEP levels are elevated. These compensate for the desensitized state of the EPI CRR response. **This explains why the presence of mild hypog is generally not identified**.

ADHD patients commonly **develop obesity and type 2 diabetes (DB2) at a relatively young age**. This occurs because CRRs elevate blood free fatty acids (FFAs) via lipolysis. Chronically activated CRRs yield chronic FFAs, which is a known cause of insulin resistance. In addition, chronic cortisol release can yield cortisol resistance, which is a known cause of obesity.

Supporting K*ADHD, **maternal obesity, DB2, and gestational diabetes increase the risk of offspring ADHD**.

ADHD patients show **dysregulations of the sympathetic nervous system (SNS) that are consistent with chronic activity and desensitization**.

KATPCs are strongly expressed at the **heart**. ADHD patients show increased cardiovascular disease, increased basal heart rate, and decreased vagal tone.

People with ADHD do not show any obvious brain pathology, but there is a delay in reaching peak cortical thickness. This may be due to repeated hypog episodes during development.

ADHD is diagnosed more in **males**. This may reflect diagnosis bias, but can also be explained by the fact that males normally have higher CRR glucose thresholds, so are more vulnerable to CRR desensitization.

Females with ADHD tend to be diagnosed as the inattentive rather than the hyperactive type. This could be because in skeletal muscle, KATP channels are expressed in type IIB (fast-twitch) fibers, and these comprise a larger area of the muscle in males than in females.

ADHD is much more common in **children** than in adults. This happens because children have higher CRR glucose thresholds than adults.

ADHD has high comorbidity with **epilepsy**. This can be explained by the fact that potassium channel dysregulations are known to be involved in epilepsy.

ADHD risk is higher in **preterm** babies. This may be because the secretion of progesterone, which delays birth, depends on KATPCs, so their impairment may cause preterm delivery. In addition, preterms develop hypog more easily.

ADHD is diagnosed more in the younger children in their classes. Beyond diagnosis bias due to less mature behavior, this can be explained by the fact that in most of the world, **the youngest children in their class are conceived in colder months** than the older children. Cold induces a sympathetic response that increases blood glucose. Cold during conception, which is a highly sensitive period, explains increased ADHD risk.

There are indications that patients with ALS have lower incidence of childhood ADHD and ADHD symptoms. K*ADHD explains this by noting that (i) Ca^{2+} is known to be a major causal agent in ALS, and (ii) Ca^{2+} inactivates KATPCs.

It should be kept in mind that ADHD symptoms are very general and could be triggered by several different causes. The KATP theory described here is a major such cause, but there could be others.

6.2 Treatment

The optimal treatment for ADHD is to slow down the opening of KATPCs. Fortunately, there is an existing class of drugs with precisely this effect. **Sulfonylureas are selective KATPC blockers that have been used for treating diabetes for decades, including in children. They are inexpensive, widely available, safe, and cross the blood-brain barrier**.

Of the sulfonylureas, gliclazide has a 16K-fold higher affinity to SUR1 over SUR2A, while glimepiride has a similar affinity to SUR1, SUR2A, and SUR2B. Gliclazide and glimepiride have a better safety profile than glibenclamide (glyburide), being associated with lower risk of insulin-induced hypog and CVD. Thus, **at this point, the first choice for treatment is gliclazide**. However, the question which of the sulfonylureas is most suitable in ADHD is an empirical one and might be personal to each patient.

Biomarker. An oral glucose tolerance test (OGTT) can expose CRR desensitization in many (but not all) patients (see detailed summary of 2 references below.)

6.3 Evidence and references

Note: references for ADHD-related facts that are assumed to be known by ADHD experts are not listed here.

Potassium. There are many excellent reviews on KATPs, including blockers and openers, relationship with CVD and diabetes, etc. [1].

Importantly for ADHD, high intracellular potassium slows down the activity of the plasma membrane sodium-potassium pump (Na^+/K^+-ATPase) [2].

Potassium channels in ADHD. A genetic analysis of ADHD found potassium channels (KCs) as one of the central pathways [3]. A mutation in the Kir6.2 KATP subunit induces ADHD (as well as other symptoms) [4]. A mutation in the SUR1 KATP subunit induces ADHD (with epilepsy and insulin-induced hypog) [5]. Mutations in the Kv1.4 (shaker) and Kv4.3 KCs induce ADHD [6, 7]. Kv10.1 and Kv2.1 knockout mice show hyperactivity [8,9].

K*ADHD explanations for some ADHD facts. ADHD is more common in males (also) because males have higher CRRs to moderate hypog [10]. ADHD is much less common in adults because CRR glucose thresholds are higher in children (i.e., children show the ADHD phenomenon more than adults) [11]. They are also much higher in DB2, explaining why almost one half of DB2 patients develop ADHD symptoms [12]. KATPCs have an important role in the secretion of progesterone in the female reproductive system and hence their impairment may be related to preterm delivery [13].

Direct SNS evidence. There is direct evidence for both increased and decreased (or desensitized) SNS activity in patients. For decreased SNS, one paper reported oral glucose tolerance test (OGTT) results in ADHD [14]. At 3-5 hours post glucose ingestion, when insulin-induced hypog occurs, EPI greatly increased in controls (as part of CRRs), but its increase in ADHD subjects was 50% lower. NEP did not change in controls but was reduced to 73% in ADHD. There was a trend for lower growth hormone and glucagon. Thus, all CRR components, especially EPI (i.e., SNS), are reduced.

Substantially lower urine EPI was reported in inattentives, with no NEP differences [15]. Children and adolescents with ADHD show significantly lower basal blood pressure, which disappears after 10y [16]. Patients show lower urinary DOPEG, a NEP metabolite of MAO in SNS neurons, largely from recently reuptaken NEP [17]. This can be due to decreased release, or increased uptake. There was also a trend for decreased urinary EPI. Patients showed decreased EPI, dopamine (DA) to cognitive stress (with higher tonic NEP, EPI) [18]. In patients, exercise yields decreased elevations of EPI, NEP, DA, and lactate. Baseline NEP is significantly lower, but both NEP and EPI are still in the normal range [19]. In a group of boys aged 13 (not diagnosed with ADHD), there was lower urinary EPI in higher aggresiveness, restlessness, concentration difficulties, and under stress [20]. In another non-diagnosed group, there was a relationship between inattention (not in patients) & lower SNS activity (longer heart pre-ejection period) [21]. In adolescent boys with externalizing problems, conduct disorder was associated with lower salivary alpha-amylase, indicating lower SNS activity [22]. Sluggish symptoms was positively associated with heart rate variability (HRV, indicating decreased SNS) [23].

Increased SNS activity was reported in many papers. Higher baseline NEP and/or EPI (with decreased EPI to cognitive stress), [18], higher heart rate in severe ADHD, and unchanged HRV [24] have been reported. Higher heart rate, activity levels, especially in the afternoon (heart also night), in unmedicated patients [25]. 2x higher NPY in plasma and urine, with markedly increased urine NEP, serotonin (SER) metabolite [26]. Increased urinary normetanephrine (NMN), the main extracellular NEP metabolite. In patients without anxiety, lower NEP/NMN, EPI/metanephrine ratios. With anxiety, increased EPI [27]. Higher urinary NEP, DA, with NEP correlating with hyperactivity [28]. Higher urinary but not plasma NEP. EPI, DA unchanged. Lower/higher urinary MHPG/metanephrine (main EPI metabolite), MAO (lower platelet), zinc, magnesium (lower), GC (lower basal salivary) [29]. Higher skin conductance, basal & under stress [30]. Significantly higher salivary alpha-amylase [31]. Significantly higher pupil dilation response, with no differerence in initial or dilated diameters [32]. Reduced task-related HRV in a meta-review [33].

Increased risk for heart problems [34], and greater fatigue and sleep problems in ADHD [35–37] also point to SNS dysregulation.

(There are many more references, including for cortisol and growth hormone, supporting chronic CRRs.)

Direct glucose evidence in patients. 17.6% lower absolute brain PET glucose metabolism was reported in hyperactive girls. Significantly decreased in 6/60 regions [38] (however, this was not replicated in another study with a small number of female patients [39]). Decreased cerebral glucose metabolism in adults with hyperactivity since childhood [40].

Higher (35.7 vs 33.9, 39 = preDB) but still normal HbA1c, with higher BMI and normal fasting blood glucose reported in 10-15yos [41]. Note that silent hypog (glucose<3 mmol/l) is possible with high HbA1c. This occurs in 24/11% of type 2 diabetes (DB2) patients with HbA1c </> = 7% [42].

Surprisingly, I found only two papers that reported oral glucose tolerance test (OGTT) results in ADHD. In the first paper, a standard 5 hour OGTT was conducted with 265 hyperkinetic children, 211 males [43]. Glucose curves were abnormal in 74%. Among these, 50% showed flat curves, 11% showed an immediate glucose decrease following ingestion, 15% showed a rapid excessive increase, and 11% showed a similar rapid increase with a slow recovery. Flat or decreasing curves (shown in 61% of the abnormal results, or 45% of the whole cohort) indicate insulin hypersensitivity, implying chronic hypog (which induces higher insulin receptor function) and/or faster insulin secretion in almost half of the patients. Rapid increase (shown in 19% of the whole cohort) indicates reduced first phase insulin secretion, supporting higher CRR thresholds. Thus, 64% showed a pattern consistent with K*ADHD. Note that faster insulin secretion indiates lower, not higher, CRR thresholds, but would still result in hypog. Chronic hypog explains the ADHD facts, but can stem from different core causes.

In the second paper [14], following a nightly fast, a standard 5h OGTT was started in 8am. Up to 3 hours post glucose ingestion, glucose and insulin behavior were similar to controls. This shows that insulin functions normally (i.e., the body knows how to handle high glucose levels). However, at 3-5hs, when insulin-induced hypog occurs, EPI greatly increased in controls as part of CRRs, but its increase in ADHD subjects was 50% lower. NEP did not change in controls but was reduced to 73% in ADHD. There was a trend for lower growth hormone and glucagon. Thus, all CRR components, especially EPI (SNS), are reduced.

Dopamine. DA is a NEP precursor, so according to K*ADHD, it is probably chronically released and desensitized in ADHD. There is evidence that this is indeed the case [44–49].

Patient diet consistent with glucose need. Patients consume more sugar-rich and saturated fat-rich food, and this correlates with symptoms [50]. Children and adolescents with ADHD consume more candy & fruit gum (sweets). Consumption is associated with hyperactivity [51]. Positive association between sugar consumption, sugar beverages & symptoms in a meta-review [52]. Higher risk with processed & snack diets, n = 14,912, China [53]. Inattention (also hyperactivity, weaker) correlates with high sugar, fat, protein, sea food diet in 18 K Swedish twins [54]. Sweetened beverage consumption associated with self-reported hyperactivity, inattention symptoms in youth [55]. Higher/lower intake of sugary, high fat foods/vegetables, fruits, protein-rich foods. n = 216, Taiwan [56]. ADHD patients show poorer dental health, higher sugary food consumption [57,58].

References

[1] A. Tinker, Q. Aziz, Y. Li, M. Specterman, ATP-sensitive potassium channels and their physiological and pathophysiological roles, Comprehensive Physiology 8 (4) (2018) 1463–1511.

[2] A.B. Knight, L.G. Welt, Intracellular potassium: a determinant of the sodium-potassium pump rate, The Journal of General Physiology 63 (3) (1974) 351–373.

[3] M.A. Mooney, S.K. McWeeney, S.V. Faraone, A. Hinney, J. Hebebrand, et al., I Consortium, Pathway analysis in attention deficit hyperactivity disorder: an ensemble approach, American Journal of Medical Genetics. Part B, Neuropsychiatric Genetics 171 (6) (2016) 815–826.

[4] P. Bowman, E. Broadbridge, B. Knight, L. Pettit, S. Flanagan, M. Reville, et al., Psychiatric morbidity in children with KCNJ 11 neonatal diabetes, Diabetic Medicine 33 (10) (2016) 1387–1391.

[5] J. Descamps, C. Ruello, K. Perge, J. de Bellescize, C. Saint-Martin, M. Nicolino, Epileptic phenotype in late-onset hyperinsulinemic hypoglycemia successfully treated by diazoxide, Journal of Pediatric Endocrinology and Metabolism 34 (5) (2021) 667–673.

[6] N. Kaya, M. Alsagob, M.C. D'Adamo, A. Al-Bakheet, S. Hasan, M. Muccioli, et al., KCNA4 deficiency leads to a syndrome of abnormal striatum, congenital cataract and intellectual disability, Journal of Medical Genetics 53 (11) (2016) 786–792.

[7] K. Smets, A. Duarri, T. Deconinck, B. Ceulemans, B.P. van de Warrenburg, S. Züchner, et al., First de novo KCND3 mutation causes severe Kv4.3 channel dysfunction leading to early onset cerebellar ataxia, intellectual disability, oral apraxia and epilepsy, BMC Medical Genetics 16 (1) (2015) 1–7.

[8] R. Ufartes, T. Schneider, L.S. Mortensen, C. de Juan Romero, K. Hentrich, H. Knoetgen, et al., Behavioural and functional characterization of Kv10.1 (Eag1) knockout mice, Human Molecular Genetics 22 (11) (2013) 2247–2262.

[9] D.J. Speca, G. Ogata, D. Mandikian, H.I. Bishop, S.W. Wiler, K. Eum, et al., Deletion of the Kv2.1 delayed rectifier potassium channel leads to neuronal and behavioral hyperexcitability, Genes, Brain and Behavior 13 (4) (2014) 394–408.

[10] S. Amiel, A. Maran, J. Powrie, A. Umpleby, I. Macdonald, Gender differences in counterregulation to hypoglycaemia, Diabetologia 36 (5) (1993) 460–464.

[11] T.W. Jones, S.D. Boulware, D.T. Kraemer, S. Caprio, R.S. Sherwin, W.V. Tamborlane, Independent effects of youth and poor diabetes control on responses to hypoglycemia in children, Diabetes 40 (3) (1991) 358–363.

[12] A.Z. Dehnavi, Y. Zhang-James, D. Draytsel, B. Carguello, S.V. Faraone, R.S. Weinstock, Association of ADHD symptoms with type 2 diabetes and cardiovascular comorbidities in adults receiving outpatient diabetes care, Journal of Clinical & Translational Endocrinology 32 (2023) 100318.

[13] J.M. Kim, K.S. Song, B. Xu, T. Wang, Role of potassium channels in female reproductive system, Obstetrics & Gynecology Science 63 (5) (2020) 565–576.

[14] N.L. Girardi, S.E. Shaywitz, B.A. Shaywitz, K. Marchione, S.J. Fleischman, T.W. Jones, et al., Blunted catecholamine responses after glucose ingestion in children with attention deficit disorder, Pediatric Research 38 (4) (1995) 539–542.

[15] G.M. Anderson, M.A. Dover, B.P. Yang, J.M. Holahan, S.E. Shaywitz, K.E. Marchione, et al., Adrenomedullary function during cognitive testing in attention-deficit/hyperactivity disorder, Journal of the American Academy of Child and Adolescent Psychiatry 39 (5) (2000) 635–643.

[16] J. Schulz, F. Huber, R. Schlack, H. Hölling, U. Ravens-Sieberer, T. Meyer, et al., The association between low blood pressure and attention-deficit hyperactivity disorder (ADHD) observed in children/adolescents does not persist into young adulthood. A population-based ten-year follow-up study, International Journal of Environmental Research and Public Health 18 (4) (2021) 1864.

[17] G.L. Hanna, E.M. Ornitz, M. Hariharan, Urinary catecholamine excretion and behavioral differences in ADHD and normal boys, Journal of Child and Adolescent Psychopharmacology 6 (1) (1996) 63–73.

[18] K. Konrad, S. Gauggel, J. Schurek, Catecholamine functioning in children with traumatic brain injuries and children with attention-deficit/hyperactivity disorder, Cognitive Brain Research 16 (3) (2003) 425–433.

[19] S.B. Wigal, D. Nemet, J.M. Swanson, R. Regino, J. Trampush, M.G. Ziegler, et al., Catecholamine response to exercise in children with attention deficit hyperactivity disorder, Pediatric Research 53 (5) (2003) 756–761.

[20] B.A. Klinteberg, D. Magnusson, Aggressiveness and hyperactive behaviour as related to adrenaline excretion, European Journal of Personality 3 (2) (1989) 81–93.

[21] S.W. Vogel, D. Bijlenga, J. Verduijn, T.I. Bron, A.T. Beekman, J.S. Kooij, et al., Attention-deficit/hyperactivity disorder symptoms and stress-related biomarkers, Psychoneuroendocrinology 79 (2017) 31–39.

[22] N. Angyal, J. Halász, G. Mészáros, J.K. Kovács, E. Kruk, Z. Nemoda, Potential salivary biomarkers and their genetic effects in a pilot study of adolescent boys with externalizing problems, Neuropsychopharmacol Hung 18 (4) (2016) 173–179.

[23] T.W. Yung, C.Y. Lai, J.Y. Chan, S.S. Ng, C.C. Chan, Neuro-physiological correlates of sluggish cognitive tempo (SCT) symptoms in school-aged children, European Child & Adolescent Psychiatry 29 (3) (2020) 315–326.

[24] T. Yüksel, Ö. Özcan, Heart rate variability as an indicator of autonomous nervous system activity in children with attention deficit hyperactivity disorder, Anadolu Psikiyatri Dergisi 19 (5) (2018) 493–500.
[25] L. Imeraj, I. Antrop, H. Roeyers, E. Deschepper, S. Bal, D. Deboutte, Diurnal variations in arousal: a naturalistic heart rate study in children with ADHD, European Child & Adolescent Psychiatry 20 (8) (2011) 381–392.
[26] R.D. Oades, R. Daniels, W. Rascher, Plasma neuropeptide-Y levels, monoamine metabolism, electrolyte excretion and drinking behavior in children with attention-deficit hyperactivity disorder, Psychiatry Research 80 (2) (1998) 177–186.
[27] S.R. Pliszka, J.W. Maas, M.A. Javors, G.A. Rogeness, J. Baker, Urinary catecholamines in attention-deficit hyperactivity disorder with and without comorbid anxiety, Journal of the American Academy of Child and Adolescent Psychiatry 33 (8) (1994) 1165–1173.
[28] M. Dvoráková, D. Jezová, P. Blazícek, J. Trebatická, I. Skodácek, J. Suba, et al., Urinary catecholamines in children with attention deficit hyperactivity disorder (ADHD): modulation by a polyphenolic extract from pine bark (pycnogenol), Nutr Neuroscience 10 (3–4) (2007) 151–157.
[29] C. Scassellati, C. Bonvicini, S.V. Faraone, M. Gennarelli, Biomarkers and attention-deficit/hyperactivity disorder: a systematic review and meta-analyses, Journal of the American Academy of Child and Adolescent Psychiatry 51 (10) (2012) 1003–1019.
[30] S. Yang, Y. Baek, The effect of stress on the subjective discomfort and skin conductance level in adults with ADHD tendency, Korean Journal of Stress Research 25 (4) (2017) 299–305.
[31] A. Krahel, E. Paszynska, A. Slopien, M. Gawriolek, J. Otulakowska-Skrzynska, S. Rzatowski, et al., Stress/immune biomarkers in saliva among children with ADHD status, International Journal of Environmental Research and Public Health 18 (2) (2021) 769.
[32] M.G. Aslan, F. Uzun, H. Fındık, M. Kaçar, M. Okutucu, Ç. Hocaoğlu, Pupillometry measurement and its relationship to retinal structural changes in children with attention deficit hyperactivity disorder, Graefe's Archive for Clinical and Experimental Ophthalmology 258 (6) (2020) 1309–1317.
[33] A. Robe, A. Dobrean, I.A. Cristea, C.R. Păsărelu, E. Predescu, Attention-deficit/hyperactivity disorder and task-related heart rate variability: a systematic review and meta-analysis, Neuroscience and Biobehavioral Reviews 99 (2019) 11–22.
[34] L. Li, H. Yao, L. Zhang, M. Garcia-Argibay, E. Du Rietz, I. Brikell, et al., Attention-deficit/hyperactivity disorder is associated with increased risk of cardiovascular diseases: a systematic review and meta-analysis, JCPP Advances (2023) e12158.
[35] S.L. Blunden, C.M. Milte, N. Sinn, Diet and sleep in children with attention deficit hyperactivity disorder: preliminary data in Australian children, Journal of Child Health Care 15 (1) (2011) 14–24.
[36] H.L. Chiang, S.S.F. Gau, H.C. Ni, Y.N. Chiu, C.Y. Shang, Y.Y. Wu, et al., Association between symptoms and subtypes of attention-deficit hyperactivity disorder and sleep problems/disorders, Journal of Sleep Research 19 (4) (2010) 535–545.
[37] D.C. Rogers, A.J. Dittner, K.A. Rimes, T. Chalder, Fatigue in an adult attention deficit hyperactivity disorder population: a trans-diagnostic approach, British Journal of Clinical Psychology 56 (1) (2017) 33–52.
[38] A.J. Zametkin, L.L. Liebenauer, G.A. Fitzgerald, A.C. King, D.V. Minkunas, P. Herscovitch, et al., Brain metabolism in teenagers with attention-deficit hyperactivity disorder, Archives of General Psychiatry 50 (5) (1993) 333–340.
[39] M. Ernst, R.M. Cohen, L.L. Liebenauer, P.H. Jons, A.J. Zametkin, Cerebral glucose metabolism in adolescent girls with attention-deficit/hyperactivity disorder, Journal of the American Academy of Child and Adolescent Psychiatry 36 (10) (1997) 1399–1406.
[40] A.J. Zametkin, T.E. Nordahl, M. Gross, A.C. King, W.E. Semple, J. Rumsey, et al., Cerebral glucose metabolism in adults with hyperactivity of childhood onset, The New England Journal of Medicine 323 (20) (1990) 1361–1366.

[41] F. Lindblad, M. Eickhoff, A.H. Forslund, J. Isaksson, J. Gustafsson, Fasting blood glucose and HbA1c in children with ADHD, Psychiatry Research 226 (2–3) (2015) 515–516.
[42] B. Engler, C. Koehler, C. Hoffmann, W. Landgraf, S. Bilz, C. Schoner, et al., Relationship between HbA1c on target risk of silent hypoglycemia and glycemic variability in patients with type 2 diabetes mellitus, Experimental and Clinical Endocrinology & Diabetes 119 (01) (2011) 59–61.
[43] L. Langseth, J. Dowd, Glucose tolerance and hyperkinesis, Food and Cosmetics Toxicology 16 (2) (1978) 129–133.
[44] N. Del Campo, S.R. Chamberlain, B.J. Sahakian, T.W. Robbins, The roles of dopamine and noradrenaline in the pathophysiology and treatment of attention-deficit/hyperactivity disorder, Biological Psychiatry 69 (12) (2011) e145-57.
[45] A. Jucaite, E. Fernell, C. Halldin, H. Forssberg, L. Farde, Reduced midbrain dopamine transporter binding in male adolescents with attention-deficit/hyperactivity disorder: association between striatal dopamine markers and motor hyperactivity, Biological Psychiatry 57 (3) (2005) 229–238.
[46] N.D. Volkow, G.J. Wang, S.H. Kollins, T.L. Wigal, J.H. Newcorn, F. Telang, et al., Evaluating dopamine reward pathway in ADHD: clinical implications, JAMA 302 (10) (2009) 1084–1091.
[47] N.D. Volkow, G.J. Wang, J. Newcorn, J.S. Fowler, F. Telang, M.V. Solanto, et al., Brain dopamine transporter levels in treatment and drug naive adults with ADHD, NeuroImage 34 (3) (2007) 1182–1190.
[48] H. Forssberg, E. Fernell, S. Waters, N. Waters, J. Tedroff, Altered pattern of brain dopamine synthesis in male adolescents with attention deficit hyperactivity disorder, Behavioral and Brain Functions 2 (1) (2006) 1–10.
[49] A.G. Ludolph, J. Kassubek, K. Schmeck, C. Glaser, A. Wunderlich, A.K. Buck, et al., Dopaminergic dysfunction in attention deficit hyperactivity disorder (ADHD), differences between pharmacologically treated and never treated young adults: a 3, 4-dihdroxy-6-[18F] fluorophenyl-l-alanine PET study, NeuroImage 41 (3) (2008) 718–727.
[50] S. Akin, F. Gultekin, O. Ekinci, A. Kanik, B. Ustundag, B.D. Tunali, et al., Processed meat products and snacks consumption in ADHD: a case–control study, Northern Clinics of İstanbul 9 (3) (2022) 266–274.
[51] N. Wolff, C. Reimelt, S. Ehrlich, H. Hölling, S. Mogwitz, V. Roessner, On the positive association between candy and fruit gum consumption and hyperactivity in children and adolescents with ADHD, Zeitschrift für Kinder- und Jugendpsychiatrie und Psychotherapie 47 (3) (2019) 228–238.
[52] A. Farsad-Naeimi, F. Asjodi, M. Omidian, M. Askari, M. Nouri, A.B. Pizarro, et al., Sugar consumption sugar sweetened beverages and attention deficit hyperactivity disorder: a systematic review and meta-analysis, Complementary Therapies in Medicine 53 (2020) 102512.
[53] S. Yan, H. Cao, C. Gu, L. Ni, H. Tao, T. Shao, et al., Dietary patterns are associated with attention-deficit/hyperactivity disorder (ADHD) symptoms among preschoolers in mainland China, European Journal of Clinical Nutrition 72 (11) (2018) 1517–1523.
[54] L. Li, M.J. Taylor, K. Bälter, R. Kuja-Halkola, Q. Chen, T.A. Hegvik, et al., Attention-deficit/hyperactivity disorder symptoms and dietary habits in adulthood: a large population-based twin study in Sweden, American Journal of Medical Genetics. Part B, Neuropsychiatric Genetics 183 (8) (2020) 475–485.
[55] D.L. Schwartz, K. Gilstad-Hayden, A. Carroll-Scott, S.A. Grilo, C. McCaslin, M. Schwartz, et al., Energy drinks and youth self-reported hyperactivity/inattention symptoms, Academic Pediatrics 15 (3) (2015) 297–304.
[56] L.J. Wang, Y.H. Yu, M.L. Fu, W.T. Yeh, J.L. Hsu, Y.H. Yang, et al., Dietary profiles, nutritional biochemistry status, and attention-deficit/hyperactivity disorder: path analysis for a case-control study, Journal of Clinical Medicine 8 (5) (2019) 709.
[57] G. Kohlboeck, D. Heitmueller, C. Neumann, C. Tiesler, J. Heinrich, R. Heinrich-Weltzien, et al., Is there a relationship between hyperactivity/inattention symptoms and poor oral health?

Results from the GINIplus and LISAplus study, Clinical Oral Investigations 17 (5) (2013) 1329–1338.

[58] P. Chandra, L. Anandakrishna, P. Ray, Caries experience and oral hygiene status of children suffering from attention deficit hyperactivity disorder, Journal of Clinical Pediatric Dentistry 34 (1) (2009) 25–29.

Chapter 7

A sympathetic nervous system theory of migraine

7.1 Introduction

Migraine (MGR) ranks second among diseases in terms of years of lost healthy life worldwide, and the first among women between the ages 15 and 49 [1]. As such, MGR is one of the most important human diseases, and the most common brain-associated disease. Although much progress has been made in recent decades in the understanding of MGR and in new drug treatment, both the cause of the disease and its mechanisms are still largely unknown [2–5].

This paper presents the first complete theory of migraine (T*MGR). It is complete in the sense that it mechanistically explains the etiology, symptoms, pathophysiology, and treatment of the disease. T*MGR is supported by overwhelming evidence, and addresses all of the salient empirical data known about the disease.

Theory overview. Briefly, T*MGR explains MGR using four simple steps. First, at the basal state, MGR involves partial saturation of the norepinephrine (NEP) branch of the sympathetic nervous system (SNS). This can be due to chronically increased activity (e.g., due to PACAP), or to inherently reduced capacity. The problem can stem from many causes, the most supported cause in MGR being higher sensitivity of the sensors triggering SNS activation.

Second, in the acute phase, MGR headache is caused by desensitization and/or excessive activation of the SNS, due to its partial saturation and to various triggers that increase SNS activity.

Third, SNS desensitization affects vascular smooth muscle cells (VSMCs) and baroreceptors (BRRs), which are continuously active to regulate blood pressure (BPR). These cells rely on the NEP SNS for their phasic function, which reduces BPR via the parasympathetic nervous system (PNS). Impaired NEP SNS function reduces their available energy, specifically impairing their Na^+/K^+-ATPase. This leads to calcium entry and hyperexcitability. Even without desensitization, excessive SNS activation can induce hyperexcitability.

Finally, the increased BRR firing and increased VSMC contractility yield oxidative and nitrosative stress, which activates TRPV1 channels. These in turn induce the release of the neuropeptide CGRP. Normally, these agents reduce BRR activation to allow for higher BPR during effort. However, hyperexcitability interferes with this normal function, causing prolonged activation instead.

The Science of the Brain. https://doi.org/10.1016/B978-0-44-345008-2.00013-8

Both TRPV1 and CGRP are strongly expressed in pain pathways, and convey pain signals to the brain. This is MGR headache.

A non-MGR contribution of T*MGR is a new physiological role for CGRP, whereby it mediates adaptation to higher stress levels. Specifically to BRRs, it mediates the phenomenon known as BRR resetting.

All four parts of this account are supported by strong bodies of evidence related to general and MGR patient data about the SNS, PACAP, the vasculature, BRRs, CGRP, TRPV1, MGR triggers and premonitory symptoms, and agents used for MGR treatment.

7.2 Theory

7.2.1 SNS and BRRs

The autonomic nervous system, comprised of the SNS and the PNS, is activated in states of deviation from homeostasis in order to help restore it [6]. The SNS is activated during deficiency states, including hypoglycemia (hypog), hypoxia, cold, pain, and psychological stress (a deficiency state because it increases the metabolic demands from the body). In these states, the SNS increases heart rate and blood pressure, increases blood glucose via lipolysis and glycogenolysis, induces thermogenesis, and induces vasodilation in performance tissues (the brain, skeletal muscle, cardiovasculature) [6]. The SNS uses both NEP and epinephrine (EPI).

A few lesser known facts about the SNS are highly relevant for MGR. First, SNS control over baroreceptors is done mainly via NEP rather than EPI [7]. Second, although sweating is known to be an exception in that it is an SNS function mediated by post-ganglionic acetylcholine (ACh) rather than NEP or EPI, NEP can in fact induce sweating [8], with heat-induced skin vasodilation partially mediated by the SNS [9]. Indeed, the superior cervical ganglion provides SNS innervation of lacrimal glands, in addition to BRRs, cranial muscle blood vessels, pupil dilators, choroid plexus, and the pineal gland. Third, the SNS not only increases blood glucose levels, it also stimulates glucose uptake by cells via insulin-independent translocation of the Glut4 transporter to the plasma membrane [10].

Desensitization. SNS responses desensitize after some time, including the responses to hypog [11], cold [12], and hypoxia [13] (for BRRs, see below). Desensitization involves endocytosis and degradation of the NEP receptors [14], and vesicle depletion (see PACAP below). Agonist-induced desensitization of beta3-NEP occurs much more slowly than that of beta1-NEP, beta2-NEP [14], and alpha1-NEP [15] (days vs. minutes to hours).

Pituitary adenylate cyclase activating polypeptide (PACAP) is recruited by strong stress [16], and increases the synthesis and release of adrenal NEPI [17]. It is essential for sustained (not initial) counterregulatory responses to hypoglycemia [18], induces brain, heart and lung vasodilation via KATP channels

[19], and promotes hyperthermia [20]. Its role is to oppose SNS desensitization via increased ligand synthesis.

Baroreceptors. BRRs are sensory neurons mainly located at the carotid bodies and heart aorta [21]. They are stretch-sensitive mechanoreceptors, firing when BPR increases. During non-stress conditions, they initiate the baroreflex, which maintains a constant BPR level via negative feedback mechanisms. BRRs directly excite neurons in the nucleus of the solitary tract (NTS), which excite GABAergic neurons in the caudal ventrolateral medulla (VLM), which in turn suppress rostral VLM (RVLM) neurons exciting sympathetic preganglionic neurons that control the heart and blood vessels [22]. Thus, the net effect of the baroreflex is to suppress the SNS and allow a parasympathetic tone, which decreases BPR and heart rate. Decreases in BPR allow SNS responses, to start a new BRR cycle.

Under effortful conditions where BPR is increased for a prolonged period of time (e.g., exercise) [23], BRRs undergo ‘resetting’ in which their activation only occurs at the new, higher BPR [24]. The precise mechanisms behind resetting are not known, but it is known to involve direct damage to mechanosensitive BRRs, loss of BRR coupling to vascular wall stretch, and increased blood vessel stiffness [24,25].

Crucially for MGR, VSMCs completely rely on lactate to provide ATP for the activation of the Na^+/K^+-ATPase [26]. In general, lactate can be produced by aerobic glycolysis and glycogenolysis, or be shuttled to neurons from astrocytes. All of these processes, and the Na^+/K^+-ATPase, are stimulated by NEP, in the brain and skeletal muscle [27–29], and in BRRs [30]. Indeed, there is rich SNS innervation of carotid and aortic BRRs [30], BRRs contain dense glycogen granules and are surrounded by cells resembling Schwann cells (the peripheral astrocytes) [31], and suppression of VSM Na^+/K^+-ATPase induces hypertension [32].

Chemoreceptors, which sense oxygen and CO2, are located in close proximity to BRRs, and also have a role in MGR, although it is smaller than that of BRRs (see below).

7.2.2 TRPV1, CGRP

TRPV1. TRPV1 is a member of the family of TRP channels, which are expressed in sensory neurons and sense heat, cold, stretch, oxidative stress, etc. [33]. In particular, BRRs express TRPV1 [34], and it is needed for their proper functioning [34]. Another TRP family member, TRPA1, is expressed in chemoreceptors [35].

TRPV1 is usually described as a heat sensor. However, it is also an oxidative stress sensor [36–41]. TRPV1 is well-known as a conveyor of pain [33], including when it is activated by oxidative stress [37–39].

TRP channels are quickly desensitized by agonists, but TRPV1 is unique in that it can be reactivated after complete desensitization by higher agonist concentrations [42].

CGRP. CGRP is a neuropeptide mainly expressed in sensory neurons, including in perivascular fibers, lungs, gut, immune cells, spinal cord, and trigeminal ganglia [43,44]. In cortex, it is expressed in pain areas [44]. Its release is stimulated by neural depolarization, including by TRPV1 in trigeminal sensory neurons [45]. Its best-known function is that of being a highly potent vasodilator (via KATP channels), and as a result, its role is usually described as being protective [43,44]. It is clearly involved in MGR (see below).

Here I introduce a new account of CGRP, where its role is to re-calibrate activation thresholds along its path in light of prolonged stress. Because the focus of the present paper is MGR, I will focus on evidence that CGRP has this role in the cardiovascular system.

The hypothesis relevant here is that **CGRP is a major mediator of BRR resetting**. As such, it reduces SNS activation during prolonged effort/stress. Indeed, CGRP release is significantly increased during exercise and heart infarction [46]. It recovers skeletal muscle excitability during muscle contraction by stimulating Na^{+}/K^{+}-ATPase activation, and maintains force development [27,47]. Importantly, CGRP knockout yields higher SNS activation (higher BPR, heart rate, BRR sensitivity, urine NEP/EPI metabolites) [48,49]. CGRP in the lower brainstem decreases BRR sensitivity [50]. CGRP opposes SNS-induced thermogenesis [51], and non-effortful SNS activation opposes CGRP release [52,53] while NEP reuptake inhibitors (simulating a high SNS activation state) increase CGRP in adrenal cathecholamine neurons [54].

7.2.3 Migraine

T*MGR is a simple theory of MGR. MGR involves an altered basal state in which the SNS is partially saturated, due to chronically increased activity (e.g., due to PACAP) or inherently reduced capacity. Headache attacks occur in two scenarios. First, they occur when triggers lead to desensitization of BRRs or of the whole NEP branch of the SNS. Because BRRs are the only place where NEP SNS is continuously used, it is also the first place to suffer the consequences of desensitization. Since VSMCs and BRRs rely on NEP to provide energy for the Na^{+}/K^{+}-ATPase, NEP desensitization leads to Na^{+}/K^{+}-ATPase failure and hence cellular hyperexcitability. This induces Ca^{2+} entry via voltage-gated calcium channels, resulting in excitotoxicity and oxidative stress [55]. Oxidative stress activates TRPV1 channels, which induce CGRP release. Both of these agents excite downstream brain pain pathways.

A second scenario in which headache can occur is via excessive activation of the SNS (due to saturation and triggers) without its desensitization. This can also lead to BRR hyperactivity and pain as described in the first scenario.

Here we will see that this account explains the properties of MGR (detailed evidence is given in the next section).

Triggers. Basically all of the conditions known to trigger MGR or claimed to do so [56,57] increase SNS activity and/or TRPV1/CGRP/PACAP. Exercise, skipping meals (hypog), stress, hypoxia and smoke directly stimulate the SNS. Dehydration increases BRR activity [58]. Heat initially decreases skin SNS activity, but this is followed by a strong increase with sweating [59]. Menstruation involves higher body temperature [60], so the effect is similar to heat. Alcohol induces hypog and exacerbates insulin-induced hypog [61]. Alcohol also directly recruits TRPV1 and CGRP [62].

Glyceryl trinitrate (GTN, nitroglycerin) has been shown to induce headache with MGR characteristics in patients [63]. GTN, and other nitric oxide donors, directly increase CGRP release (4x in rat trigeminal ganglia) and CGRP promoter activity [64]. The induction of MGR attacks by vasodilators (GTN, KATP openers) [65] can also be explained via strong stimulation of BRRs.

Premonitory symptoms. MGR attacks are commonly preceded by so-called premonitory symptoms. All of these symptoms indicate either higher SNS activity or its ongoing desensitization.

Thirst is a very common premonitory symptom [66]. It is induced by many stimuli that induce renin release, including the SNS, carotid artery vasoconstriction (BRRs), and NEP/EPI [67]. Hunger and food craving are due to activation of the counter-regulatory responses to hypog, which include the SNS [11]. Nausea and vomiting are known symptoms of the postural tachycardia syndrome (POTS), a dysautonomia that involves SNS hyperactivation [68]. Urination [66] is an SNS-mediated response. Tiredness and concentration difficulties [66] indicate that SNS desensitization is underway. Neck pain or stiffness occur in more than half of MGR patients [66,69], showing that this location is central to MGR headache.

Nature of pain. MGR headache is unique among headaches in that it is described as 'throbbing' (pulsing). This happens because it is generated by repeated BRR cellular firing. It has been argued [5] that since the throbbing pain rate is not synchronized with the arterial pulse rate [70], the vasculature is not involved in MGR pain. However, MGR pain involves cellular hyperexcitability, so the rate of pain transmission is indeed expected to be different from that of heart beats.

Timeline of pain. MGR headache can build up over days, and takes hours to days to pass. This occurs when the problem and/or the triggers focus on the beta3-NEP receptor (supporting thermogenesis), which requires this time frame to desensitize and resensitize [14].

Aura. A subset of MGR patients experience aura symptoms during (and before) attacks, mainly including flashes of light and blind spots. T*MGR explains aura as follows. The SNS affects visual inputs to the brain via beta3-NEP receptors expressed in retinal blood vessels [71]. SNS desensitization disrupts normal visual processing, inducing hyperactivity as in BRRs. Indeed, human visual cortex shows elevated activity during aura [72]. Aura is a special case of the next item.

Sensory hypersensitivity. Vision is not the only modality that shows sensory hypersensitivity in MGR. In fact, the idea that MGR is basically a sensory hypersensitivity disease has been raised [5]. Virtually all low-level sensory pathways are affected by the SNS and express TRPV1 and CGRP.

7.3 Evidence

To support T*MGR, we need evidence from MGR patients showing partial SNS saturation, why this might happen, SNS desensitization or excessive activation right before and during attacks, BRR dysfunction, and high oxidative stress, TRPV1, and CGRP in the MGR paths. All of this evidence already exists in the literature and is listed below.

7.3.1 Basal state

Partial SNS saturation (SNS hypofunction). A large number of papers have used a battery of tests to assess SNS and PNS function at the pain-free (interictal) period, including SNS/PNS responses to quick standing, the tilt test, deep breathing, handgrip, the Valsalva maneuver, thermal (cold pain) sensitivity, psychological stress, skin sweating (SCR), heart rate variability, and hyperCO2. The vast majority (but not all [73]) of these papers report SNS hypofunction [74–97].

This indicates that the SNS is close to saturation. The most likely reasons are that it is already active at a higher capacity than normal, so that its capacity to respond to rapid challenges is decreased, or that it is already partially desensitized. However, an inherent hypofunction, supported by some evidence [98,99], is also possible.

The data above can also be interpreted to show higher PNS activity, which dominates the SNS. However, the PNS generally also shows hypofunction in MGR [100] (also shown in some of the tests cited above), which accords with SNS hypofunction because PNS activity is largely driven by SNS reflexes.

MGR is comorbid with several diseases associated with impaired SNS function, including respiratory diseases (asthma and chronic obstructive pulmonary disease) [101,102], anxiety, obesity, sleep problems [103], coronary heart disease [104], angina pectoris, myocardial infarction [105], syncope [106], and POTS [107].

MGR patients show brain glucose deficiency, mainly in pain areas, supporting impaired SNS/NEP function [108]. When waking up with a headache, patients show increased NEP and cortisol 3 hours before waking [109]. This supports hypog, since NEP and cortisol are part of the response to hypog. Patients also show brain ATP depletion [110], which can be due to hypog or to hyperexcitability.

Recall that PACAP increases SNS ligand synthesis and release, thus pushes the SNS closer to desensitization. It induces migraine headache in 72% of subjects, with premonitory symptoms in 48% (but not in subjects who developed an attack) [111]. Its levels are increased in the cranial circulation following painful stimuli, sumatriptan (MGR drug) decreases its levels, levels are lower interictally, and intravenous injections induce attacks [112]. PACAP KO significantly decreases trigeminal NTG-induced photophobia [113].

Small fiber neuropathy has been demonstrated in patient skin, showing peripheral autonomic damage [114].

BRR, BPR. In addition to the general SNS saturation noted above, there is also specific evidence for altered BRR sensitivity in MGR [115,116], and for SNS neck hypofunction [117]. In addition, decreased BRR sensitivity predicts chronic headache [116]. BRR-mediated BPR responses are reduced in MGR [118]. Patients show higher resting diastolic BPR [119]. Following NEP injection, patients take 5x as long until BPR recovery vs. controls, showing BRR dysfunction [98]. Reduced NEP in BRRs has been demonstrated via exaggerated BPR responses to an alpha1-NEP agonist [120].

All drugs that lower BPR decrease headache frequency [121,122]. More than 75% of patients show comorbidities, hypertension being one of the most common ones [103]. Other common ones include other conditions associated with chronic SNS, such as anxiety disorders and back pain.

Two large epidemiologic studies found an association between increased systolic BPR and *reduced* MGR (and other headache) risk [123]. The apparent contradiction with the other evidence can be explained as follows. On one hand, high basal SNS activity induces high BPR as explained above. On the other hand, low BPR may indicate that SNS desensitization is already taking place, in which case high BPR can be viewed as protective. We expect higher BPR at periods far from headache attacks (unless the SNS is chronically desensitized), and higher or lower BPR at periods closer to the attacks. BPR alone is not a reliable biomarker for MGR.

Cerebral blood flow (CBF) is another unreliable marker for MGR. The SNS response under effort/stress includes increased heart rate and vasodilation, which increase CBF. Thus, as in BPR, basal CBF or CBF reactivity can be higher far from attacks. However, if the SNS is already desensitized, patients would show low basal CBF, and they might show high or low CBF close to attacks. The evidence is indeed inconclusive, showing all of these states [124–127].

Hyperexcitability. As mentioned above, MGR patients show sensory hyperexcitability. For example, visually and auditory evoked potentials show reduced habituation [128], photophobia thresholds are significantly reduced, which correlates with blunted autonomic responses [129], and there is increased visual cortex and plasma lactate [130,131].

Oxidative and nitrosative stress. MGR patients show increased oxidative and nitrosative stress. Lipid peroxidation metabolites and nitric acid are increased in patient urine [132], and patients with high frequency MGR have low serum anti-oxidants and high lipid peroxidation [133].

Genetics. According to T*MGR, the main mechanistic account of MGR is a saturated SNS. However, a complete account of the etiology of the disease needs to explain why this happens. There is some genetic evidence pointing to the sensors that trigger SNS activation.

The strongest genes identified in GWAS are those encoding TRPM8, PRDM16, and TASK2 [134]. TRPM8 is a cold sensor, with a SNP that reduces its expression and attenuates cold pain sensation being protective against MGR [135]. This shows that reduced recruitment of the SNS reduces MGR risk.

MGR is associated with a SNP in the PRDM16 gene [136], which promotes development of brown adipose tissue (BAT). BAT supports thermogenesis and is an important SNS target tissue. TASK2 (encoded by KCNK5) is an acid sensor that participates in the hyperCO2 responses.

Evidence from a large twin study points to the ATP1A2 gene, which encodes subunit 2 of the Na^{+}/K^{+}-ATPase [137]. However, there is also a negative result for this gene [138].

Living in high altitudes increases the hypoxia SNS responses and is associated with higher MGR risk [139]. It is known that the human genome shows adaptations to high altitude [140], but this has not been shown specifically in MGR.

A significant MGR association was found with 5 insulin receptor SNPs, which may stimulate compensating SNS hyperactivity [141]. SNPs were also found in the glutathione anti-oxidant pathway [142].

7.3.2 Acute headache state

Attacks are induced by desensitization of BRRs and possibly of other locations of SNS function, or by excessive SNS activation. Thus, the evidence should mainly show BRR hypofunction, but it can also show hyperactivity, and activity in other parts of the SNS can be increased or decreased. Indeed, most reports show SNS desensitization during and after attacks [77,88,93,117,143–149].

The reduced visual and auditory habituation normalizes just before attacks, showing desensitization [128]. Some papers report high SNS activity right before and during attacks, both non-cardiovascular [150–153] and cardiovascular [154–157].

The pons is activated during attacks [158–160], supporting the involvement of BRR targets. There is increased CGRP release [161] and nitrovasive and oxidative stress during attacks [162]. Carotid arteriography induced attacks in 9/13 patients [143], showing that the BRR location is a highly sensitive pain spot. In addition, the neck shows pain during attacks [163].

Pain relievers. Many medications for treating acute headache, including ergots and triptans, mimic the effects of the SNS (e.g., vasoconstriction) without relying on it [164]. This supports SNS desensitization as a causative pain factor. Magnesium, which decreases cellular calcium influx, can also relieve pain [165].

7.4 Treatment

According to T*MGR, enhancing the SNS should be preventive in MGR. Indeed, exercise has a positive effect on the frequency and severity of headaches

[166], and beta blockers, which oppose SNS desensitization, are probably the most effective preventive drugs [2].

Botox inhibits TRPV1 and CGRP, thereby opposing the development of pain [167].

TRPV1 agonists quickly desensitize TRPV1. Indeed, intranasal civamide (TRPV1 agonist) strongly helps acute pain [168], and the classical TRPV1 agonist capsaicin helps in chronic MGR [169]. As noted above, many sympatomimetics relieve acute pain.

Most recently, CGRP-based drugs have been approved for treatment. Receptor antagonists (gepants) are moderately effective for prevention but not for acute treatment [170]. This is not surprising, given that TRPV1 is expressed along all of the pain path and can convey pain even without CGRP. Moreover, CGRP calibrates the SNS and BRRs to higher workloads, and as such it should be protective in MGR in the long-term. Indeed, prolonged usage of CGRP inhibitors (gepants or CGRP antibodies) may be associated with cardiovascular risk [171].

As we have seen above, increased PACAP could be one reason for faster SNS desensitization. Indeed, a single iv of 750 mg LuAG09222 (PACAP ligand antibody) was better than placebo in decreasing MGR frequency over the subsequent 4 weeks [172].

Chocolate is claimed by some to be helpful, and by others to be a trigger [57]. It is a trigger because it may yield insulin-induced hypog, and it may be acutely helpful by providing BRRs and other cells with glucose. However, sugars are generally not expected to provide quick effective acute treatment, because it takes time for the desensitized NEP receptors to recuperate.

One paper reported effective acute treatment via a partial rebreathing device that increases brain oxygen, opposing hypoxia [173].

An acute treatment direction that has not been attempted yet is lactate infusions. This sounds paradoxical in light of the basal increased lactate levels in patients (see above). However, lactate is increased at the basal state due to chronic SNS activation, while infusions during attacks may provide BRRs with the energy they need for proper Na^+/K^+-ATPase activation.

7.5 Discussion

This chapter presented the first complete theory of MGR. T*MGR is very simple, relying on established biological processes, and all of its components are supported by large bodies of evidence. Moreover, T*MGR addresses all of the supported evidence gathered about MGR.

Other theories. There is currently no complete theory of MGR, and it is widely agreed that the cause and mechanisms of MGR are unknown [2–5]. Over the years, there have been several ideas with growing and then diminishing popularity, including cortical spreading depression (a transient wave of cortical neural depolarization), trigeminovascular system, and vasodilation [2]. A central question in past theories was whether the pain origin is central or peripheral. The former has been convincingly ruled out [174], in favor of intra- and extra-cranial perivascular origin (so with some overlap with T*MGR). However, again, detailed mechanisms have not been presented.

The two theories closest to T*MGR focus on NEP and oxidative stress. MGR has been hypothesized to involve chronic SNS dysfunction with relative NEP depletion and increased release of cotransmitters dopamine, prostaglandins, ATP, and adenosine [164]. This theory overlaps T*MGR with respect to chronic SNS dysfunction, but without any mechanistic overlap or insight. A second theory presented MGR as a disease of brain energy deficiency that yields oxidative stress [175]. Again, there is some shallow overlap with T*MGR, without detailed mechanisms.

A great achievement of MGR research is the identification of the importance of CGRP, which has resulted in several approved CGRP-based drugs. However, as discussed above, it is not clear to what extent these drugs are better than other treatments.

Other headaches. It is not difficult to extend T*MGR to explain other types of headaches in addition to MGR. This was not done here in order to keep the paper focused. Nonetheless, a few words are in order. First, T*MGR trivially explains tension-type headaches, which are different from MGR by being bilateral and with a pressing rather than throbbing pain [176]. The pain mechanisms in T*MGR can be evoked without the BRR desensitization that lends MGR its throbbing pain aspect.

Second, T*MGR includes a sibling theory explaining cluster headache. Cluster headache prefers men (vs. MGR, which prefers women), and it always involves cranial autonomic symptoms (vs. MGR, where these occur in many but not all patients). The main distinction between the diseases (except pain strength, which is higher in cluster headache) is probably the duration of the pain, since cluster headache attacks last between 15 and 180 minutes, and those of MGR 4-72 hours [177]. According to T*MGR, cluster headache parallels MGR in that it involves the chemoreceptor paths (alpha1-NEP) rather than baroreceptors. This theory will hopefully be detailed elsewhere.

List of abbreviations

alpha1-NEP: alpha1 adrenergic receptor.
BAT: brown adipose tissue.
beta1/2/3-NEP: beta1/2/3/ adrenergic receptor.
BPR: blood pressure.
BRR: baroreptor.
CSD: Cortical spreading depression.
GWAS: genome-wide association studies.

MGR: migraine.
NEP: norepinephrine (noradrenaline).
NTS: nucleus of the solitary tract.
PNS: parasympatheric nervous system.
KATP channels: ATP-inactivated potassium channels.
POTS: postural tachycardia syndrome.
RVLM: rostral ventrolateral medulla.
SCR: skin conductance response.
SNP: single-nucleotide polymorphism.
SNS: sympathetic nervous system.
TRPA1: transient receptor potential cation channel subfamily A member 1.
TRPM8: transient receptor potential cation channel subfamily M member 8.
TRPV1: transient receptor potential cation channel subfamily V member 1.
VLM: ventrolateral medulla.
VSMC: vascular smooth muscle cell.

Acknowledgment

I would like to thank Prof. Messoud Ashina for his comments on a previous drafts of this paper.

References

[1] T. Steiner, L. Stovner, R. Jensen, D. Uluduz, Z. Katsarava, The Global Campaign against Headache LTB. Migraine remains second among the world's causes of disability, and first among young women: findings from GBD2019, Springer, 2020.
[2] M.D. Ferrari, P.J. Goadsby, B. Rami, T. Kurth, A. Cenk, A. Charles, et al., Migraine (Primer), Nature Reviews Disease Primers 8 (1) (2022).
[3] M. Ashina, The New England Journal of Medicine 383 (2020) 1866–1876.
[4] K.A. Haanes, L. Edvinsson, Pathophysiological mechanisms in migraine and the identification of new therapeutic targets, CNS Drugs 33 (6) (2019) 525–537.
[5] P.J. Goadsby, P.R. Holland, M. Martins-Oliveira, J. Hoffmann, C. Schankin, S. Akerman, Pathophysiology of migraine: a disorder of sensory processing, Physiological Reviews 97 (2) (2017) 553–622.
[6] E.E. Benarroch, The autonomic nervous system: basic anatomy and physiology, CONTINUUM: Lifelong Learning in Neurology 13 (6) (2007) 13–32.
[7] S.F. Morrison, Differential control of sympathetic outflow, American Journal of Physiology. Regulatory, Integrative and Comparative Physiology 281 (3) (2001) R683–R698.
[8] K.R. Chémali, R. Gorodeski, T.C. Chelimsky, α-adrenergic supersensitivity of the sudomotor nerve in complex regional pain syndrome, Annals of Neurology 49 (4) (2001) 453–459.
[9] G.J. Hodges, W.A. Kosiba, K. Zhao, J.M. Johnson, The involvement of heating rate and vasoconstrictor nerves in the cutaneous vasodilator response to skin warming, American Journal of Physiology. Heart and Circulatory Physiology 296 (1) (2009) H51–H56.
[10] N. Dehvari, D.S. Hutchinson, J. Nevzorova, O.S. Dallner, M. Sato, M. Kocan, et al., β2-Adrenoceptors increase translocation of GLUT4 via GPCR kinase sites in the receptor C-terminal tail, British Journal of Pharmacology 165 (5) (2012) 1442–1456.
[11] Z.M. Kakall, M.M. Kavurma, E.M. Cohen, P.R. Howe, P.E. Nedoboy, P.M. Pilowsky, Repetitive hypoglycemia reduces activation of glucose-responsive neurons in C1 and C3 medullary brain regions to subsequent hypoglycemia, American Journal of Physiology: Endocrinology and Metabolism 317 (2) (2019) E388–E398.

[12] H. Cernecka, C. Sand, M.C. Michel, The odd sibling: features of β3-adrenoceptor pharmacology, Molecular Pharmacology 86 (5) (2014) 479–484.
[13] W. Long, L. Zhang, L.D. Longo, Fetal and adult cerebral artery KATP and KCa channel responses to long-term hypoxia, Journal of Applied Physiology 92 (4) (2002) 1692–1701.
[14] K. Okeke, S. Angers, M. Bouvier, M.C. Michel, Agonist-induced desensitisation of β3-adrenoceptors: Where, when, and how?, British Journal of Pharmacology 176 (14) (2019) 2539–2558.
[15] M. Maze, C.K. Spiss, G. Tsujimoto, B.B. Hoffman, Epinephrine infusion induces hyporesponsiveness of vascular smooth muscle, Life Sciences 37 (17) (1985) 1571–1578.
[16] N. Stroth, B. Kuri, T. Mustafa, S.A. Chan, L. Eiden, PACAP controls adrenomedullary catecholamine secretion and expression of catecholamine biosynthetic enzymes at high splanchnic nerve firing rates characteristic of stress transduction in male mice, Endocrinology 154 (1) (2013) 330–339.
[17] C. Tönshoff, L. Hemmick, M.J. Evinger, Pituitary adenylate cyclase activating polypeptide (PACAP) regulates expression of catecholamine biosynthetic enzyme genes in bovine adrenal chromaffin cells, Journal of Molecular Neuroscience 9 (1997) 127–140.
[18] C. Hamelink, O. Tjurmina, R. Damadzic, W.S. Young, E. Weihe, H.W. Lee, et al., Pituitary adenylate cyclase-activating polypeptide is a sympathoadrenal neurotransmitter involved in catecholamine regulation and glucohomeostasis, Proceedings of the National Academy of Sciences 99 (1) (2002) 461–466.
[19] A. Baron, D. Monnier, A. Roatti, A.J. Baertschi, Pituitary adenylate cyclase-activating polypeptide activates KATP current in rat atrial myocytes, American Journal of Physiology. Heart and Circulatory Physiology 280 (3) (2001) H1058–H1065.
[20] I. Pataki, Á. Adamik, M. Jászberényi, M. Mácsai, G. Telegdy, Pituitary adenylate cyclase-activating polypeptide induces hyperthermia in the rat, Neuropharmacology 39 (7) (2000) 1303–1308.
[21] J.E. Hall, M.E. Hall, Guyton and Hall Textbook of Medical Physiology, 14th Edition, Elsevier Health Sciences, 2020.
[22] A.M. Schreihofer, P.G. Guyenet, The baroreflex and beyond: control of sympathetic vasomotor tone by GABAergic neurons in the ventrolateral medulla, Clinical and Experimental Pharmacology & Physiology 29 (5–6) (2002) 514–521.
[23] J. Liu, N. Song, Y. Wang, J. Walker, J. Yu, A single baroreceptor unit consists of multiple sensors, Scientific Reports 11 (1) (2021) 23111.
[24] E.A. Wehrwein, M.J. Joyner, Regulation of blood pressure by the arterial baroreflex and autonomic nervous system, Handbook of Clinical Neurology 117 (2013) 89–102.
[25] R.A. Dampney, Resetting of the baroreflex control of sympathetic vasomotor activity during natural behaviors: description and conceptual model of central mechanisms, Frontiers in Neuroscience 11 (2017) 461.
[26] J. Shi, Y. Yang, A. Cheng, G. Xu, F. He, Metabolism of vascular smooth muscle cells in vascular diseases, American Journal of Physiology. Heart and Circulatory Physiology (2020).
[27] T. Clausen, K. Overgaard, The role of K+ channels in the force recovery elicited by Na+-K+ pump stimulation in Ba2+-paralysed rat skeletal muscle, The Journal of Physiology 527 (2) (2000) 325–332.
[28] M.E. Gibbs, D.S. Hutchinson, R.J. Summers, Role of β-adrenoceptors in memory consolidation: β3-adrenoceptors act on glucose uptake and β2-adrenoceptors on glycogenolysis, Neuropsychopharmacology 33 (10) (2008) 2384–2397.
[29] R. Jensen, J. Nielsen, N. Ørtenblad, Inhibition of glycogenolysis prolongs action potential repriming period and impairs muscle function in rat skeletal muscle, The Journal of Physiology 598 (4) (2020) 789–803.
[30] G. Akoev, Catecholamines, acetylcholine and excitability of mechanoreceptors, Progress in Neurobiology 15 (4) (1980) 269–294.
[31] J. Tranum-Jensen, The ultrastructure of the sensory end-organs (baroreceptors) in the atrial endocardium of young mini-pigs, Journal of Anatomy 119 (Pt 2) (1975) 255.

[32] K. Sekine, K. Yamakawa, E. Ogata, Na+ K+-ATPase Activity and Responsiveness of Vascular Smooth Muscle to Norepinephrine, Angiotensin II and Calcium Ionophore A23187 in Guinea Pig Aortic Strips, Clinical and Experimental Hypertension Part A: Theory and Practice 6 (7) (1984) 1267–1280.

[33] B. Nilius, A. Szallasi, Transient receptor potential channels as drug targets: from the science of basic research to the art of medicine, Pharmacological Reviews 66 (3) (2014) 676–814.

[34] H. Sun, D.P. Li, S.R. Chen, W.N. Hittelman, H.L. Pan, Sensing of blood pressure increase by transient receptor potential vanilloid 1 receptors on baroreceptors, The Journal of Pharmacology and Experimental Therapeutics 331 (3) (2009) 851–859.

[35] Y.Y. Wang, R.B. Chang, E.R. Liman, TRPA1 is a component of the nociceptive response to CO2, The Journal of Neuroscience 30 (39) (2010) 12958–12963.

[36] A. Starr, R. Graepel, J. Keeble, S. Schmidhuber, N. Clark, A. Grant, et al., A reactive oxygen species-mediated component in neurogenic vasodilatation, Cardiovascular Research 78 (1) (2008) 139–147.

[37] N. Nishio, W. Taniguchi, Y. Sugimura, N. Takiguchi, M. Yamanaka, Y. Kiyoyuki, et al., Reactive oxygen species enhance excitatory synaptic transmission in rat spinal dorsal horn neurons by activating TRPA1 and TRPV1 channels, Neuroscience 247 (2013) 201–212.

[38] X. Chen, Z. Chen, G. Ma, J. Sha, S. Zhao, Z. Liu, et al., Reactive Oxygen Species Induced Upregulation of TRPV1 in Dorsal Root Ganglia Results in Low Back Pain in Rats, Journal of Inflammation Research (2024) 2245–2256.

[39] M. Ibi, K. Matsuno, D. Shiba, M. Katsuyama, K. Iwata, T. Kakehi, et al., Reactive oxygen species derived from NOX1/NADPH oxidase enhance inflammatory pain, The Journal of Neuroscience 28 (38) (2008) 9486–9494.

[40] S. Negri, P. Faris, G. Tullii, M. Vismara, A.F. Pellegata, F. Lodola, et al., Conjugated polymers mediate intracellular Ca2+ signals in circulating endothelial colony forming cells through the reactive oxygen species-dependent activation of Transient Receptor Potential Vanilloid 1 (TRPV1), Cell Calcium 101 (2022) 102502.

[41] B. Kievit, A.D. Johnstone, J. Gibon, P.A. Barker, Mitochondrial reactive oxygen species mediate activation of TRPV1 and calcium entry following peripheral sensory axotomy, Frontiers in Molecular Neuroscience 15 (2022) 852181.

[42] K. Novakova-Tousova, L. Vyklicky, K. Susankova, J. Benedikt, A. Samad, J. Teisinger, et al., Functional changes in the vanilloid receptor subtype 1 channel during and after acute desensitization, Neuroscience 149 (1) (2007) 144–154.

[43] R. King, S.J. Smillie, X. Kodji, S. Brain, Calcitonin gene-related peptide: physiology and pathophysiology, Physiological Reviews 94 (4) (2014) 1099–1142.

[44] A.F. Russo, D.L. Hay, CGRP physiology, pharmacology, and therapeutic targets: migraine and beyond, Physiological Reviews 103 (2) (2023) 1565–1644.

[45] S. Akerman, H. Kaube, P. Goadsby, Vanilloid type 1 receptors (VR1) on trigeminal sensory nerve fibres play a minor role in neurogenic dural vasodilatation and are involved in capsaicin-induced dural dilation, British Journal of Pharmacology 140 (4) (2003) 718–724.

[46] P. Lechleitner, C. Haring, J. Mair, N. Genser, C.J. Wiedermann, F. Dienstl, et al., Exercise-induced increase in plasma concentrations of calcitonin gene-related peptide in patients with coronary heart disease and healthy controls, International Journal of Angiology 3 (01) (1994) 16–19.

[47] Effects of calcitonin gene-related peptide on rat soleus muscle excitability: mechanisms and physiological significance, American Journal of Physiology. Regulatory, Integrative and Comparative Physiology 295 (4) (2008) R1214–R1223.

[48] Y. Oh-hashi, T. Shindo, Y. Kurihara, T. Imai, Y. Wang, H. Morita, et al., Elevated sympathetic nervous activity in mice deficient in αCGRP, Circulation Research 89 (11) (2001) 983–990.

[49] T.H. Mai, J. Wu, A. Diedrich, E.M. Garland, D. Robertson, Calcitonin gene-related peptide (CGRP) in autonomic cardiovascular regulation and vascular structure, Journal of the American Society of Hypertension 8 (5) (2014) 286–296.

[50] S. Kim, Y. Ouchi, H. Sekiguchi, H. Fujikawa, K. Shimada, K. Yagi, Endogenous calcitonin gene-related peptide modulates tachycardiac but not bradycardiac baroreflex in rats, American Journal of Physiology. Heart and Circulatory Physiology 274 (5) (1998) H1489–H1494.
[51] A. Kobayashi, Y. Namba, O. Ezaki, S. Inoue, S. Kimura, T.H. Lee, Temperature- and capsaicin-sensitive nerve fibers in brown adipose tissue attenuate thermogenesis in the rat, Pflügers Archiv 437 (1998) 36–42.
[52] W. Bowles, C. Flores, D. Jackson, β2-Adrenoceptor regulation of CGRP release from capsaicin-sensitive neurons, Journal of Dental Research 82 (4) (2003) 308–311.
[53] B.A. Marichal-Cancino, A. González-Hernández, E. Muñoz-Islas, C.M. Villalón, Monoaminergic receptors as modulators of the perivascular sympathetic and sensory CGRPergic outflows, Current Neuropharmacology 18 (9) (2020) 790–808.
[54] G. Höfle, R. Weiler, R. Fischer-Colbrie, C. Humpel, A. Laslop, T. Wohlfarter, et al., Stimulation of rat adrenal medulla can induce differential changes in the peptide and mRNA levels of chromogranins, neuropeptides and other constituents of chromaffin granules, Regulatory Peptides 32 (3) (1991) 321–331.
[55] N.M. Connolly, J.H. Prehn, The metabolic response to excitotoxicity–lessons from single-cell imaging, Journal of Bioenergetics and Biomembranes 47 (1–2) (2015) 75–88.
[56] The triggers or precipitants of the acute migraine attack, Cephalalgia 27 (5) (2007) 394–402.
[57] E.C. Gross, M. Lisicki, D. Fischer, P.S. Sándor, J. Schoenen, The metabolic face of migraine–from pathophysiology to treatment, Nature Reviews Neurology 15 (11) (2019) 627–643.
[58] N. Charkoudian, J.R. Halliwill, B.J. Morgan, J.H. Eisenach, M.J. Joyner, Influences of hydration on post-exercise cardiovascular control in humans, The Journal of Physiology 552 (2) (2003) 635–644.
[59] D. Gagnon, C.G. Crandall, Sweating as a heat loss thermoeffector, Handbook of Clinical Neurology 156 (2018) 211–232.
[60] F.C. Baker, F. Siboza, A. Fuller, Temperature regulation in women: effects of the menstrual cycle, Temperature 7 (3) (2020) 226–262.
[61] C. Oba-Yamamoto, J. Takeuchi, A. Nakamura, R. Takikawa, A. Ozaki, H. Nomoto, et al., Combination of alcohol and glucose consumption as a risk to induce reactive hypoglycemia, Journal of Diabetes Investigation 12 (4) (2021) 651–657.
[62] M. Trevisani, M. Manconi, R. Gatti, G.D. Siena, J. Capone, Ethanol causes neurogenic vasodilation by TRPV1 activation and CGRP release in the trigeminovascular system of the guinea pig, Cephalalgia 28 (1) (2008) 9–17.
[63] J. Van Der Grond, R. Van Der Geest, G. Terwindt, M. Ferrari, Migraine headache is not associated with cerebral or meningeal vasodilatation-a 3T magnetic resonance angiography study, Brain 131 (8) (2008) 2192–2200.
[64] J. Bellamy, E.J. Bowen, A.F. Russo, P.L. Durham, Nitric oxide regulation of calcitonin gene-related peptide gene expression in rat trigeminal ganglia neurons, European Journal of Neuroscience 23 (8) (2006) 2057–2066.
[65] M.A.M. Al-Karagholi, J.M. Hansen, S. Guo, J. Olesen, M. Ashina, Opening of ATP-sensitive potassium channels causes migraine attacks: a new target for the treatment of migraine, Brain 142 (9) (2019) 2644–2654.
[66] N. Giffin, L. Ruggiero, S. Silberstein, J. Tvedskov, J. Olesen, J. Altman, et al., Premonitory symptoms in migraine: an electronic diary study, Neurology 60 (6) (2003) 935–940.
[67] J.T. Fitzsimons, The renin-angiotensin system and drinking behavior, Progress in Brain Research 42 (1975) 215–233.
[68] C. Shibao, C. Arzubiaga, L.J. Roberts, S. Raj, B. Black, P. Harris, et al., Hyperadrenergic postural tachycardia syndrome in mast cell activation disorders, Hypertension 45 (3) (2005) 385–390.
[69] J. Blau, E. MacGregor, Migraine and the neck, Headache: The Journal of Head and Face Pain 34 (2) (1994) 88–90.
[70] A.H. Ahn, On the temporal relationship between throbbing migraine pain and arterial pulse, Headache: The Journal of Head and Face Pain 50 (9) (2010) 1507–1510.

[71] A. Mori, T. Miwa, K. Sakamoto, T. Nakahara, K. Ishii, Pharmacological evidence for the presence of functional β 3-adrenoceptors in rat retinal blood vessels, Naunyn-Schmiedeberg's Archives of Pharmacology 382 (2010) 119–126.
[72] N. Hadjikhani, M. Sanchez del Rio, O. Wu, D. Schwartz, D. Bakker, B. Fischl, et al., Mechanisms of migraine aura revealed by functional MRI in human visual cortex, Proceedings of the National Academy of Sciences 98 (8) (2001) 4687–4692.
[73] G. Pierangeli, P. Parchi, G. Barletta, M. Chiogna, E. Lugaresi, P. Cortelli, Power spectral analysis of heart rate and diastolic blood pressure variability in migraine with and without aura, Cephalalgia 17 (7) (1997) 756–760.
[74] R.A. Cohen, D.A. Williamson, J.E. Monguillot, P.C. Hutchinson, J. Gottlieb, W.F. Waters, Psychophysiological response patterns in vascular and muscle-contraction headaches, Journal of Behavioral Medicine 6 (1983) 93–107.
[75] P.D. Drummond, Vascular responses in headache-prone subjects during stress, Biological Psychology 21 (1) (1985) 11–25.
[76] L.S. Rubin, D. Graham, R. Pasker, W. Calhoun, Autonomic nervous system dysfunction in common migraine, Headache: The Journal of Head and Face Pain 25 (1) (1985) 40–48.
[77] P. Cortelli, P. De Carolis, A. Sturani, A. Ligabue, R. Agati, A. Baldrati, et al., Cardiovascular and biochemical assessment in migraine patients submitted to tilt test, Functional Neurology 1 (3) (1986) 285–290.
[78] H. Havanka-Kanniainen, U. Tolonen, V. Myllylä, Autonomic dysfunction in adult migraineurs, Headache: The Journal of Head and Face Pain 26 (8) (1986) 425–430.
[79] H. Havanka-Kanniainen, K. Juujärvi, U. Tolonen, V. Myllylä, Cardiovascular reflexes and plasma noradrenaline levels in migraine patients before and during nimodipine medication, Headache: The Journal of Head and Face Pain 27 (1) (1987) 39–44.
[80] S. Gomi, F. Gotoh, S. Komatsumoto, Y. Ishikawa, N. Araki, J. Hamada, Sweating function and retinal vasomotor reactivity in migraine, Cephalalgia 9 (3) (1989) 179–185.
[81] M. Tabata, T. Takeshima, N. Burioka, T. Nomura, K. Ishizaki, N. Mori, et al., Cosinor analysis of heart rate variability in ambulatory migraineurs, Headache: The Journal of Head and Face Pain 40 (6) (2000) 457–463.
[82] C. Harer, R. Von Kummer, Cerebrovascular CO2 reactivity in migraine: assessment by transcranial Doppler ultrasound, Journal of Neurology 238 (1991) 23–26.
[83] R. Martín, C. Ribera, J.M. Moltó, C. Ruiz, L. Galiano, J. Matías-Guiu, Cardiovascular reflexes in patients with vascular headache, Cephalalgia 12 (6) (1992) 360–364.
[84] T. Pogacnik, S. Sega, B. Pecnik, T. Kiauta, Autonomic function testing in patients with migraine, Headache: The Journal of Head and Face Pain 33 (10) (1993) 545–550.
[85] G. Fiermonte, F. Pierelli, F. Pauri, F. Cosentino, R. Soccorsi, P. Giacomini, Cerebrovascular CO2 reactivity in migraine with aura and without aura. A transcranial D oppler study, Acta Neurologica Scandinavica 92 (1995) 166–169.
[86] A. Mosek, V. Novak, T.L. Opfer-Gehrking, J.W. Swanson, P.A. Low, Autonomic dysfunction in migraineurs. Headache, The Journal of Head and Face Pain 39 (2) (1999) 108–117.
[87] F. Vernieri, F. Tibuzzi, P. Pasqualetti, C. Altamura, P. Palazzo, P. Rossini, Increased cerebral vasomotor reactivity in migraine with aura: an autoregulation disorder? A transcranial Doppler and near-infrared spectroscopy study, Cephalalgia 28 (7) (2008) 689–695.
[88] S. Yildiz, N. Yildiz, B. Korkmaz, Sympathetic skin responses from frontal region in migraine headache: a pilot study, Cephalalgia 28 (7) (2008) 696–704.
[89] R. Venkatesan, P. Naveen, M. Bedi, V. Varshney, S. Venkidusamy, A study of autonomic functions in the patients of episodic migraine, National Journal of Physiology, Pharmacy and Pharmacology 4 (2) (2014) 171.
[90] M. Cambron, H. Maertens, K. Paemeleire, L. Crevits, Autonomic function in migraine patients: ictal and interictal pupillometry, Headache: The Journal of Head and Face Pain 54 (4) (2014) 655–662.
[91] O.V. Mamontov, L. Babayan, A.V. Amelin, R. Giniatullin, A.A. Kamshilin, Autonomous control of cardiovascular reactivity in patients with episodic and chronic forms of migraine, The Journal of Headache and Pain 17 (2016) 1–8.

[92] J. Koenig, D.P. Williams, A.H. Kemp, J.F. Thayer, Vagally mediated heart rate variability in headache patients—a systematic review and meta-analysis, Cephalalgia 36 (3) (2016) 265–278.
[93] M.G. Miglis, Migraine and autonomic dysfunction: which is the horse and which is the jockey?, Current Pain and Headache Reports 22 (2018) 1–7.
[94] L. Zhang, S. Qiu, C. Zhao, P. Wang, S. Yu, Heart rate variability analysis in episodic migraine: A cross-sectional study, Frontiers in Neurology 12 (2021) 647092.
[95] S.K. Kavuncu, P. Nalçacıoğlu, N.H. Güneş, D. Özkoyuncu, C. Kara, A shift of the pupillary balance towards the parasymphathetic system in migraine patients with aura, Archives of Neuropsychiatry 59 (4) (2022) 268.
[96] M. Shi, D. Luo, J. Guo, D. Yang, Z. Li, H. Zhao, The function of the autonomic nervous system in Asian patients with chronic migraine, Frontiers in Neuroscience 16 (2022) 773321.
[97] A.R. Pavelić, K. Zebenholzer, C. Wöber, Reconceptualizing autonomic function testing in migraine: a systematic review and meta-analysis, The Journal of Headache and Pain 25 (1) (2024) 54.
[98] F. Gotoh, S. Komatsumoto, N. Araki, S. Gomi, Noradrenergic nervous activity in migraine, Archives of Neurology 41 (9) (1984) 951–955.
[99] K. Mikamo, T. Takeshima, K. Takahashi, Cardiovascular sympathetic hypofunction in muscle contraction headache and migraine, Headache: The Journal of Head and Face Pain 29 (2) (1989) 86–89.
[100] L.L. Thomsen, H.K. Iversen, F. Boesen, J. Olesen, Transcranial Doppler and cardiovascular responses during cardiovascular autonomic tests in migraineurs during and outside attacks, Brain 118 (5) (1995) 1319–1327.
[101] G. Davey, P. Sedgwick, W. Maier, G. Visick, D.P. Strachan, H.R. Anderson, Association between migraine and asthma: matched case-control study, British Journal of General Practice 52 (482) (2002) 723–727.
[102] L.L. Kang, P.E. Chen, T.H. Tung, C.W. Chien, Association between asthma and migraine: a systematic review and meta-analysis of observational studies, Frontiers in Allergy 2 (2021) 741135.
[103] V. Caponnetto, M. Deodato, M. Robotti, M. Koutsokera, V. Pozzilli, C. Galati, et al., Comorbidities of primary headache disorders: a literature review with meta-analysis, The Journal of Headache and Pain 22 (2021) 1–18.
[104] D.N. Kalkman, E.G. Couturier, A. El Bouziani, J. Dahdal, J. Neefs, J. Woudstra, et al., Migraine and cardiovascular disease: what cardiologists should know, European Heart Journal 44 (30) (2023) 2815–2828.
[105] K. Rose, A. Carson, C. Sanford, P. Stang, C. Brown, A. Folsom, et al., Migraine and other headaches: associations with Rose angina and coronary heart disease, Neurology 63 (12) (2004) 2233–2239.
[106] R.K. Khurana, Syncope and headache, Current Pain and Headache Reports 22 (2018) 1–8.
[107] B.R. Mueller, J. Robinson-Papp, Postural orthostatic tachycardia syndrome and migraine: A narrative review, Headache: The Journal of Head and Face Pain 62 (7) (2022) 792–800.
[108] J. Kim, S. Kim, S. Suh, S. Koh, K. Park, K. Oh, Interictal metabolic changes in episodic migraine: a voxel-based FDG-PET study, Cephalalgia 30 (1) (2010) 53–61.
[109] L. Hsu, A. Crisp, J. Koval, C. Chen, M. Carruthers, K. Zilkha, Early morning migraine: nocturnal plasma levels of catecholamines, tryptophan, glucose, and free fatty acids and sleep encephalographs, The Lancet 309 (8009) (1977) 447–451.
[110] K. Paemeleire, J. Schoenen, 31P-MRS in migraine: fallen through the cracks, Headache 53 (4) (2013) 676–678.
[111] S. Guo, A.L. Vollesen, J. Olesen, M. Ashina, Premonitory and nonheadache symptoms induced by CGRP and PACAP38 in patients with migraine, Pain 157 (12) (2016) 2773–2781.
[112] L. Edvinsson, Pituitary adenylate cyclase activating polypeptide (PACAP) in migraine pathophysiology, Pituitary Adenylate Cyclase Activating Polypeptide—PACAP (2016) 609–615.

[113] A. Markovics, V. Kormos, B. Gaszner, A. Lashgarara, E. Szoke, K. Sandor, et al., Pituitary adenylate cyclase-activating polypeptide plays a key role in nitroglycerol-induced trigeminovascular activation in mice, Neurobiology of Disease 45 (1) (2012) 633–644.
[114] M. Stillman, L. Zhou, R. Shields, N. Thompson, F. Jaeger, K. Mayuga, et al., Autonomic Dysfunction among migraineurs with and without complaints of orthostatic intolerance: Evidence for small fiber nerve damage, Annals of Headache Medicine Journal 6 (01) (2021).
[115] D.M. Rossi, H.C.D. de Souza, D. Bevilaqua-Grossi, A.C.C. Vendramim, S.V. Philbois, G.F. Carvalho, et al., Impairment on cardiovascular autonomic modulation in women with migraine, International Journal of Environmental Research and Public Health 20 (1) (2022) 763.
[116] B.R. Mueller, C. Ray, A. Benitez, J. Robinson-Papp, Reduced cardiovagal baroreflex sensitivity is associated with postural orthostatic tachycardia syndrome (POTS) and pain chronification in patients with headache, Frontiers in Human Neuroscience 17 (2023) 1068410.
[117] B. Korkmaz, S. Yildiz, N. Yildiz, Sympathetic skin responses from the neck area in patients with unilateral migraine, Nöro Psikiyatri Arşivi 52 (2) (2015) 151.
[118] E. Sanya, C. Brown, C. Von Wilmowsky, B. Neundörfer, M. Hilz, Impairment of parasympathetic baroreflex responses in migraine patients, Acta Neurologica Scandinavica 111 (2) (2005) 102–107.
[119] A. Shechter, W.F. Stewart, S.D. Silberstein, R.B. Lipton, Migraine and autonomic nervous system function: a population-based, case-control study, Neurology 58 (3) (2002) 422–427.
[120] M. Boccuni, M. Alessandri, B. Fusco, F. Cangi, The pressor hyperresponsiveness to phenylephrine unmasks sympathetic hypofunction in migraine, Cephalalgia 9 (4) (1989) 239–245.
[121] M. Law, J.K. Morris, R. Jordan, N. Wald, Headaches and the treatment of blood pressure: results from a meta-analysis of 94 randomized placebo-controlled trials with 24 000 participants, Circulation 112 (15) (2005) 2301–2306.
[122] C. Carcel, F. Haghdoost, J. Shen, P. Nanda, Y. Bai, E. Atkins, et al., The effect of blood pressure lowering medications on the prevention of episodic migraine: a systematic review and meta-analysis, Cephalalgia 43 (6) (2023) 03331024231183166.
[123] E. Tronvik, L. Stovner, K. Hagen, J. Holmen, J. Zwart, High pulse pressure protects against headache: prospective and cross-sectional data (HUNT study), Neurology 70 (16) (2008) 1329–1336.
[124] G. Micieli, D. Bosone, A. Cavallini, P. Bellantonio, F. Rossi, G. Nappi, Increased cerebral blood flow velocity induced by cold pressor test in migraine: a possible basis for pathogenesis?, Cephalalgia 15 (6) (1995) 494–498.
[125] C. Weiller, A. May, M. Jüptner, H. Kaube, R. Schayck, H. Coenen, et al., Brain stem activation in spontaneous human migraine attacks, Nature Medicine 1 (7) (1995) 658–660.
[126] G. De Benedittis, G. Da Passano CF Granata, A. Lorenzetti, R. Giuffre, CBF changes during headache-free periods and spontaneous/induced attacks in migraine with and without aura: a TCD and SPECT comparison study, Journal of Neurosurgical Sciences 43 (2) (1999) 141.
[127] J.M. Hansen, C.J. Schankin, Cerebral hemodynamics in the different phases of migraine and cluster headache, Journal of Cerebral Blood Flow and Metabolism 39 (4) (2019) 595–609.
[128] A. Judit, P. Sandor, Habituation of visual and intensity dependence of auditory evoked cortical potentials tends to normalize just before and during the migraine attack, Cephalalgia 20 (8) (2000) 714–719.
[129] M.M. Cortez, N.A. Rea, L.A. Hunter, K.B. Digre, K. Brennan, Altered pupillary light response scales with disease severity in migrainous photophobia, Cephalalgia 37 (8) (2017) 801–811.
[130] H. Watanabe, T. Kuwabara, M. Ohkubo, S. Tsuji, T. Yuasa, Elevation of cerebral lactate detected by localized sup 1 H-magnetic resonance spectroscopy in migraine during the interictal period, Neurology 47 (4) (1996) 1093–1095.
[131] T. Aczél, T. Körtési, J. Kun, P. Urbán, W. Bauer, R. Herczeg, et al., Identification of disease- and headache-specific mediators and pathways in migraine using blood transcriptomic and metabolomic analysis, The Journal of Headache and Pain 22 (2021) 1–18.

[132] I. Ciancarelli, M. Tozzi-Ciancarelli, C.D. Massimo, C. Marini, A. Carolei, Urinary nitric oxide metabolites and lipid peroxidation by-products in migraine, Cephalalgia 23 (1) (2003) 39–42.

[133] E.C. Gross, N. Putananickal, A.L. Orsini, D.R. Vogt, P.S. Sandor, J. Schoenen, et al., Mitochondrial function and oxidative stress markers in higher-frequency episodic migraine, Scientific Reports 11 (1) (2021) 4543.

[134] D. Pietrobon, Ion channels in migraine disorders, Current Opinion in Physiology 2 (2018) 98–108.

[135] N.R. Gavva, R. Sandrock, G.E. Arnold, M. Davis, E. Lamas, C. Lindvay, et al., Reduced TRPM8 expression underpins reduced migraine risk and attenuated cold pain sensation in humans, Scientific Reports 9 (1) (2019) 19655.

[136] V. Siokas, I. Liampas, A.M. Aloizou, M. Papasavva, C. Bakirtzis, E. Lavdas, et al., Deciphering the role of the rs2651899, rs10166942, and rs11172113 polymorphisms in migraine: A meta-analysis, Medicina 58 (4) (2022) 491.

[137] D.R. Nyholt, K.I. Morley, M.A. Ferreira, S.E. Medland, D.I. Boomsma, A.C. Heath, et al., Genomewide significant linkage to migrainous headache on chromosome 5q21, American Journal of Human Genetics 77 (3) (2005) 500–512.

[138] C. Netzer, U. Todt, A. Heinze, J. Freudenberg, V. Zumbroich, T. Becker, et al., Haplotype-based systematic association studies of ATP1A2 in migraine with aura, American Journal of Medical Genetics. Part B, Neuropsychiatric Genetics 141 (3) (2006) 257–260.

[139] L. Edvinsson, Migraine associated with altitude: results from a population-based study in Nepal, European Journal of Neurology 24 (8) (2017) 1055–1061.

[140] A.W. Bigham, F.S. Lee, Human high-altitude adaptation: forward genetics meets the HIF pathway, Genes & Development 28 (20) (2014) 2189–2204.

[141] L.C. McCarthy, D.A. Hosford, J.H. Riley, M.I. Bird, N.J. White, D.R. Hewett, et al., Single-nucleotide polymorphism alleles in the insulin receptor gene are associated with typical migraine, Genomics 78 (3) (2001) 135–149.

[142] K. Ishizaki, H. Kowa, Y. Adachi, T. Takeshima, F. Sakai, K. Nakashima, Glutathione S-transferase polymorphisms: susceptibility to migraine without aura, European Neurology 49 (4) (2003) 218–222.

[143] M. Lauritzen, T.S. Olsen, N.A. Lassen, O.B. Paulson, Changes in regional cerebral blood flow during the course of classic migraine attacks, Annals of Neurology: Official Journal of the American Neurological Association and the Child Neurology Society 13 (6) (1983) 633–641.

[144] Disturbances in ocular sympathetic function and facial blood flow in unilateral migraine headache, Journal of Neurology, Neurosurgery and Psychiatry 53 (2) (1990) 121–125.

[145] J. Van Hilten, M. Ferrari, J. Van der Meer, H. Gijsman, B. Looij Jr, Plasma interleukin-1, tumour necrosis factor and hypothalamic-pituitary-adrenal axis responses during migraine attacks, Cephalalgia 11 (2) (1991) 65–67.

[146] B. Sperling, J. Olesen, H. Iversen, Migraine pain associated with middle cerebral artery dilatation: reversal by sumatriptan, The Lancet 338 (8758) (1991) 13–17.

[147] V. Mylius, H.J. Braune, K. Schepelmann, Dysfunction of the pupillary light reflex following migraine headache, Clinical Autonomic Research 13 (2003) 16–21.

[148] N. Fabre, P. Payoux, F. Chollet, G. Geraud, Posterior cerebral hypoperfusion in migraine without aura, Cephalalgia 28 (8) (2008) 856–862.

[149] G. Bugdayci, S. Yildiz, B. Altunrende, N. Yildiz, S. Alkoy, Salivary alpha amylase activity in migraine patients, Autonomic Neuroscience 155 (1–2) (2010) 121–124.

[150] S. Shaw, R. Johnson, H. Keogh, Metabolic changes during glucose tolerance tests in migraine attacks, Journal of the Neurological Sciences 33 (1–2) (1977) 51–59.

[151] R. Burstein, D. Yarnitsky, I. Goor-Aryeh, B.J. Ransil, Z.H. Bajwa, An association between migraine and cutaneous allodynia, Annals of Neurology 47 (5) (2000) 614–624.

[152] M. Obermann, M. Yoon, P. Dommes, J. Kuznetsova, M. Maschke, C. Weimar, et al., Prevalence of trigeminal autonomic symptoms in migraine: a population-based study, Cephalalgia 27 (6) (2007) 504–509.

[153] D.G. Zhang, F.M. Amin, S. Guo, M.B. Vestergaard, A. Hougaard, M. Ashina, Plasma glucose levels increase during spontaneous attacks of migraine with and without aura, Headache: The Journal of Head and Face Pain 60 (4) (2020) 655–664.
[154] F. Cirignotta, T. Sacquegna, R. DÀlessandro, A. Baldrati, P. De Carolis, G. Coccagna, et al., Systemic arterial pressure and heart rate changes during migraine and cluster headaches: preliminary study, Headache: The Journal of Head and Face Pain 22 (1) (1982) 35–37.
[155] A. Perciaccante, A. Fiorentini, R. Valente, M. Granata, L. Tubani, Migraine and heart rate variability, Archives of Internal Medicine 167 (20) (2007) 2264.
[156] M.S. Asghar, A.E. Hansen, F.M. Amin, R. van der Geest, P. van der Koning, H.B. Larsson, et al., Evidence for a vascular factor in migraine, Annals of Neurology 69 (4) (2011) 635–645.
[157] F. Frank, M. Faulhaber, K. Messlinger, C. Accinelli, M. Peball, A. Schiefecker, et al., Migraine and aura triggered by normobaric hypoxia, Cephalalgia 40 (14) (2020) 1561–1573.
[158] M.S. Matharu, T. Bartsch, N. Ward, R.S. Frackowiak, R. Weiner, P.J. Goadsby, Central neuromodulation in chronic migraine patients with suboccipital stimulators: a PET study, Brain 127 (1) (2004) 220–230.
[159] S.K. Afridi, N.J. Giffin, H. Kaube, K.J. Friston, N.S. Ward, R.S. Frackowiak, et al., A positron emission tomographic study in spontaneous migraine, Archives of Neurology 62 (8) (2005) 1270–1275.
[160] S. Afridi, M. Matharu, L. Lee, H. Kaube, K. Friston, R. Frackowiak, A PET study exploring the laterality of brainstem activation in migraine using glyceryl trinitrate, Brain 128 (4) (2005) 932–939.
[161] P. Goadsby, L. Edvinsson, R. Ekman, Vasoactive peptide release in the extracerebral circulation of humans during migraine headache, Annals of Neurology: Official Journal of the American Neurological Association and the Child Neurology Society 28 (2) (1990) 183–187.
[162] G. Yilmaz, H. Sürer, L.E. Inan, Ö. Coskun, D. Yücel, Increased nitrosative and oxidative stress in platelets of migraine patients, The Tohoku Journal of Experimental Medicine 211 (1) (2007) 23–30.
[163] P. Tfelt-Hansen, I. Lous, J. Olesen, Prevalence and significance of muscle tenderness during common migraine attacks, Headache: The Journal of Head and Face Pain 21 (2) (1981) 49–54.
[164] S.J. Peroutka, Migraine: a chronic sympathetic nervous system disorder, Headache: The Journal of Head and Face Pain 44 (1) (2004) 53–64.
[165] U. Gröber, J. Schmidt, K. Kisters, Magnesium in prevention and therapy, Nutrients 7 (9) (2015) 8199–8226.
[166] L. Machado-Oliveira, Y.O. da Silva Gauto, F.J. de Santana Neto, M.G. da Silva, A.H. Germano-Soares, P.R.B. Diniz, Effects of different exercise intensities on headache: a systematic review, American Journal of Physical Medicine & Rehabilitation 99 (5) (2020) 390–396.
[167] X. Zhang, A.M. Strassman, V. Novack, M.F. Brin, R. Burstein, Extracranial injections of botulinum neurotoxin type A inhibit intracranial meningeal nociceptors' responses to stimulation of TRPV1 and TRPA1 channels: Are we getting closer to solving this puzzle?, Cephalalgia 36 (9) (2016) 875–886.
[168] S. Diamond, F. Freitag, S. Phillips, J. Bernstein, J. Saper, Intranasal civamide for the acute treatment of migraine headache, Cephalalgia 20 (6) (2000) 597–602.
[169] G. Barzoi, F. Agro, Repeated intranasal capsaicin applications to treat chronic migraine, British Journal of Anaesthesia 90 (6) (2003) 812.
[170] C. Altamura, N. Brunelli, M. Marcosano, L. Fofi, F. Vernieri, Gepants-a long way to cure: a narrative review, Neurological Sciences 43 (9) (2022) 5697–5708.
[171] E. Rivera-Mancilla, C.M. Villalón, A. MaassenVanDenBrink, CGRP inhibitors for migraine prophylaxis: a safety review, Expert Opinion on Drug Safety 19 (10) (2020) 1237–1250.
[172] M. Ashina, R. Phul, M. Khodaie, E. Löf, I. Florea, A monoclonal antibody to PACAP for migraine prevention, The New England Journal of Medicine 391 (9) (2024) 800–809.

[173] C.H. Fuglsang, T. Johansen, K. Kaila, H. Kasch, F.W. Bach, Treatment of acute migraine by a partial rebreathing device: A randomized controlled pilot study, Cephalalgia 38 (10) (2018) 1632–1643.
[174] J. Olesen, R. Burstein, M. Ashina, P. Tfelt-Hansen, Origin of pain in migraine: evidence for peripheral sensitisation, The Lancet Neurology 8 (7) (2009) 679–690.
[175] J.M. Borkum, Brain energy deficit as a source of oxidative stress in migraine: a molecular basis for migraine susceptibility, Neurochemical Research 46 (8) (2021) 1913–1932.
[176] D. Onan, S. Younis, W.D. Wellsgatnik, F. Farham, S. Andruškevičius, A. Abashidze, et al., Debate: differences and similarities between tension-type headache and migraine, The Journal of Headache and Pain 24 (1) (2023) 92.
[177] M.A.M. Al-Karagholi, K.P. Peng, A.S. Petersen, I. De Boer, G.M. Terwindt, M. Ashina, Debate: are cluster headache and migraine distinct headache disorders?, The Journal of Headache and Pain 23 (1) (2022) 151.

Chapter 8

A ceramide theory of multiple sclerosis

8.1 Introduction

Multiple sclerosis (MS) is a debilitating disease involving demyelination, impaired movement, vision, spinal cord functions (e.g., bladder control), and cognition [1]. It is the most prevalent chronic inflammatory disease of the central nervous system [1], affecting more than 2M people worldwide, with a prevalence of more than 1% in North America and Europe and 0.2% in East Asia and sub-Saharan Africa [2]. The efficacy of current MS therapies is moderate at best [1], and they do not stop disease progression.

MS is commonly perceived as an autoimmune disease mainly involving T cells [3]. However, the evidence for T cell autoimmunity, including for myelin-derived antigens, is circumstantial and weak [4,5]. There is epidemiological [6] and pathological [7] evidence supporting a major role for Epstein-Barr virus (EBV) infection, which affects B cells, in MS, and additional considerations (e.g., the efficacy of B cell depletion treatment) supporting a major role for B cells [3]. However, no convincing mechanisms have been described so far [8].

This chapter presents a novel theory (T*MS) as to how activated B cells induce the myelin damage seen in MS. The theory relies on well-known biological mechanisms, and is supported by diverse preclinical and clinical evidence.

Theory overview. T*MS explains the mechanisms of MS in four simple steps. First, what causes the disease is strong persistent activation of B cells, as often happens with reactivated EBV infection. Second, activated B cells release cytokines, including tumor necrosis factor alpha (TNFa), whose role is to promote immune cell migration and tissue penetration. Third, a major way through which TNFa attains its role is by acting on ceramide products. It induces the breakdown of sphingomyelin (SPM) and galactosylceramide (GalCer) and the liberation of arachidonic acid, thereby destabilizing membrane lipids. It also stimulates immune cell migration into blood and their penetration into tissues.

Finally, crucially, SPM and GalCer are essential for the maintenance of brain myelin sheaths, and their breakdown leads to demyelination. It does not impair myelin synthesis and non-terminal differentiation of myelin-producing cells, explaining the unique trajectory of MS lesions over time, specifically, the common relapsing-remitting course of the disease.

The Science of the Brain. https://doi.org/10.1016/B978-0-44-345008-2.00014-X

All aspects of this theory are supported by evidence. T*MS explains the often dramatical improvements achieved by B cell depletion, the efficacy of fingolimod (an inhibitor of the signaling of one of the main ceramide products), and the relative lack of benefit of other treatment approaches.

8.2 Theory

8.2.1 Background

Ceramide and its products. Ceramides are lipids containing sphingosine and fatty acids. Ceramide participates in four main pathways [9]. First, it is used to generate sphingosine (via acid ceramidase, with the inverse reaction mediated by ceramide synthase). Sphingosine generates sphingosine 1-phosphate (S1P) via sphingosine kinases 1 and 2.

Second, ceramide and ATP form ceramide 1-phosphate (C1P) and ADP via ceramide kinase (CERK).

Third, ceramide and phosphocholine form sphingomyelin (SPM) via SPM synthase (SMS). SPM breakdown is mediated by sphingomyelin phosphodiesterase (SMase, sphingomyelinase), which has two main forms, acid (aSMAse) and neutral (nASmase). SMase promotes the shedding of extracellular vesicles via SPM breakdown [10].

Finally, ceramide is the backbone of cerebrosides (mainly galactosylceramide (GalCer) and glucosylceramide (GlcCer), ceramide glycosylated with a galactose/glucose residue, respectively). GalCer is cleaved to ceramide and galactose by galacosylceramidase (GALC). The lysosomal enzymes saposinA and saposinC are coactivators of GALC to promote GalCer degradation [11], and this is assisted by cathepsinB, which mediates cleavage of prosaposin [12].

SPM and GalCer are major components in cell membranes, including myelin (see below), the blood-brain barrier (BBB), and endothelial cells in general, while S1P and C1P are major signaling molecules. S1P is abundant in the circulation and promotes immune cell migration, including exit from lymph nodes [13]. C1P promotes tissue destabilization and immune tissue penetration by stimulating cytosolic phospholipase A2, which liberates membrane arachidonic acid to destabilize membranes and produce prostaglandins (PGs) [14]. GalCer strongly promotes B cell proliferation, differentiation, and activation via the CD1d B cell receptor [15].

Myelin. Myelin sheaths are oligodendrocyte (OLG) processes that wrap around axons, mainly to support rapid electrical conduction [16]. In humans, about 70% of myelin is comprised of lipids, with cholesterol (>27%) and GalCer (>22%) being the main components. Sphingomyelin (>11%) and sulfatide (sulfated GalCer, 3.8%) are also important components [17]. GalCer and sulfatide are not essential for myelin formation, but are essential for its maintenance and stability [18]. OLG precursor cells (OPCs) and OLGs express GalCer and sulfatide only at terminal differentiation [19].

Remyelination is an ongoing process in adult brain [20]. New OLGs can be generated from a quiescent OPC pool to replace lost myelin.

EBV. EBV affects B cells. Transformed cells express high levels of TNFa, TNFb, and TGFb mRNA. Conversely, TNFa and TNFb enhance B cells after EBV [21]. EBV transformation increases galactosylation by 15-1225% in rheumatoid arthritis B cells [22].

EBV can infect astrocytes to enhance brain infiltration by peripheral blood lymphocytes [23]. It also affects epithelial cells [24], decreasing their exit from the cell cycle [25].

The expression of CD23 is greatly increased in the cell surface of EBV-transformed B cells [26]. CD23 stimulates growth and adhesion among B cells [27].

Humans are the only natural host for EBV [28]. Note that MS is a strictly human disease. It does not affect non-human primates [29].

TNFa. TNFa has two forms, soluble and transmembrane, which act on two receptors. It is released by macrophages, B cells, T cells, natural killer cells, dendritic cells, monocytes, microglia, astrocytes, and even neurons [30]. In particular, CD23, which marks activated B cells, induces TNFa release [31], and there is high TNFa in EBV-positive peripheral T cell lymphomas [32,33]. Periodontitis lesions show very high levels of TNF, which are even higher in EBV-positive lesions [34].

TNFa activates all of the ceramide-based pathways involved in membrane destabilization. It activates SMase [35–38] decreasing myelin SPM [39]. It activates CERK (which induces C1P) [37], liberating arachidonic acid [40], and activates sphingosine kinase (to produce S1P) [41]. It increases the translation and activity of cathepsinB [42,43], which promotes GalCer degradation.

Myelin contains TNFa receptors (but mainly p75) [39]. TNF opposes myelin not only via ceramide products. Lipopolysaccharides kill OPCs by inducing TNFa release from microglia [44]. Reactive astrocytes inhibit OPC survival and differentiation via secreted TNFa that acts on OPC TNFR1 [45].

We need to keep in mind that TFN signaling is far from being completely understood. Although the new phrasing of its role presented in this chapter (immune migration and tissue penetration) is definitely supported by the evidence, there are aspects of its signaling that are still puzzling. Specifically, TNF is known to promote both cell survival (by opposing apoptosis and necrosis) and death [46]. This may be because the survival effects act on immune cells while the negative effects are due to immune responses.

8.2.2 Multiple sclerosis

MS. The above data about ceramide, myelin, TNFa, and EBV give rise to a simple theory of MS. MS occurs in situations where B cells (or other immune cells) are persistently activated, as is the case with some reactivated EBV infections. Activated immune cells induce TNFa release. TNFa promotes immune cell migration and tissue penetration, and a major tool through which this is done is by acting on ceramide products. TNFa promotes S1P, which stimulates immune migration, and promotes the degradation of SPM, GalCer, and arachidonic acid, all with the effect of degrading and destabilizing membranes. TNF's tissue penetration effects occur in the brain as well, promoting brain infiltration of immune cells. The main location of expression of SPM and GalCer in the brain is myelin, and their degradation impairs the proper maintenance of existing myelin sheaths.

Disease types. The most common MS type (about 85% of patients) is relapsing-remitting MS [1]. Here, relapses are followed by long (months to years) periods of relative quiet without new disease activity. Deficits that occur during attacks are fixed in about 60%. T*MS explains this seemingly strange state as follows. The damage induced by TNFa is mainly limited to SPM and GalCer, which are needed for myelin maintenance, thereby causing lesions. Myelin synthesis is not impaired, explaining why the brain manages to execute substantial fixing processes. After causing a lesion, immune cells do not necessarily stay at the vicinity of the lesion, which can allow full recovery.

The second common disease type is primary progressive MS. Here, there is no remission after the initial symptoms. This happens when the initial disease drive (immune activation) is stronger, possibly involving several immune cell types, and with a wider spatial extent, which does not leave the brain time and space to recuperate.

Most (65%) relapsing-remitting patients switch at some point to a progressive course (termed secondary progressive). This can be explained by the presence of the problem continuously attracting immune cells into the brain and to existing lesions, even if they are small. Although immune activity can be helpful (e.g., by removing myelin debris), at some point, its persistent activation is likely to become toxic.

Peripheral damage. Myelin in the peripheral nervous system is damaged in MS, albeit to a lesser extent that central myelin [47]. T*MS explains this by noting that peripheral myelin has less GalCer and much more SPM than central myelin [48].

Pregnancy. MS relapse rates diminish during pregnancy [49]. T*MS explains this by noting that the first pregnancy trimester is characterized by a complete lack of TNFa. TNFa then increases to labor, with very high production at the onset of spontaneous abortions [50].

Sex differences. The prevalence of MS among women has increased in the last decades to be 2-3 higher than that in men [2]. Women have lower sphingolipids (including ceramide and SPM) between the ages 18-39yo. This is reversed at ages 56-70, but the MS age of onset is 31-33yo $\pm$10 [51].

Vitamin D. Vitamin D deficiency is one of the few established risk factors for MS [49]. Vitamin D decreases TNFa signaling [52].

Altitude. Living at higher altitudes is associated with an earlier age of onset of MS [53]. UV irradiation (which is higher at higher altitudes) is associated with aSMase activation [54], and ionizing radiation has been shown to induce rapid SPM hydrolysis to ceramide [55].

Smoking. Smoking is a well-established environmental risk factor in MS [49,56]. Smoking is associated with increased TNFa (but not always) [57], and activates nSMase in lung cell death [58]. In addition, smoking increases COX2 expression and PG synthesis (i.e., arachidonic acid liberation and membrane degradation) in human urinary bladder cancer [59]. On the other hand, active smoking was reported to decrease PG synthesis in human gut musoca [60]. If this is the case, then the high smoking rates in MS could be a form of self-treatment.

8.3 Evidence

B cells and EBV in MS. The involvement of B cells [3,61] and EBV [6,62] in MS pathogenesis has been reviewed at depth, so we will not repeat the evidence here. A recent result not included in these reviews is that expanded CSF T cells are specific to EBV-infected B cells [63].

TNFa in MS. There is strong evidence for TNFa involvement in MS. Increased blood TNFa preceded the exacerbation of symptoms in relapsing-remitting patients by at most two weeks [64]. The increase has normalized in many cases, with symptoms appearing only when it persisted. Blood mononuclear cells in relapsing but not stable patients showed higher TNFa and lymphotoxin mRNA [65]. Increased TNFa and IgG in peripheral mononuclear cells were reported, with increased soluble CD23 (B cell growth/activation marker) correlating with IgG [66]. TNFa production in intrathecal cells was reported, with CSF TNFa correlating with disease activity and with poor outcome [67]. MS lesions showed high TNFa, associated with astrocytes and macrophages [68,69]. Significantly high TNFa was reported in chronic active lesions [70].

TNFa was included in the 20 highest markers in a Belgium population GWAS [71].

Additional TNF data is discussed under treatment below.

Ceramides in MS. There is overwhelming evidence for ceramide abnormalities in MS. Increased ceramide and ceramide products (indicating degradation of ceramide products) were reported in patient CSF, serum and lymphocytes [72,73]. Ceramide accumulates in reactive astrocytes in active lesions [74]. Significantly increased ceramide metabolizing enzymes were found in plasma [75].

Serum aSMase activity was significantly higher in MS [76]. Patient CSF shows higher aSMase-enriched & total exosomes, significantly higher aSMase activity, and lower SPMs [77]. Increased aSMase activity was detected in active MS lesions, possibly driven by reactive astrocytes. Fingolimod, which acts on the S1P and C1P paths (see below), decreases this and ceramide-induced immune infiltration [78]. CSF SPM was identified as a fast, sensitive, fast, simple peripheral demyelination biomarker [79]. TNFa induced exosomal ceramide and SPM release in an OLG-related cell line [80].

Experimental autoimmune encephalomyelitis (EAE) is a popular MS model in which demyelination is induced by a stimulated immune response. EAE is blocked by inhibition of aSMase [81]. The cuprizone model of MS uses copper chelation to yield OLG death. In this model, aSMase deficiency enhances myelin repair [82]. Knockout of nSMase (but not aSMase) prevented oxidative stress-induced OLG death [83].

Plaques show decreased sulfatides and cerebrosides [84]. Decreased cerebrosides are an early white matter change [85]. Patients show decreased myelin sulfatides [86,87], and increased total cerebrosides in serum [86]. Patient plasma extracellular vesicles contain sulfatides [88]. Sulfatide was decreased by 60% in plaque matter, and by 25% in adjacent normal-appearing white matter [89]. Normal-appearing white matter showed significantly reduced sulfatide [90]. Increased lysosomal hydrolase activity, especially of sulfatide, was seen in plaques, which was more extensive in acute cases [91].

In chronic progressive MS patients, GalCer is undetectable in serum, indicating very strong on-going breakdown. In relapsing-remitting patients, GalCer elevation positively correlated with relapses [92]. Similarly, plasma contained no GalCer in patients with unspecified disease type [93]. Plaques contained only 1% of GalCer, GlcCer, & sulfatide vs normal- appearing white matter. Periplaques showed intermediate amounts [94].

Patient CSF shows significantly increased cathepsinB (promoting GalCer degradation), in MS, chronic inflammatory demyelinating polyneuropathy, and Guillain-Barre syndrome (where the immune system targets muscles) [95].

CSF antibodies against sulfatide have been reported [96,97].

In normal-appearing white and grey matter in active patients, higher phospholipids and lower sphingolipids were found [98]. Normal lipid composition in normal-appearing white matter has also been reported [99].

C1P stimulates cPLA2, which liberates arachidonic acid for the synthesis of prostaglandins. MS patients show higher CSF [100] and leukocyte [101] prostaglandin E2. A sharp increase occurred in patients with active symptoms right before symptom onset [101]. COX inhibitors (which prevent prostaglandin E2 synthesis) are beneficial in MS [102].

Patient white matter and plaques showed increased sphingosine (the S1P path) [103].

In summary, ceramide definitely shows abnormalities in MS, with the evidence focusing mainly on increased degradation of SPM and GalCer, the two leading ceramide products in myelin, which are important for myelin maintenance.

Risk factors. The risk factors discussed above (smoking, vitamin D, altitude), and pregnancy protection, also constitute supporting evidence for T*MS.

8.4 Treatment

Classical MS treatments are described in the reviews cited above. Our focus in B cells, EBV, and TNFa.

Depletion therapy. The new focus on B cells is largely driven by the impressive success of B cell-based therapy by targeting CD20 [104].

CD20 depletion targets the mature naive and memory mature B cells, but does not affect immature and plasma cells. Although memory B cells and long-lived plasma cells are increased in MS CNS, it is possible that anti-CD20 therapy only depletes memory B cells [3]. This should decrease the effect of EBV-infected B cells.

Ceramide-based. Fingolimod is a structural analogue of sphingosine, phosphorylated by sphingosine kinase and acting on S1PR1, probably negatively regulating its signaling. It constitutes one of the more effective treatments in MS (relapsing-remitting, not progressive). Fingolimod blocks the exit of lymphocytes (not effector memory T cells) from lymph nodes [105], thereby reducing B and T cell migration and tissue penetration.

There are small molecule aSMase inhibitors (FIASMA) approved for treating other conditions [106]. Their use in MS needs to be examined. One such molecule has been shown to be beneficial in MS [107].

TNF. In apparent opposition to T*MS, although successful in animal models, TNFa inhibitors were harmful in MS trials, and triggered demyelination when used for treating various diseases, mainly rheumatoid arthritis [30]. This is explained as follows. As noted above, TNF is capable of inducing completely opposite effects, both pro- and anti-survival [46]. The drugs used in trials and treatment are non-selective, and although their main effect is antagonism, they can also serve as agonists [30]. Selective inhibition of soluble TNF was protective in EAE, increasing myelination, while non-selective inhibition with RA drugs was not [108]. Non-selective inhibition increased memory B cells in rheumatoid factor positive RA patients [109]. These are the cells depleted by the beneficial B cell depletion therapy. In addition, TNF knockout yields prolonged expansion of activated memory T cells, which exacerbates EAE [110].

Thus, it seems that the non-selective TNFa inhibitors that are approved and used for treating non-MS conditions act mainly to enhance memory B cells (which is not surprising, given that a major role of TNFa is to promote B cell function), which has a negative effect in MS.

COX. COX inhibitors, which oppose TNF-C1P action by preventing PG E2 synthesis, are beneficial in MS [102].

8.5 Discussion

This chapter presented the first theory of MS that explains its pathological mechanisms. Contrary to the prevailing dominating T cell dogma, T*MS posits that the main phenomenon in MS is driven by ceramide products. T*MS shows how activated B cells (e.g., as a result of reactivated EBV) can cause demyelination by secreting cytokines, mainly TNFa, that break down myelin lipids essential for myelin maintenance. This novel account provides evidence for the causal role of B cell activation and EBV in MS etiology, and explains various perplexing properties of MS, the main one being why a relapsing-remitting disease course is so common.

T cells, B cells. T cells are involved in MS, and have been historically viewed as the primary participants in MS immunity and pathology, with the role of B cells being that of presenting antigens to T cells [3,111]. This can probably be attributed to the association of MS with an inflammatory T help profile, and the central role of T cells in models of demyelinating disease [61]. However, as cited above, the evidence for T cell autoimmunity in MS is actually weak [4,5], and no convincing mechanisms for T cell-induced myelin damage have been described. Recently, it has become clear that B cells play a major role, mainly due to the dramatic benefit of B cell depletion therapies [3,61]. Nonetheless, the precise role of B cells in MS, and the etiology of MS, are unknown at present [3,61]. The present paper closes this gap. People should stop describing MS as a T cell disease and start describing it as a B cell disease. T cells are certainly activated, but their role is secondary.

Other theories. In general, the demyelination mechanisms in MS are currently considered to be unknown [8]. The idea that myelin lipids are central in the disease has been raised [17], without the presentation of detailed mechanisms. A hypothesis in the direction of the present account has been presented in the previous century [112]. It identified TNFa as a major factor, but did not go further. Likewise, the possible role of immune cytokines, including TNF family members, in brain penetration by immune cells has been previously discussed [113].

Autoimmunity. The account here resolves one of the major puzzles of MS: the lack of evidence for antigens attacking myelin. MS is not a classical autoimmune disease in this sense, but it is an autoimmune disease in the literal sense, because the disease pathology is indeed induced by agents abnormally released by immune cells. These agents are not released as part of the final immune response, but mainly as part of the initial immune response, where immune cells destabilize membranes so that they could penetrate tissues to do their job (although memory B cells seem to be strongly involved).

Cancer. The account in this chapter can be easily extended to provide a novel account of several types of cancer. B cell lymphomas invoke similar mechanisms to those described in this chapter to disseminate themselves and penetrate tissue. Cancer has not been discussed in this chapter in order to keep it focused. It will hopefully be described elsewhere.

Strengths and weaknesses. The main strength of the current theory is that it finally describes a convincing coherent biological account of what causes demyelination in MS. Its main weakness is that it does not fully explain the effects of non-selective TNFa inhibitors (although the fact that they enhance memory B cells does provide a good account).

T*MS is not a complete theory of MS, because there are some important EBV-related questions that it does not answer (and does not purport to answer). First, it is not clear why EBV reactivation induces MS in some people, but does not do so in other people. Symptomatic EBV infection manifested as infectious mononucleosis dramatically increases MS risk [49], but most patients do not get MS. Second, it is not clear whether reactivated EBV is a necessary condition for MS, or whether it is possible to get MS via other means (e.g., persistent non-EBV immune activation). Third, it is not clear why some people with EBV get cancers, while others get MS. Fourth, it is not clear why EBV specifically affects GalCer and SPM more than other ceramide products. The answer might be related to the fact that EBV cell entry is mediated by glycoproteins (the protein equivalent of cerebrosides) [114]. It can be speculated that EBV hijacks the galactose stores in GalCer to expediate its cellular entry. Finally, it can be asked why the main damage is in the brain and not in other tissues (ignoring EBV lymphomas). This might be related to special properties of EBV, or to tissue lipid composition (the previous point).

Theory predictions. A bold prediction is that there should be a ceramide-based treatment that dramatically improves patient state and prevents relapse. Treatment that directly targets ceramide products might be more effective that TNF-based treatment, because although TNFa is the central focus in the untreated state, other immune-related cytokines can also probably drive the disease, certainly in its progressive form.

List of abbreviations

aSMase: acid sphingomyelin phosphodiesterase.
BBB: blood-brain barrier.
C1P: ceramide 1-phosphate.
COX: cyclooxygenase.
EBV: Epstein-Barr virus.
EAE: Experimental autoimmune encephalomyelitis.
GalCer: alpha-galactosylceramide (a cerebroside).
GlcCer: glucosylceramide (a cerebroside).
MS: multiple sclerosis.
nSMase: neutral sphingomyelin phosphodiesterase.
OLG: oligodendrocyte.
OPC: oligodendrocyte precursor cell.
RA: rheumatoid arthritis.

PG: prostaglandin.
S1P: sphingosine 1-phosphate.
SPM: sphingomyelin.
SMase: sphingomyelin phosphodiesterase.
sulfatide: sulfated GalCer.
TNFa: tumor necrosis factor alpha.

References

[1] D.S. Reich, C.F. Lucchinetti, P.A. Calabresi, Multiple Sclerosis, The New England Journal of Medicine 378 (2018) 169–180, available from https://api.semanticscholar.org/CorpusID:26576337.
[2] E. Leray, T. Moreau, A. Fromont, G. Edan, Epidemiology of multiple sclerosis, Revue Neurologique 172 (1) (2016) 3–13.
[3] C. Baecher-Allan, B.J. Kaskow, H.L. Weiner, Multiple sclerosis: mechanisms and immunotherapy, Neuron 97 (4) (2018) 742–768.
[4] A. Chaudhuri, P.O. Behan, Multiple sclerosis is not an autoimmune disease, Archives of Neurology (2004) 10:1610–2, available from https://api.semanticscholar.org/CorpusID:2370622.
[5] B. Wootla, M. Eriguchi, M. Rodriguez, Is multiple sclerosis an autoimmune disease?, Autoimmune Diseases 2012 (1) (2012) 969657.
[6] K. Bjornevik, C. Münz, J.I. Cohen, A. Ascherio, Epstein–Barr virus as a leading cause of multiple sclerosis: mechanisms and implications, Nature Reviews Neurology 19 (3) (2023) 160–171.
[7] B. Serafini, B. Rosicarelli, D. Franciotta, R. Magliozzi, R. Reynolds, P. Cinque, et al., Dysregulated Epstein-Barr virus infection in the multiple sclerosis brain, The Journal of Experimental Medicine 204 (12) (2007) 2899–2912.
[8] H. Lassmann, Multiple sclerosis: lessons from molecular neuropathology, Experimental Neurology 262 (2014) 2–7.
[9] Y.A. Hannun, L.M. Obeid, Sphingolipids and their metabolism in physiology and disease, Nature Reviews. Molecular Cell Biology 19 (3) (2018) 175–191.
[10] G. Van Niel, G. d'Angelo, G. Raposo, Shedding light on the cell biology of extracellular vesicles, Nature Reviews. Molecular Cell Biology 19 (4) (2018) 213–228.
[11] K. Harzer, B.C. Paton, H. Christomanou, M. Chatelut, T. Levade, M. Hiraiwa, et al., Saposins (sap) A and C activate the degradation of galactosylceramide in living cells, FEBS Letters 417 (3) (1997) 270–274.
[12] M.J. Kim, H. Jeong, D. Krainc, Lysosomal ceramides regulate cathepsin B-mediated processing of saposin C and glucocerebrosidase activity, Human Molecular Genetics (2022).
[13] A.A. Baeyens, S.R. Schwab, Finding a way out: S1P signaling and immune cell migration, Annual Review of Immunology 38 (1) (2020) 759–784.
[14] N. Presa, A. Gomez-Larrauri, I.G. Rivera, M. Ordoñez, M. Trueba, A. Gomez-Muñoz, Regulation of cell migration and inflammation by ceramide 1-phosphate, Biochimica et Biophysica Acta (BBA)-Molecular and Cell Biology of Lipids 1861 (5) (2016) 402–409.
[15] Q. Chen, K.L. Mosovsky, A.C. Ross, Retinoic acid and α-galactosylceramide regulate the expression of costimulatory receptors and transcription factors responsible for B cell activation and differentiation, Immunobiology 218 (12) (2013) 1477–1487.
[16] C. Stadelmann, S. Timmler, A. Barrantes-Freer, M. Simons, Myelin in the central nervous system: structure, function, and pathology, Physiological Reviews (2019).
[17] M. Podbielska, E. Hogan, Molecular and immunogenic features of myelin lipids: incitants or modulators of multiple sclerosis?, Multiple Sclerosis Journal 15 (9) (2009) 1011–1029.
[18] J.M. Boggs, Role of galactosylceramide and sulfatide in oligodendrocytes and CNS myelin: formation of a glycosynapse, in: Glycobiology of the Nervous System, Springer, 2014, pp. 263–291.

[19] N. Jackman, A. Ishii, R. Bansal, Oligodendrocyte development and myelin biogenesis: parsing out the roles of glycosphingolipids, Physiology 24 (5) (2009) 290–297.

[20] D. Kremer, P. Göttle, H.P. Hartung, P. Küry, Pushing forward: remyelination as the new frontier in CNS diseases, Trends in Neurosciences 39 (4) (2016) 246–263.

[21] R. Rochford, M.J. Cannon, R.E. Sabbe, K. Adusumilli, G. Picchio, J.M. Glynn, et al., Common and idiosyncratic patterns of cytokine gene expression by Epstein-Barr virus transformed human B cell lines, Viral Immunology 10 (4) (1997) 183–195.

[22] I. Wilson, F. Platt, D. Isenberg, T. Rademacher, Aberrant control of galactosyltransferase in peripheral B lymphocytes and Epstein-Barr virus transformed B lymphoblasts from patients with rheumatoid arthritis, Journal of Rheumatology 20 (8) (1993) 1282–1287.

[23] S. Jakhmola, H.C. Jha, Glial cell response to Epstein-Barr Virus infection: A plausible contribution to virus-associated inflammatory reactions in the brain, Virology 559 (2021) 182–195.

[24] L.M. Hutt-Fletcher, The long and complicated relationship between Epstein-Barr virus and epithelial cells, Journal of Virology 91 (1) (2017) 10–1128.

[25] M.R. Eichelberg, R. Welch, J.T. Guidry, A. Ali, M. Ohashi, K.R. Makielski, et al., Epstein-Barr virus infection promotes epithelial cell growth by attenuating differentiation-dependent exit from the cell cycle, MBio 10 (4) (2019) 10–1128.

[26] S. Kijimoto-Ochiai, A. Noguchi, T. Ohnishi, Y. Araki, Complex formation of CD23/surface immunoglobulin and CD23/CD81/MHC class II on an EBV-transformed human B cell line and inferable role of tetraspanin, Microbiology and Immunology 48 (5) (2004) 417–426.

[27] J. Gordon, CD23 and B cell activation, Clinical and Experimental Allergy 22 (2) (1992).

[28] S. Fujiwara, H. Nakamura, Animal models for gammaherpesvirus infections: recent development in the analysis of virus-induced pathogenesis, Pathogens 9 (2) (2020) 116.

[29] R.M. Bove, Why monkeys do not get multiple sclerosis (spontaneously) An evolutionary approach, Evolution, Medicine, and Public Health 2018 (1) (2018) 43–59.

[30] E. Kemanetzoglou, E. Andreadou, CNS demyelination with TNF-α blockers, Current Neurology and Neuroscience Reports 17 (2017) 1–15.

[31] S. Lecoanet-Henchoz, J.F. Gauchat, J.P. Aubry, P. Graber, P. Life, N. Paul-Eugene, et al., CD23 regulates monocyte activation through a novel interaction with the adhesion molecules CD11b-CD18 and CD11c-CD18, Immunity 3 (1) (1995) 119–125.

[32] J.D. Lay, C.J. Tsao, J.Y. Chen, M.E. Kadin, I.J. Su, Upregulation of tumor necrosis factor-alpha gene by Epstein-Barr virus and activation of macrophages in Epstein-Barr virus-infected T cells in the pathogenesis of hemophagocytic syndrome, The Journal of Clinical Investigation 100 (8) (1997) 1969–1979.

[33] J. Ho, R. Liang, G. Srivastava, Differential cytokine expression in EBV positive peripheral T cell lymphomas, Molecular Pathology 52 (5) (1999) 269.

[34] K. Hernádi, E. Gyöngyösi, B. Mészáros, L. Szakács, A. Szalmás, E. Csoma, et al., Elevated tumor necrosis factor-alpha expression in periapical lesions infected by Epstein-Barr virus, Journal of Endodontics 39 (4) (2013) 456–460.

[35] Inhibition of TSH-induced hydrogen peroxide production by TNF-alpha through a sphingomyelinase signaling pathway, American Journal of Physiology: Endocrinology and Metabolism 273 (3) (1997) E638.

[36] C.J. Clarke, T.G. Truong, Y.A. Hannun, Role for neutral sphingomyelinase-2 in tumor necrosis factor α-stimulated expression of vascular cell adhesion molecule-1 (VCAM) and intercellular adhesion molecule-1 (ICAM) in lung epithelial cells: p38 MAPK is an upstream regulator of nSMase2, Journal of Biological Chemistry 282 (2) (2007) 1384–1396.

[37] B.M. Barth, S.J. Gustafson, J.L. Hankins, J.M. Kaiser, J.K. Haakenson, M. Kester, et al., Ceramide kinase regulates TNFα-stimulated NADPH oxidase activity and eicosanoid biosynthesis in neuroblastoma cells, Cellular Signalling 24 (6) (2012) 1126–1133.

[38] A.A. Shamseddine, M.V. Airola, Y.A. Hannun, Roles and regulation of neutral sphingomyelinase-2 in cellular and pathological processes, Advances in Biological Regulation 57 (2015) 24–41.

[39] G. Chakraborty, S. Ziemba, A. Drivas, R. Ledeen, Myelin contains neutral sphingomyelinase activity that is stimulated by tumor necrosis factor-α, Journal of Neuroscience Research 50 (3) (1997) 466–476.

[40] X. Yang, W. Sheng, D. Ridgley, M. Haidekker, G. Sun, J. Lee, Astrocytes regulate α-secretase-cleaved soluble amyloid precursor protein secretion in neuronal cells: Involvement of group IIA secretory phospholipase A2, Neuroscience 300 (2015) 508–517.

[41] R.K. Barr, H.E. Lynn, P.A. Moretti, Y. Khew-Goodall, S.M. Pitson, Deactivation of sphingosine kinase 1 by protein phosphatase 2A, Journal of Biological Chemistry 283 (50) (2008) 34994–35002.

[42] M.E. Guicciardi, J. Deussing, H. Miyoshi, S.F. Bronk, P.A. Svingen, C. Peters, et al., Cathepsin B contributes to TNF-α–mediated hepatocyte apoptosis by promoting mitochondrial release of cytochrome c, The Journal of Clinical Investigation 106 (9) (2000) 1127–1137.

[43] L. Foghsgaard, D. Wissing, D. Mauch, U. Lademann, L. Bastholm, M. Boes, et al., Cathepsin B acts as a dominant execution protease in tumor cell apoptosis induced by tumor necrosis factor, The Journal of Cell Biology 153 (5) (2001) 999–1010.

[44] S. Kim, A.J. Steelman, H. Koito, J. Li, Astrocytes promote TNF-mediated toxicity to oligodendrocyte precursors, Journal of Neurochemistry 116 (1) (2011) 53–66.

[45] Z. Su, Y. Yuan, J. Chen, Y. Zhu, Y. Qiu, F. Zhu, et al., Reactive astrocytes inhibit the survival and differentiation of oligodendrocyte precursor cells by secreted TNF-α, Journal of Neurotrauma 28 (6) (2011) 1089–1100.

[46] L. Probert, TNF and its receptors in the CNS: The essential, the desirable and the deleterious effects, Neuroscience 302 (2015) 2–22.

[47] E. Oudejans, A. Luchicchi, E.M. Strijbis, J.J. Geurts, A.M. van Dam, Is MS affecting the CNS only? Lessons from clinic to myelin pathophysiology, Neurology: Neuroimmunology & Neuroinflammation 8 (1) (2021) e914.

[48] P. Morell (Ed.), Myelin, 2nd ed., Springer Science & Business Media, 1984.

[49] K.A. McKay, S. Jahanfar, T. Duggan, S. Tkachuk, H. Tremlett, Factors associated with onset, relapses or progression in multiple sclerosis: a systematic review, Neurotoxicology 61 (2017) 189–212.

[50] S. Daher, F. Fonseca, O.G. Ribeiro, C.C. Musatti, M. Gerbase-DeLima, Tumor necrosis factor during pregnancy and at the onset of labor and spontaneous abortion, European Journal of Obstetrics & Gynecology and Reproductive Biology 83 (1) (1999) 77–79.

[51] M. Muilwijk, N. Callender, S. Goorden, F.M. Vaz, I.G. van Valkengoed, Sex differences in the association of sphingolipids with age in Dutch and South-Asian Surinamese living in Amsterdam, the Netherlands, Biology of Sex Differences 12 (2021) 1–14.

[52] K. Zwerina, W. Baum, R. Axmann, G.R. Heiland, J.H.W. Distler, J.S. Smolen, et al., Vitamin D receptor regulates TNF-mediated arthritis, Annals of the Rheumatic Diseases 70 () (2011) 1122–1129, available from https://api.semanticscholar.org/CorpusID:10781969.

[53] C. Tao, S. Simpson, I. Van Der Mei, L. Blizzard, E. Havrdova, D. Horakova, et al., Higher latitude is significantly associated with an earlier age of disease onset in multiple sclerosis, Journal of Neurology, Neurosurgery and Psychiatry 87 (12) (2016) 1343–1349.

[54] M. Komatsu, T. Takahashi, T. Abe, I. Takahashi, H. Ida, G. Takada, Evidence for the association of ultraviolet-C and H2O2-induced apoptosis with acid sphingomyelinase activation, Biochimica et Biophysica Acta (BBA)-Molecular and Cell Biology of Lipids 1533 (1) (2001) 47–54.

[55] Ionizing radiation acts on cellular membranes to generate ceramide and initiate apoptosis, The Journal of Experimental Medicine 180 (2) (1994) 525–535.

[56] L. Belbasis, V. Bellou, E. Evangelou, J.P. Ioannidis, I. Tzoulaki, Environmental risk factors and multiple sclerosis: an umbrella review of systematic reviews and meta-analyses, The Lancet Neurology 14 (3) (2015) 263–273.

[57] D.G. Yanbaeva, M.A. Dentener, E.C. Creutzberg, G. Wesseling, E.F. Wouters, Systemic effects of smoking, Chest 131 (5) (2007) 1557–1566.

[58] M. Levy, E. Khan, M. Careaga, T. Goldkorn, Neutral sphingomyelinase 2 is activated by cigarette smoke to augment ceramide-induced apoptosis in lung cell death, American Journal of Physiology. Lung Cellular and Molecular Physiology 297 (1) (2009) L125–L133.
[59] A.F. Badawi, S.L. Habib, M.A. Mohammed, A.A. Abadi, M.S. Michael, Influence of cigarette smoking on prostaglandin synthesis and cyclooxygenase-2 gene expression in human urinary bladder cancer, Cancer Investigation 20 (5–6) (2002) 651–656.
[60] G.F. Quimby, C.A. Bonnice, S.H. Burstein, G.L. Eastwood, Active smoking depresses prostaglandin synthesis in human gastric mucosa, Annals of Internal Medicine 104 (5) (1986) 616–619.
[61] M.T. Cencioni, M. Mattoscio, R. Magliozzi, A. Bar-Or, P.A. Muraro, B cells in multiple sclerosis – from targeted depletion to immune reconstitution therapies, Nature Reviews Neurology 17 (2021) 399–414, available from https://api.semanticscholar.org/CorpusID:235272257.
[62] M.P. Pender, The essential role of Epstein-Barr virus in the pathogenesis of multiple sclerosis, The Neuroscientist 17 (4) (2011) 351–367.
[63] A. Gottlieb, H.P.T. Pham, J.G. Saltarrelli, J.W. Lindsey, Expanded T lymphocytes in the cerebrospinal fluid of multiple sclerosis patients are specific for Epstein-Barr-virus-infected B cells, Proceedings of the National Academy of Sciences 121 (3) (2024) e2315857121.
[64] J. Beck, P. Rondot, L. Catinot, E. Falcoff, H. Kirchner, J. Wietzerbin, Increased production of interferon gamma and tumor necrosis factor precedes clinical manifestation in multiple sclerosis: do cytokines trigger off exacerbations?, Acta Neurologica Scandinavica 78 (4) (1988) 318–323.
[65] P. Rieckmann, M. Albrecht, B. Kitze, T. Weber, H. Tumani, A. Broocks, et al., Cytokine mRNA levels in mononuclear blood cells from patients with multiple sclerosis, Neurology 44 (8) (1994) 1523.
[66] M. Zaffaroni, L.G. Stampino, A. Ghezzi, S.M. Baldini, A. Zibetti, In vitro cytokine, sCD23 and IgG secretion in multiple sclerosis, Journal of Neuroimmunology 61 (1) (1995) 1–5.
[67] M.K. Sharief, R. Hentges, Association between tumor necrosis factor-α and disease progression in patients with multiple sclerosis, The New England Journal of Medicine 325 (7) (1991) 467–472.
[68] F. Hofman, D. Hinton, K. Johnson, J. Merrill, Tumor necrosis factor identified in multiple sclerosis brain, The Journal of Experimental Medicine 170 (2) (1989) 607–612.
[69] K. Selmaj, C.S. Raine, B. Cannella, C.F. Brosnan, Identification of lymphotoxin and tumor necrosis factor in multiple sclerosis lesions, The Journal of Clinical Investigation 87 (3) (1991) 949–954.
[70] B. Cannella, C.S. Raine, The adhesion molecule and cytokine profile of multiple sclerosis lesions, Annals of Neurology: Official Journal of the American Neurological Association and the Child Neurology Society 37 (4) (1995) 424–435.
[71] A. Goris, S. Sawcer, K. Vandenbroeck, H. Carton, A. Billiau, E. Setakis, et al., New candidate loci for multiple sclerosis susceptibility revealed by a whole genome association screen in a Belgian population, Journal of Neuroimmunology 143 (1–2) (2003) 65–69.
[72] B.A. Sela, G. Konat, H. Offner, Elevated ganglioside concentration in serum and peripheral blood lymphocytes from multiple sclerosis patients in remission, Journal of the Neurological Sciences 54 (1) (1982) 143–148.
[73] A. Kułakowska, M. Żendzian-Piotrowska, M. Baranowski, T. Konończuk, W. Drozdowski, J. Górski, et al., Intrathecal increase of sphingosine 1-phosphate at early stage multiple sclerosis, Neuroscience Letters 477 (3) (2010) 149–152.
[74] S. Kim, A.J. Steelman, Y. Zhang, H.C. Kinney, J. Li, Aberrant upregulation of astroglial ceramide potentiates oligodendrocyte injury, Brain Pathology 22 (1) (2012) 41–57.
[75] J. Kurz, R. Brunkhorst, C. Foerch, L. Blum, M. Henke, L. Gabriel, et al., The relevance of ceramides and their synthesizing enzymes for multiple sclerosis, Clinical Science 132 (17) (2018) 1963–1976.

[76] C. Leurs, M.L. Pinheiro, L. Wierts, S. den Hoedt, M. Mulder, A. Eijlers, et al., Acid sphingomyelinase: No potential as a biomarker for multiple sclerosis, Multiple Sclerosis and Related Disorders 28 (2019) 44–49.
[77] D. Pieragostino, I. Cicalini, P. Lanuti, E. Ercolino, M. di Ioia, M. Zucchelli, et al., Enhanced release of acid sphingomyelinase-enriched exosomes generates a lipidomics signature in CSF of Multiple Sclerosis patients, Scientific Reports 8 (1) (2018) 1–12.
[78] R. van Doorn, P.G. Nijland, N. Dekker, M.E. Witte, M.A. Lopes-Pinheiro, B. van het Hof, et al., Fingolimod attenuates ceramide-induced blood–brain barrier dysfunction in multiple sclerosis by targeting reactive astrocytes, Acta Neuropathologica 124 (3) (2012) 397–410.
[79] G. Capodivento, D. Visigalli, M. Garnero, R. Fancellu, M.D. Ferrara, A. Basit, et al., Sphingomyelin as a myelin biomarker in CSF of acquired demyelinating neuropathies, Scientific Reports 7 (1) (2017) 1–9.
[80] M. Podbielska, Z.M. Szulc, E. Kurowska, E.L. Hogan, J. Bielawski, A. Bielawska, et al., Cytokine-induced release of ceramide-enriched exosomes as a mediator of cell death signaling in an oligodendroglioma cell line, Journal of Lipid Research 57 (11) (2016) 2028–2039.
[81] K.A. Becker, R. Halmer, L. Davies, B.D. Henry, R. Ziobro-Henry, Y. Decker, et al., Blockade of experimental multiple sclerosis by inhibition of the acid sphingomyelinase/ceramide system, Neurosignals 25 (1) (2017) 88–97.
[82] M. Chami, R. Halmer, L. Schnoeder, K. Anne Becker, C. Meier, K. Fassbender, et al., Acid sphingomyelinase deficiency enhances myelin repair after acute and chronic demyelination, PLoS ONE 12 (6) (2017) e0178622.
[83] A. Jana, K. Pahan, Oxidative stress kills human primary oligodendrocytes via neutral sphingomyelinase: implications for multiple sclerosis, Journal of Neuroimmune Pharmacology 2 (2) (2007) 184–193.
[84] R. Wilson, D.R. Tocher, Lipid and fatty acid composition is altered in plaque tissue from multiple sclerosis brain compared with normal brain white matter, Lipids 26 (1) (1991) 9–15.
[85] B. Gerstl, L. Eng, M. Tavaststjerna, J. Smith, S. Kruse, Lipids and proteins in multiple sclerosis white matter, Journal of Neurochemistry 17 (5) (1970) 677–689.
[86] J. Clausen, I.B. Hansen, Myelin constituents of human central nervous system: studies of phospholipid, glycolipid, and fatty acid pattern in normal and multiple sclerosis brains, Acta Neurologica Scandinavica 46 (1) (1970) 1–17.
[87] H. Woelk, P. Borri, Lipid and fatty acid composition of myelin purified from normal and MS brains, European Neurology 10 (4) (1973) 250–260.
[88] A.L. Moyano, G. Li, A.I. Boullerne, D.L. Feinstein, E. Hartman, D. Skias, et al., Sulfatides in extracellular vesicles isolated from plasma of multiple sclerosis patients, Journal of Neuroscience Research 94 (12) (2016) 1579–1587.
[89] B.N. Marbois, K.F. Faull, A.L. Fluharty, S. Raval-Fernandes, L.H. Rome, Analysis of sulfatide from rat cerebellum and multiple sclerosis white matter by negative ion electrospray mass spectrometry, Biochimica et Biophysica Acta 1 (2000) 59–70, available from https://api.semanticscholar.org/CorpusID:30224338.
[90] C. Alling, L. Svennerholm, et al., Lipid alterations in apparently normal white matter in multiple sclerosis, Brain Research 35 (2) (1971) 325–336.
[91] M.L. Cuzner, A. Davison, Changes in cerebral lysosomal enzyme activity and lipids in multiple sclerosis, Journal of the Neurological Sciences 19 (1) (1973) 29–36.
[92] C. Lubetzki, Y.T. PharmD, A.G. PharmD, O. Lyon-Caen, F. Lhermitte, B. Zalc, Galactosylceramide: a reliable serum index of demyelination in multiple sclerosis, Annals of Neurology: Official Journal of the American Neurological Association and the Child Neurology Society 26 (3) (1989) 407–409.
[93] N. Baumann, M. Lemonnier, C. Jacque, R. Marteau, M. Harpin, F. Lhermitte, Plasma galactocerebrosides in multiple sclerosis, Biomedicine/[publiee Pour l'AAICIG] 23 (9) (1975) 387–390.
[94] S. Yahara, N. Kawamura, Y. Kishimoto, T. Saida, W.W. Tourtellotte, A change in the cerebrosides and sulfatides in a demyelinating nervous system: development of the methodology and

study of multiple sclerosis and Wallerian degeneration, Journal of the Neurological Sciences 54 (2) (1982) 303–315.

[95] A. Nagai, Y. Murakawa, M. Terashima, K. Shimode, N. Umegae, H. Takeuchi, et al., Cystatin C and cathepsin B in CSF from patients with inflammatory neurologic diseases, Neurology 55 (12) (2000) 1828–1832.

[96] J.L. Kanter, S. Narayana, P.P. Ho, I. Catz, K.G. Warren, R.A. Sobel, et al., Lipid microarrays identify key mediators of autoimmune brain inflammation, Nature Medicine 12 (1) (2006) 138–143.

[97] A.A. Ilyas, Z.W. Chen, S.D. Cook, Antibodies to sulfatide in cerebrospinal fluid of patients with multiple sclerosis, Journal of Neuroimmunology 139 (1–2) (2003) 76–80.

[98] D. Wheeler, V.V.R. Bandaru, P.A. Calabresi, A. Nath, N.J. Haughey, A defect of sphingolipid metabolism modifies the properties of normal appearing white matter in multiple sclerosis, Brain 131 (11) (2008) 3092–3102.

[99] K. Suzuki, S. Kamoshita, Y. Eto, W.W. Tourtellotte, J.O. Gonatas, Myelin in multiple sclerosis: composition of myelin from normal-appearing white matter, Archives of Neurology 28 (5) (1973) 293–297.

[100] N. Mattsson, M. Yaong, L.E. Rosengren, K. Blennow, J.E. Månsson, O. Andersen, et al., Elevated cerebrospinal fluid levels of prostaglandin E2 and 15-(S)-hydroxyeicosatetraenoic acid in multiple sclerosis, Journal of Internal Medicine (2009) 265, available from https://api.semanticscholar.org/CorpusID:43130433.

[101] P. Dore-Duffy, J.O. Donaldson, T. Koff, M. Longo, W.B. Perry, Prostaglandin release in multiple sclerosis: correlation with disease activity, Neurology 36 (1986) 1587, available from https://api.semanticscholar.org/CorpusID:2727439.

[102] M. Hoxha, E. Spahiu, E. Prendi, B. Zappacosta, A systematic review on the role of arachidonic acid pathway in multiple sclerosis, CNS & Neurological Disorders Drug Targets (2020), available from https://api.semanticscholar.org/CorpusID:221327341.

[103] L.G. Miller, J.A. Young, S.K. Ray, G. Wang, S. Purohit, N.L. Banik, et al., Sphingosine toxicity in EAE and MS: evidence for ceramide generation via serine-palmitoyltransferase activation, Neurochemical Research 42 (2017) 2755–2768.

[104] M. Margoni, P. Preziosa, M. Filippi, M.A. Rocca, Anti-CD20 therapies for multiple sclerosis: current status and future perspectives, Journal of Neurology 269 (3) (2022) 1316–1334.

[105] D. Pelletier, D.A. Hafler, Fingolimod for multiple sclerosis, The New England Journal of Medicine 366 (4) (2012) 339–347.

[106] J. Skácel, B.S. Slusher, T. Tsukamoto, Small molecule inhibitors targeting biosynthesis of ceramide, the central hub of the sphingolipid network, Journal of Medicinal Chemistry 64 (1) (2021) 279–297.

[107] J. Mostert, F. Admiraal-Behloul, J. Hoogduin, J. Luyendijk, D. Heersema, M. Van Buchem, et al., Effects of fluoxetine on disease activity in relapsing multiple sclerosis: a double-blind, placebo-controlled, exploratory study, Journal of Neurology, Neurosurgery and Psychiatry 79 (9) (2008) 1027–1031.

[108] R. Brambilla, J.J. Ashbaugh, R. Magliozzi, A. Dellarole, S. Karmally, D.E. Szymkowski, et al., Inhibition of soluble tumour necrosis factor is therapeutic in experimental autoimmune encephalomyelitis and promotes axon preservation and remyelination, Brain 134 (9) (2011) 2736–2754.

[109] P. Roll, K. Muhammad, M. Schumann, S. Kleinert, H. Tony, RF positivity has substantial influence on the peripheral memory B-cell compartment and its modulation by TNF inhibition, Scandinavian Journal of Rheumatology 41 (3) (2012) 180–185.

[110] G. Kassiotis, G. Kollias, Uncoupling the proinflammatory from the immunosuppressive properties of tumor necrosis factor (TNF) at the p55 TNF receptor level: implications for pathogenesis and therapy of autoimmune demyelination, The Journal of Experimental Medicine 193 (4) (2001) 427–434.

[111] V.K. Kuchroo, H.L. Weiner, How does Epstein-Barr virus trigger MS?, Immunity 55 (3) (2022) 390–392.

[112] R.W. Ledeen, G. Chakraborty, Cytokines, signal transduction, and inflammatory demyelination: review and hypothesis, Neurochemical Research 23 (1998) 277–289.
[113] C. Larochelle, J.I. Alvarez, A. Prat, How do immune cells overcome the blood–brain barrier in multiple sclerosis?, FEBS Letters 585 (23) (2011) 3770–3780.
[114] C. Shannon-Lowe, Rowe M. Epstein, Barr virus entry, kissing and conjugation, Current Opinion in Virology 4 (2014) 78–84.

Chapter 9

A calcium channel $\alpha 2\delta$ subunit theory of amyotrophic lateral sclerosis and frontotemporal dementia

9.1 Introduction

Amyotrophic lateral sclerosis (ALS) is a fatal disease involving the degeneration of motor neurons (MTNs) [1,2]. Most patients exhibit sporadic ALS (sALS), whose etiology is not known, while 10% of the patients show a familial form (fALS) that involves identified genetic mutations. In both variants, approved treatments only have a marginal benefit, and death occurs a few years after diagnosis. There is substantial overlap between ALS and frontotemporal dementia (FTD), especially its behavioral variant (FTDbv), which is associated with TDP43 [3].

Beyond a few initial hypotheses [4], there is currently no theory that addresses the major facts of sALS, fALS or FTD. Here I present a new theory of ALS and FTDbv that explains their etiology, pathophysiology, and clinical symptoms. The main thesis is that sALS is caused by an impairment of the $\alpha 2\delta$ (a2d) subunit of high voltage-activated voltage-gated calcium channels (H-VGCCs), most likely due to autoimmune targeting. This results in chronically higher calcium entry throughout life, which eventually yields toxicity that causes the disease symptoms, cellular stress and degeneration. The mutations associated with fALS also induce chronic calcium, with similar downstream consequences.

Section 9.2 provides general background on VGCCs and the a2d subunit, including its role in synapse development, signaling, and maintenance. Section 9.3 explains the reasons for suspecting a2d, and presents an account of the specific calcium and a2d impairment in ALS. Section 9.4 details evidence supporting the theory, including calcium dysregulation in ALS, the explanatory power of chronic calcium for the facts known about ALS, a2d evidence, and insulin-related evidence. Section 9.5 discusses autoimmunity in ALS, and Section 9.6 discusses FTD.

The Science of the Brain. https://doi.org/10.1016/B978-0-44-345008-2.00015-1

9.2 Voltage-gated calcium channels (VGCCs)

General background. The family of VGCCs includes high voltage-activated VGCCs (H-VGCC) and the low voltage-activated T-type VGCC, which is not involved in ALS. H-VGCCs are comprised of a pore alpha1 (a1) subunit, an auxiliary beta subunit, and an auxiliary a2d subunit [5–8]. Each of these has several gene variants and some have alternative splicing variants. H-VGCCs include L-VGCC (L-type, Cav1), P/Q-VGCC (Cav2.1), N-VGCC (Cav2.2), and R-VGCC (Cav2.3). H-VGCCs are activated in relatively depolarized membrane potentials and support transmitter release and sustained execution.

Cav1.1 is expressed in skeletal muscle, where it promotes voltage sensing, calcium outflux from the sarcoplasmic reticulum, and excitation-contraction coupling. Cav1.2 is expressed in neurons, the cardiovascular system, pancreas beta cells, adrenal chromaffin cells [9], and skin [10]. Cav1.3 is expressed in metabolism and valence areas, including the extended amygdala, hypothalamus nuclei, and brainstem [11]. Cav2.1 is expressed in neurons, including MTN axons (presynaptically) and cerebellar Purkinje cells. Cav2.2 is highly expressed throughout the brain during development, with high cortex and hippocampus expression remaining in adulthood [12]. Cav2.3 is expressed in neurons, cardiac and smooth muscle, and beta cells [7]. L-VGCC-like channels are expressed in immune cells, including B cells and T cells [13–17].

The a2d subunits. The a2d subunit is present in L-VGCC, P/Q-VGCC, and N-VGCC [6]. There are four a2d genes, a2d1-4. The subunit is generated by a single gene whose product is cleaved into two disulfide-bonded polypeptides. This cleavage is essential for its function [18]. The subunit is extracellular, glycosylated, and GPI-anchored at the membrane [19].

With respect to distribution, a2d1 is widely expressed in the brain, mainly in excitatory neurons, including in the hippocampus, hypothalamus, the insula, olfactory areas, and dorsal root ganglia [20,21]. It is less strongly expressed in frontal areas. It is expressed in skeletal muscle [22], the heart, smooth muscle [6] and pancreatic beta cells, where it is the main a2d subunit [23]. a2d2 is mainly expressed in inhibitory neurons and in the cerebellum [20]. It is also expressed in immune T cells [17]. a2d3 is expressed in MTNs and caudate-putamen (i.e., the motor system) [20,21], and also in the retina [24]. a2d4 is limited to the retina [25].

Physiological roles of a2d. Both of the auxiliary H-VGCC subunits, beta and a2d, promote VGCC trafficking to the plasma membrane [26]. A specific role of the a2d subunit is to promote channel anchoring in stable membrane sites, including neural synapses [27]. There is unequivocal evidence that a2d promotes synapse formation, maintenance and neurotransmission [28–35]. a2d supports high amplitude synaptic calcium entry, both via VGCC activation and via association with NMDA receptors and promotion of their surface trafficking [36–38]. The subunit supports anchoring of VGCC in lipid rafts [19,39,40], and synaptic adhesion [41–44]. These roles are highly preserved: invertebrate a2d homologs are expressed at the neuromuscular junction (NMJ), where they are involved in synaptogenesis and presynaptic morphology [45,46].

We particularly emphasize the role of a2d within the larger plasticity picture of adhesion molecules such as neuroligin/neurexin and LRRTM. Such proteins connect pre- and postsynaptic sites to improve synapse stability and signaling [47]. The a2d subunit participates with these proteins in trans-synaptic nanocolumns that are connected to the cytoskeleton and restrict the spatial propagation of neurotransmitters, allowing strong and rapid downstream signaling [47].

9.3 Proposed calcium & a2d impairment in ALS

9.3.1 Motivation

Calcium evidence. The involvement of high calcium and calcium channels in ALS pathology is well-known and supported by overwhelming evidence given in Section 9.4. The present paper is the first to propose a causal role for a2d impairment. There are several reasons to focus on a2d as the main culprit in ALS, summarized here.

Suspect by subcellular location. The role of a2d is to support synapses, and synaptic impairment at the NMJ is the major pathological feature in ALS [48–52], with axon degeneration preceding MTN death.

Suspect by membrane location. a2d is located extracellularly, making it accessible to antibodies, immune cells, and other circulating factors. The beta subunits are intracellular, and the a1 subunits are transmembrane proteins.

Suspect by elimination. The antibody evidence listed in Section 9.4 clearly demonstrates autoimmune targeting of H-VGCCs in ALS. However, it does not point to any specific channel or protein, with positive results regarding the involvement of L-, P/Q-, and N-VGCCs, which have different a1 subunits. This lack of specificity with respect to a1 seems to point to the target being the a2d and/or the beta subunits (although Section 9.5 explains why this argument actually does not rule out the L-VGCC a1 subunit). However, the target could also be a region of genetic overlap between several a1 subunits. Naturally, there may also be several disease variants, each targeting a different subunit.

9.3.2 Calcium part of the theory

My account of calcium in ALS is as follows. Usually starting in early life, most likely as a result of a channelopathy or autoimmune targeting, H-VGCCs calcium metabolism is excessively active in ALS. This high basal activity provides ALS patients with physical and mental strength that are commonly higher than in other people (e.g., ALS is known to be associated with sports).

Calcium can induce toxicity, and this is eventually what it does in ALS. At some point in life, some of the tissues expressing H-VGCC start showing decreased function. There are three major such tissues, MTNs, skeletal muscle (SKM), and insulin-releasing pancreas beta cells (in FTD, it is specific areas of the brain). Cardiorespiration is also damaged, as seen by the most common death cause.

As is the case for many biological agents, healthy calcium signaling involves strong (high amplitude) influx that is rapidly terminated and cleared via negative feedback (negFB) mechanisms [53–56]. In addition, healthy signaling occurs in restricted nanodomains where the Ca^{2+} signal is boosted [57]. In ALS, due to calcium channel subunit impairment, at disease onset we have the opposite situation, prolonged and weaker signaling. This is what the term **chronic** commonly refers to. Thus, our premise is that ALS involves strong cellular calcium that at some point turns to be chronic and toxic.

9.3.3 a2d part of the theory

How does a2d impairment cause excessive calcium throughout life, which turns into chronic calcium at disease onset? The main role of a2d is to anchor the channel at stable membrane sites where it supports signaling nanodomains. Without a functioning a2d, the beta subunit still supports channel trafficking, but it is not anchored properly at the membrane. Without nanodomains, more calcium enters the cell.

Moreover, it is reasonable to assume that part of the action of a2d is to exert negative feedback on channel transcription and trafficking, because stable anchoring at the membrane is the last step needed for channel formation. Without a functioning a2d, the number of a1 subunits would be larger, which induces larger calcium entry.

A simple complementary mechanims whereby reduced a2d function can yield chronicity is by increasing the channel's lateral mobility [58], which can decouple it from the synapse and yield similar consequences as reduced negative feedback.

Which a2d? As there are four a2d genes, a theory that points to a2d needs to address their respective roles in the disease. There are at least three possible hypotheses. First, each a2d could give rise to a different disease. a2d3, which is expressed in skeletal muscle and MTNs, would be responsible for ALS; a2d1, with its cortical expression, would be the target in FTD; a2d2, with its cerebellum expression, would be involved in some variants of autoimmune cerebellum ataxia (some of which are known to attack VGCCs) [59]; and a2d4 might be involved in some autoimmune retinal diseases (see below). A problem with this (too) elegant proposal is that beta cell impairment is fundamental to ALS (see Section 9.4), and beta cells mainly express a2d1.

Another hypothesis is that the main culprit in ALS is a2d1, since it is strongly expressed in the tissues most affected in ALS (the motor system, brain, and beta cells). Yet another possibility is that all a2d subunits can be affected, since they possess considerable genetic overlap.

At present, all of these hypotheses are possible, since there is insufficient evidence to arbitrate between them. The last two seem more likely than the first for ALS, but the role of a2d2 and a2d4 in the first hypothesis may be valid.

In summary, impaired a2d function can induce chronically higher calcium entry into cells throughout life. At some point, this results in calcium toxicity that yields degeneration and death.

9.4 ALS evidence

9.4.1 Calcium

Serum, Ig, CSF evidence. There is overwhelming direct and indirect evidence that patient antibodies, serum, and CSF interact with calcium channels in ALS. A thorough search found 36 papers [60–95].

In 18 of these papers, the interaction directly involved increased calcium. Patient antibodies and sera induce the following effects: (most of these results are MTNs) increased P-VGCC currents (and open time) in cerebellum Purkinje cells [67], extracellular calcium-dependent cell death in MTN-neuroblastoma hybrid cell line (VCS4.1), prevented by N- or P-VGCC (but not L-VGCC) antagonists [68], increased calcium and vesicle number in spinal MTNs [72], increased Ca^{2+} currents in a hybrid MTN VCS4.1 cells [71], increased extracellular calcium entry via VGCCs leading to higher intracellular calcium in hybrid MTN VCS4.1 cells [77], increased Ca^{2+} influx via P/Q-VGCC, N-VGCC (only weakly via L-VGCC) in cortical synaptosomes [81], development of L-VGCC (but not P/Q-VGCC-)-induced transmitter release in the neuromuscular junction (NMJ) [84], increased presynaptic Ca^{2+} in MTNs, along with golgi patholgoy and increased golgi Ca^{2+} [82], faster H-VGCC current activation in MTNs [85], MTN degeneration and significantly increased number of Ca^{2+}-containing golgi, mitochondria, and rough endoplasmic reticulum (ER) [86], potentiation of transmitter release from MTN via influx through N-VGCC [88], necrosis, MTN degeneration, swelling and Ca^{2+} of golgi endoplasmic reticulum, mitochondria [87], increased muscle miniature end-plate potential frequency, NMJ ACh release, which are significantly decreased in P/Q-VGCC (but not N-VGCC) KO [89], intracellular Ca^{2+} release in astrocytes via IP3 (intracellular stores) [91], high rather than oscillating L-VGCC-mediated intracellular Ca^{2+} in mouse islets (in ALS patients with type 2 diabetes) [92], MTN degeneration, inclusion-like IgG accumulation, increased intracellular Ca^{2+} [93], increased number of synaptic and Ca^{2+} elevation in MTN terminals [94], and increased cytoplasmic calcium, cell death in mice MTNs [95] (the last two results are with serum of patients with identified mutations).

In 8 of the 36 papers, the interaction resulted in directly decreased Ca^{2+}. This includes decreased charge movement, peak calcium current, and slower channel inactivation in skeletal muscle L-VGCCs [63], decreased mean skeletal muscle L-VGCC open time with stabilization to a smaller amplitude [65], decreased peak L-VGCC current with increased tail current deactivation rate in mammalian skeletal muscle fibers [66], decreased charge movement and peak L-VGCC currents in isolated muscle fibers [70], depressed inward Ba^{2+}-mediated (high threshold) VGCC currents in rat cerebellum granule culture [69], suppressed intracellular Ca^{2+} increase via P/Q-VGCCs (but not N-, L-VGCC) influx in cultured neurons [74], decreased H-VGCC peak and faster and more hyperpolarized inactivation in mice DRG neurons [76], and inhibition of L-VGCC-mediated dopamine release [79].

In 8 of the 36 papers, the reported results indirectly support increased calcium, including increased NMJ presynaptic ACh release frequency following 4 hours and 4-12 week incubation [60,61], increased NMJ miniature end-plate potential frequency (resting quantal ACh release) [62], enhanced excitatory transmission in hippocampus culture via presynaptic glutamate release [75], increased CSF glutamate [78], increased NMJ spontaneous transmitter release and quantal content, with similar effects produced by caffeine via Ca^{2+} [80], increased spontaneous NMJ ACh release in 3/4 cases [83] (this paper also reported decreased spontaneous NMJ ACh release in some cases, indirectly supporting decreased calcium), and endoplasmic reticulum stress in spinal MTNs [90] (this result is with sALS CSF). These results only provide indirect support, because although increased neurotransmitter release can stem from increased calcium, it can also be due to other reasons.

The presence of VGCC antibodies was reported in several papers, including antibodies to L-VGCC [64,70,83] and P-, Q-, and N-VGCC [73]. Patient IgGs were found to be present in MTN axon terminals [96].

Many of these results were done in the same lab (Appel), but more than half of them were done by unrelated labs, over more than two decades. A technical argument was raised against the initial wave of these results [97], but it has been refuted [87].

It should be emphasized that this evidence is from ALS patients, not from animal models, which are not valid for sALS (according to the present paper).

Direct MTN evidence. There is direct and indirect evidence for calcium involvement in ALS beyond calcium-related antibody/serum effects. Calcium is significantly increased in patient muscle nerve terminals [98].

Drug evidence. Taking VGCC blockers or ACE inhibitors (which decrease intracellular Ca^{2+} [99]) against hypertension is associated with decreased ALS risk [100–102].

Genetic evidence. MTNs induced from pluripotent stem cells of patients with all major fALS-associated genes (C9orf72, SOD1, TDP43, FUS) show higher Ca^{2+} (basal and transients) [103]. In SOD1 mutants, increased MTN calcium and sodium persistent inward currents is early postnatal change [104].

Other tissue. It can be argued that a general H-VGCC impairment cannot be the core cause of ALS, because this would cause a much wider impairment than the MTN one seen in ALS. However, ALS patients actually do show wide impairment, which overlaps the distribution of H-VGCCs. In addition to MTNs and skeletal muscle issues, ALS patients show cognitive deficits [105,106], cardiorespiratory and cardiovascular damage [107–112], skin neuropathy [113–115], pain in all disease stages, sometimes before motor symptoms [116], impaired insulin secretion [117,118], Purkinje cell damage [119], and immune system dysregulation (excessive inflammation coupled with inefficient immune responses) [120]. The affected tissues are precisely those with high H-VGCC expression. In addition, calcium is significantly increased in patient blood lymphocytes [121].

The beta cell evidence is especially relevant. Like the calcium evidence, both increased and decreased insulin release have been reported [117]. The decrease is of early phase secretion [118].

The question why MTNs are more sensitive than the other tissues is discussed below.

In summary, there is overwhelming evidence for calcium dysregulation in ALS, pointing to chronic calcium.

9.4.2 Explanatory power for ALS facts

Studying the sALS literature, several major pathological phenomena can be identified: muscle use problems, muscle wasting, muscle spasms (fasciculation, twitches) (the three main clinical symptoms); symptom appearance with aging (the main epidemiological datum); degeneration of spinal or bulbar (but not ocular) MTNs (the main pathological datum); aggregation of the TDP43 protein [122], oxidative stress [123–129], and mitochondria dysfunction [130] (the main cellular data); hypermetabolism in motor areas [131] (the main imaging datum); and toxicity of patient serum/Ig/CSF (much of it related to calcium, as detailed above).

Chronic intracellular calcium can explain all of these data points. It can cause muscle spasms because intracellular Ca^{2+} elevation is what induces muscle contractions [132]. Hypermetabolism is identified using PET via increased glucose uptake capacity. Chronic calcium would yield a chronic activation of calcium pumps (PMCA, SERCA), which consume ATP [133]. Relative ATP deficiency activates AMPK, which increases Glut4 translocation to the cell surface [134] and thus glucose uptake capacity. Increased activated AMPK is indeed present in patient MTNs [135,136]. Chronically high ATP consumption can also account for muscle wasting (see also insulin discussion below).

Chronic calcium induces oxidative stress (mainly H2O2), mitochondria permeability pore opening, and ER stress [137–142]. Oxidative stress and H2O2 induce and are enhanced by the cellular stress responses, including the unfolded protein and heat shock responses, and can lead to apoptosis [143–145]. TDP43 is a major protein recruited by cellular stress responses [122]. Cellular stress and oxidative stress (specifically H2O2) induce TDP43 aggregation, and its localization in stress granules [146–151]. TDP43 is strongly related to ALS, both due to intracellular aggregates in almost all patients [152,153] and to mutations in 10% of fALS patients [122]. In our view, it is not causal in sALS, since the parsimonious account of its aggregation is chronic activation by stress responses. Chronic cellular stress eventually activates the death arms of cellular stress responses [154,155], explaining MTN degeneration and muscle use problems.

The late onset age of ALS can be explained by the fact that normal aging involves increased calcium currents [156,157] and reduced calcium buffering [158], making aged cells more susceptible to abnormal Ca^{2+}.[1]

The specific vulnerability of non-ocular MTNs in ALS has been explained by the fact that these MTNs express very low levels of calcium binding proteins [159,160] (although there are also conflicting results [161]). Eye movements and the cerebellum might be relatively preserved because the level of these proteins in oculomotor neurons and Pukinje cells are 5-6 and 15 times higher, respectively [160,162]. Moreover, sensitive MTNs (tongue) express 3 fold higher levels of H-VGCC currents than ocular MTNs [163]. In addition, MTNs have long axons and high energy requirements, making them more sensitive to chronic ATP consumption and oxidative stress.

High pre-onset physical activity is strongly associated with increased ALS risk [164–170] (although there are also neutral results [171,172]). High calcium increases muscle contraction capacity and performance, explaining this datum.

In summary, chronic calcium is toxic to cells and can account for the salient data of ALS.

9.4.3 a2d

There is some evidence for the a2d hypothesis. It is small compared to the strong evidence implicating H-VGCCs, but sufficient for lending credibility to the theory.

Patient IgG interacts with a2d, with the predicted effects. There is one direct evidence supporting the hypothesis. In a study with ALS patients comorbid with type 2 diabetes (DB2), in 60% of the patients, serum induced high rather than oscillating L-VGCC-mediated intracellular Ca^{2+} in mouse pancreas beta cells. The ALS-DB2 serum induced 2.4x higher basal insulin release, and somewhat lower glucose-stimulated insulin secretion than DB2 serum. Crucially, this was shown to be mediated by IgG targeting the a2d1 subunit [92]. IgGs from ALS patients not diagnosed with DB2 were not tested.

Thus, patient IgG contains a2d1 antibodies, and these induce effects that are similar to those induced by chronic calcium (increased release with a smaller amplitude).

a2d is decreased in ALS. The a2d1 subunit was shown to be significantly decreased in patient MTNs (8 vs. 3 controls) and in familial iPSCs-derived MTNs

[1] A more specific mechanism for disease onset is impaired insulin signaling (see below), which also occurs with aging.

(24 vs. 18) [173]. However, the same project reported similar results for a large number of other proteins.

a2d suppression increases risk. Gabapentin and pregabalin are a2d ligands that disrupt channel function and are routinely used for treating epilepsy and pain. Suppression of a2d should enhance the a2d impairment present in ALS and exacerbate the state of ALS patients. Indeed, a regional census study in Italy found that usage of antiepileptic drugs 5-6 years prior to ALS diagnosis was associated with increased ALS risk [174]. In about half of these patients, the drug was gabapentin.

a2d suppression accelerates symptoms. Respiration problems are a hallmark of ALS. In a clinical trial of gabapentin in ALS, it exacerbated patient condition by accelerating respiration (forced vital capacity) decline [175]. Gabapentin therapy can also induce recurrent hypoventilation and respiratory failure in non-ALS patients [176,177].

a2d suppression is associated with motor diseases. Gabapentin can induce severe myopathy and other muscle problems (myositis, rhabdomyolysis) [178–184]. It can also induce myoclonus (twitches, spasms, fasciculations), a core feature of ALS [185–188].

Myasthenia gravis (MG) is an autoimmune disease involving antibodies targeting the NMJ (mainly nicotinic receptors) [189]. There is some evidence that gabapentin may be harmful in MG [190], showing that suppression of a2d can be involved in NMJ damage.

Animal models. Mice with a2d2 mutations display impaired motor performance [191]. Two non-lethal a2d knockout mouse models have been reported, with a2d1 KOs showing no apparent motor deficits [192], and a2d4 KOs being hyperactive [25]. The latter model shows again that a2d impairment can result in increased physical activity, but a2d4 is not expressed in relevant tissue in humans. The former model does not support the a2d hypothesis, but it does not refute it either. Mice do not exhibit the neurodegenerative diseases associated with aging in humans, so the a2d1 model might be a model of pre- but not post-onset human ALS.

9.4.4 Insulin

The fact that a paper presenting a theory of ALS contains a section on insulin may be surprising, since insulin is not mentioned at all in neurology textbooks and general ALS reviews [1,2,193], and is mentioned very little even in focused reviews of metabolism in ALS [194,195].

In my view, insulin is fundamental to the disease [117]. Not only is insulin function impaired by the causal processes of ALS, it is this impairment that serves as a major trigger of disease symptoms. Here I summarize results from a companion paper focusing on insulin in ALS [117], and add new evidence specific to calcium channels and cholesterol.

Insulin impairment. There is a large body of evidence from glucose tolerance tests showing that insulin secretion and/or signaling are impaired in ALS. However, this is usually not detected: although some ALS patients are diagnosed with diabetes (DB), most of them are not, because patient glucose levels are inside the normal range. My explanation for this is that chronic calcium induces excessive insulin-independent glucose uptake (IIGU) that masks the insulin problem. As detailed above, chronic calcium can explain the ALS hypermetabolism results via excessive ATP consumption, activated AMPK, and Glut4 membrane translocation, resulting in increased glucose uptake capacity that compensates for reduced insulin. Moreover, intracellular calcium directly induces IIGU, even at amounts below the muscle contraction threshold.

Insulin and ALS processes. Insulin and the detrimental processes taking place in ALS mutually oppose each other. Insulin promotes the growth mode of cellular stress responses, and opposes their death mode. It promotes protein synthesis, opposes degeneration, and reduces excessive H2O2 and intracellular calcium. Conversely, the harmful modes of cellular stress responses induce insulin resistance [117].

Insulin and diabetes. Early diabetes (usually type 1 (DB1)) is associated with increased risk for ALS, which we explain in two complementary ways. First, the VGCC impairment that causes ALS also damages beta cells, and this can manifest as early DB. Second, the lifelong impairment in insulin shown in DB1 is difficult to control even with modern medicine, yielding an earlier onset in people with ALS. In the former, the two diseases have the same core cause, while in the latter, insulin deficiency increases risk. Indeed, DB1 patients and mouse models exhibit early MTN loss and impaired muscle function [196–198].

Late diabetes (type 2 (DB2)) is associated with decreased ALS risk, which seems to contradict our view that insulin impairment is the trigger for disease symptoms. However, DB2 involves elevated levels of blood insulin, and many patients are given insulin-based treatment. The theory here predicts insulin to be protective, and indeed, there is epidemiological evidence showing that taking insulin-based drugs reduces ALS risk [117]. DB2 also involves higher blood glucose, which was recently shown to be associated with lower TDP43 pathology in normal aging [199].

Trajectories. Insulin and body mass index (BMI) trajectories are detailed in the companion paper [117].

Calcium. Insulin's beneficial effect on acute (non-chronic) calcium signaling is detailed in the companion paper [117]. For example, insulin rapidly activates Akt, ERK1/2, and CaMKII [200,201]. Crucially, L-VGCC or CaMKII inhibitors significantly decrease insulin-stimulated glucose uptake in SKM [202]. As long as insulin release is OK, it manages to cover up for the ALS problem. As it starts deteriorating, disease symptoms erupt.

Cholesterol. Insulin is a major factor in cholesterol synthesis via the Akt/mTOR/SREBP axis [203,204]. Cholesterol is in turn an essential component of lipid rafts, which are crucial for synaptic receptors, including nicotinic receptors at the NMJ [205,206], and for cytoskeleton health during both axonal growth and neurite maintenance [207,208]. Indeed, ALS patients show cholesterol dysregulation [209,210]. However, cholesterol does not seem to be a major factor in the disease, in light of the quite small effect exerted by statins [211]. Insulin's protective effect occurs via calcium metabolism much more than with lipid metabolism.

9.5 Autoimmunity

In addition to the calcium-related antibody evidence cited above, it has long been recognized that ALS shows elevated circulating immune complexes [212–214] and spinal cord infiltration by T cells [215]. More recently, reduced numbers of regulatory T cells were shown to correlate with disease progression [216,217]. Impaired blood-spinal and blood-brain barriers in ALS were reported [218]. Thus, the immune system is clearly active in ALS [120,219], and immune T cells express a2d, in T cells [17].

Immune involvement in a neurodegeneration disease is not surprising, since degenerating cells recruit immune (and glia) cells. Here I present the case for autoimmune reactivity being actually causal in ALS.

Calcium-related antibodies. The strongest body of evidence for autoimmunity is the one detailed above with respect to the presence and effect of patient antibodies interacting with calcium channels. While such antibodies can result from degeneration or injury that are due to other reasons (e.g., an inherent born VGCC abnormality, or traumatic brain injury, which is indeed associated with increased ALS risk [166,167,220]), autoimmunity trivially explains their existence. Moreover, the physically fit lifetime phenotype of ALS supports an early event rather than a relatively late injury.

Immune complement. The classical pathway of complement activation is by antigen-antibody complexes [221], and the complement terminal pathway induces neurodegeneration and cell death. Among the four IgG subclasses, only IgG1 and IgG3 bind complement effectively [222], and IgG3 is the subclass of 1B50-1, an a2d1 antibody [223]. There is substantial evidence for classical complement activation in ALS [212,213,224–227], including in spinal cord and motor end-plates [228–230]. Activation in motor end-plates includes ones that are still innervated [230].

Complement provides strong evidence to an active antibody-mediated process that contributes to or is responsible for NMJ deinnervation, and the antibodies are of the type that can target a2d.

Association with autoimmune diseases. General support for ALS being related to autoimmunity (but not specifically to a2d) comes from its disproportional pre-onset association with autoimmune diseases, including in an all-England study

[231], an all-Sweden study [232], a large Netherlands study [233], and the FDA adverse event reporting system [234].

Association with myasthenia gravis (MG). As mentioned above, MG is an autoimmune disease that targets nicotinic receptors in the NMJ [189]. ALS in associated with MG beyond chance levels [235–237]. A possible scenario here is that the NMJ impairment in MG triggers the autoimmune reaction against VGCCs, inducing ALS symptoms.

Muscular autoimmune diseases targeting VGCCs. There are several autoimmune diseases that target VGCCs. The most relevant one is Lambert-Eaton myasthenic syndrome (LEMS), which is a neuromuscular disease. LEMS involves antibodies against the a1, beta or a2d subunits of P/Q-VGCC, but not antibodies to a2d alone [238]. Thus, an autoimmune disease that targets a2d can be expected, but has not been found yet.

NMJ exposure. Above, we explained the specific vulnerability of non-ocular MTNs in ALS via reduced calcium buffering and increased VGCC currents. A simpler account is that the NMJ lies outside the blood-brain barrier, exposing it to circulating antibodies and immune cells.

Ocular MTNs. The well known ocular immune privilege [239] can be argued to provide another explanation for the relative protection of ocular MTNs, supporting autoimmunity in ALS. However, this account is not that convincing, given that ocular MTNs are damaged in the autoimmune diseases LEMS and MG [189].

The retina strongly expresses a2d4 [25] and also some a2d3 [24]. It can be speculated that these are the targets in the minority of LEMS and MG patients that do not exhibit the antibodies usually associated with these diseases. However, I am not aware of any evidence supporting this idea.

Adaptive immune trajectories in ALS. If ALS is caused by autoimmunity, both active adaptive immune cells and antibodies should be detected, which is indeed the case. However, there is a factor that complicates the situation: immune cells themselves, including B and T cells, express L-VGCCs or L-VGCC-like channels [13,15,240,241]. In particular, L-VGCCs are crucial for B cell proliferation and their transition into plasma cells, which are the ones secreting antibodies [14,242–244]. Plasma cells also express L-VGCCs [241], and a2d2 is essential for the proper function of Th2 T cells [17]. This means that an immune reaction against H-VGCCs could target immune cells themselves, eventually resulting in decreasing antibody and lymphocyte levels.

This observation supports the theory instead of opposing it, since it can explain why serum/Ig-VGCC interaction was not identified in all ALS patients.

There is some evidence supporting this model. IgG levels were reported to be normal at early disease stages, and strongly decrease with disease progression, along with CD4 T cell activation [245]. IgG levels were significantly higher in male patients than in controls, but negatively correlated with disease severity and duration [225]. Serum circulating immune complexes, mainly composed of IgG, were significantly elevated on diagnosis, but decreased to control levels at the 2nd visit (although IgG remained high) [214]. A recent meta-analysis found that lower IgG is associated with early- vs. late-onset patients, indicating that disease severity negatively correlates with IgG levels [226]. In addition, B cells were reported to be completely absent from spinal cord infiltrates [246], and lymphocytes were markedly decreased in early stage ALS [247].

In summary, there is some support for autoimmunity being causal in ALS, but most of the evidence is also consistent with immunity being recruited by other causal factors, e.g., genetic mutations or injury.

9.6 Frontotemporal dementia (FTD)

Background. FTD has substantial overlap with ALS. 40% of FTD patients show MTN dsyfunction [248], and 50% of ALS patients show FTD symptoms, with many meeting diagnosis criteria [249]. FTD has two main variants, tau-positive and tau-negative, and the tau-negative variant involves pathological TDP43 as in ALS [152,153]. As in ALS, most TDP43 inclusions colocate with stress granules [250]. There are also FTD variants distinguished by symptoms (e.g., with certain types of language damage). For simplicity, I will focus on the TDP43 variant (roughly FTDbv) here.

FTD is classified as a dementia because it eventually involves degeneration and memory loss. However, it is very different from other dementias. Symptoms manifest as executive dysfunction, apathy, behavioral disinhibition, hypereating, and lack of empathy, with relative sparing of episodic memory [251,252].

Theory. Due to the tight link with ALS, our starting point is that the underlying cause is similar, a VGCC impairment. As in ALS, we need to ask whether there are neurons that are particularly vulnerable, and why. It turns out that the von-economo neurons (VENs) in the insula and ACC are specifically vulnerable [253,254], and that their anatomical and molecular profile [255] is very similar to that of MTNS: they have large axons and low expression of calcium buffer proteins [256]. Thus, **in both ALS and FTD, the main damage is in neurons that are more sensitive to calcium overload.**

To complete the picture, we need to show that VEN impairment can explain the major FTD symptoms. It has been shown that lesions of the anterior insula (but not ACC) impair the capacity of identifying others' pain [257], explaining the lack of empathy and the behavioral disinhibition in FTD. Feeling your own pain is known to be essential for empathy for others' pain [258], and gray matter loss in the right insula and anterior temporal cortex is associated with blunted pain in FTD [259]. Relatedly, the anterior insula is the major site of interoceptive heart inputs to the brain, with blunted heart reactivity to emotional stimuli in FTDbv [260].

As in ALS, there is a link between the appearance of symptoms and low insulin-induced glucose uptake. Regardless of FTD, self control is known to be lowest when brain glucose is low [261]. The symptoms of insulin-induced hypoglycemia are well-known and include rudeness, violence, abnormal sexual behavior, exhiliration, asociality, perseveration, impulsivity, slowness, speech difficulties, and even hallucinations [262]. Hypereating and sweet craving in FTD can simply be explained by the brain sensing a deficiency in insulin-induced glucose uptake. Further supporting metabolism involvement, excessive eating is correlated to hypothalamus atrophy [263,264].

FTD apathy can be explained via blunted facial EMG responses due to right insula damage [265].

Insula lesions yield swallowing problems, which may directly explain swallowing problems in many ALS patients (in addition to the classical accounts) [266].

Glucose evidence. In addition to the evidence cited above with respect to the damage in FTD focusing on frontal areas and VENs, there is a large body of evidence showing 'hypometabolism' in FTD in these areas [267,268]. This is generally shown using FDG-PET, where decreased PET ligand binding is interpreted as hypometabolism. However, what decreased PET ligand binding shows is reduced expression of glucose transporters, which implies higher utilization (ligand binding can also show higher occupancy, which has the same effect due to negative feedback). Thus, it is not that the vulnerable areas utilize less glucose, they in fact uptake more glucose. This we explain exactly as in ALS – chronic activation of VGCCs induces excessive insulin-independent glucose uptake, where glucose is not used for protein synthesis and anti-oxidant defenses, promoting degeneration.

Insulin is involved in these results. FTD involves increased fasting insulin, HOMA-IR (indicating insulin resistance), triglycerides, and lower HDL [269]. DB type 2 occurs in 39% vs. 23% in controls [270]. C-peptide, indicating insulin, is increased, with 5y earlier onset with higher levels [271]. Note that higher C-peptide is associated with regional cortical thinning in cognitively healthy people [272].

There are other indications of hypoglycemia, including dysregulation of CRH, ACTH, and cortisol [273]. A coarse trend was found where CSF glucose was lower and with a lower standard deviation than all other groups tested [274].

Calcium evidence. As in ALS, FTD shows calcium pathology. The calcium binding protein calbindinD28 is dramatically decreased in frontal cortex in patients with both ALS and FTD [275]. Patients CSF is toxic to mouse spinal GABA and calbindinD28 neurons [276].

Interestingly, the brain distribution of L-VGCC (Cav1.2) includes valence (amygdala) and motor areas, but not the hippocampus [11], supporting our account of the difference between FTD and dementias involving episodic memory.

Serum calcium binding proteins (9, 10) are decreased in FTD [277]. FTD patients show significantly increased serum calcium [278]. iPSCs from FTD-tau patients also show dysregulated Ca^{2+} elevation after electrical stimulation

[279]. There is Ca^{2+} damage with oxidative stress biomarkers [280]. In one case, P/Q-VGCC, and N-VGCC antibodies caused FTD symptoms in a patient with rheumatoid arthritis and thyroid history [281].

Autoimmunity evidence. FTD shows a wide range of antibodies compared to other dementias [282]. In 41/175 (23%) of patients, serum has anti-GluA3 antibodies [283]. FTD shows blood-brain barrier dysfunction, with significantly higher CSF IgGs. This shows more in ALS-FTD than ALS and is associated with worse prognosis [284]. FTD patients had about 25% more autoimmune diseases than controls (lowest in FTD with C9orf72 mutation) [285].

Additional VEN and areal evidence. In FTD patients, loss of VENs and of GABA theta subunit-expressing pyramidal neurons is associated with TDP43 and FUS pathology [286]. Frontoinsular VENs and fork cells show early, disproportionate TDP43 aggregation, correlating with symptom severity and empathy loss [287].

Obviously, VENs are not the only vulnerable neurons. All frontal areas around them show early atrophy, including ACC, mPFC [288], insula, orbital frontal cortex [289], bilateral inferior frontal gyrus, temporal pole, and the rest of the insula [290].

We also note that aging and high BMI involve hypoperfusion specifically in the insula and limbic brainstem, respectively [291]. Diabetes predicts brain hypoperfusion only in the insula, with higher brain hypoperfusion in insula in diabetes vs. obesity [291]. Thus, the insula is specifically vulnerable to gluocse metabolism possibly even without calcium impairment. Hypoglycemia events double dementia risk, and vice versa [292].

9.7 Discussion

In this chapter I presented the first complete theory of ALS and FTD, a theory that explains their etiology and pathology. The theory has three components. First, the fundamental problem is in H-VGCCs. Second, the specific subunit that is most likely involved in most (or all) cases is a2d (although we did leave open which of a2d1-a2d4 are more involved). Third, the source of the problem could be genetic or autoimmune-induced.

TDP43. A large part of the research done in ALS focuses on the TDP43 protein. In my view, it is not a core cause of the disease, since TDP43 aggregates simply indicate chronic metabolic cellular stress. I think that it is a mistake to focus so much research priority on TDP43 instead of on more fundamental topics.

Calcium. I think that the centrality of calcium in ALS would be easily accepted by the readers, due to the fact that calcium dysregulation has been so thoroughly demonstrated [293,294]. The challenge with calcium in ALS has turned out to be the identification of the specific subunit(s) involved, due to contradictory results produced by the early set of papers. The present paper is the first to raise the idea that the a2d subunit is the core one. This makes sense for a large number of reasons detailed above. (Naturally, other subunits can also trigger the detrimental processes described here in various constellations.)

We should remember that the a2d subunit is cleaved, folded, glycosylated, GPI-anchored in lipid rafts, and uses disulfide bonds. It seems that antibodies only bind it in this state, causing null results in experiments with denatured proteins. This is an empirical issue to be resolved, and it trivially explains some negative results.

Autoimmunity. We have presented the case that the a2d impairment in ALS stems from autoimmunity. It should be emphasized that it is possible that it stems from some genetic (or epigenetic) cause. At present, there is no evidence supporting this direction, but given that mutations in many relevant genes are strongly associated with ALS (fALS), this is a possibility that needs to be examined.

ALS cells are stronger than normal throughout life, because they enjoy more calcium. At some point, calcium gets chronic and toxic, and this self-amplifying process rapidly damages cells, eventually killing them. This model holds for MTNs, beta cells, skeletal muscle cells, and possibly immune cells. The turning point commonly (but surely not always) occurs when insulin function is reduced to such an extent that it cannot support the ATP, anti-oxidative stress, and protein synthesis requirements of the affected cells.

These results are consistent with a model in which antibodies target immune cell VGCCs throughout life, without noticeable damage (or maybe even improving their reactivity). At some point cells cannot contain this state, setting in motion a detrimental process that does not depend on antibodies anymore. Chronic calcium is self-amplifying (since it involves the suppression of negFB), and perfectly fits the properties of such a detrimental process.

Insulin. As explained above, the collapse of insulin signaling is a strong candidate for what actually triggers the eruption of the disease. At present, this view is not shared by anybody (in fact, it is actively disputed by many people I have contacted). It is not clear to me why physicians assume that if patient blood glucose levels are at the normal range, this indicates healthy insulin function. About half of cellular glucose uptake is insulin-independent, and it is known to be triggered by calcium. This excessive calcium masks the insulin problem in ALS, and can easily be identified via the initial stages of the OGTT, which can show decreased insulin secretion. The OGTT is a common and easy test and should be administered to all ALS patients.

FTD. FTD is a simple parallel of ALS in which the vulnerable cells are prefrontal VENs and their neighbors, which have properties similar to MTNs. I have shown how this simple model can naturally explain the various FTD symptoms, including lack of empathy and disinhibition.

Theory predictions. As far as I know, the basic experiment to support or refute the a2d direction has not been conducted. No study has reported testing ALS

IgGs against the a2d subunit (any of them) alone. Studies widely report testing against the a1 subunit, but not against the auxiliary subunits.

The most relevant reported result is Shi et al. [92]. They studied ALS patients with DB2, showing that in 60% of them IgGs target the a2d1 subunit when it is expressed in cells. It should not be too difficult to extend this result to the general sALS population.

I believe that insulin treatment may be disease-modifying in ALS if started early enough, and this is one of my theory predictions.

Treatment. In addition to insulin, the theory implies that available immune-based therapies might be beneficial in sALS, since they directly target the disease's causal processes. For example, spectacular results have been recently achieved with CAR T therapy targeting B cells (CD19) against lupus [295]. However, it could be that the damage in ALS has already been done and that B cells are already deficient.

It may be thought that gabapentin and pregabalin, L-VGCC blockers, could help. However, gabapentin impairs a2d membrane trafficking [296].

Acknowledgments

I thank Gilad Jacobson, PhD., for commenting on a draft of this chapter.

References

[1] O. Hardiman, A. Al-Chalabi, A. Chio, E.M. Corr, G. Logroscino, W. Robberecht, et al., Amyotrophic lateral sclerosis, Nature Reviews Disease Primers 3 (1) (2017) 1–19.

[2] N. Leigh, J. Sreedharan, L. Wijesekera, Motor neuron disease: amyotrophic lateral sclerosis, in: Neuroscience in the 21st Century: From Basic to Clinical, second edition, Springer, New York, 2016, pp. 3799–3841.

[3] G.D. Rabinovici, B.L. Miller, Frontotemporal lobar degeneration: epidemiology, pathophysiology, diagnosis and management, CNS Drugs 24 (2010) 375–398.

[4] L. Van Den Bosch, Amyotrophic lateral sclerosis: mechanisms and therapeutic strategies, in: Disease-Modifying Targets in Neurodegenerative Disorders, Elsevier, 2017, pp. 277–296.

[5] W.A. Catterall, Voltage-gated calcium channels, Cold Spring Harbor Perspectives in Biology 3 (8) (2011) a003947.

[6] A.C. Dolphin, Voltage-gated calcium channels and their auxiliary subunits: physiology and pathophysiology and pharmacology, The Journal of Physiology 594 (19) (2016) 5369–5390.

[7] J. Striessnig, A. Pinggera, G. Kaur, G. Bock, P. Tuluc, L-type Ca2+ channels in heart and brain, Wiley Interdisciplinary Reviews: Membrane Transport and Signaling 3 (2) (2014) 15–38.

[8] S. Geisler, C.L. Schöpf, G.J. Obermair, Emerging evidence for specific neuronal functions of auxiliary calcium channel $\alpha2\delta$ subunits, General Physiology and Biophysics 34 (2) (2015) 105.

[9] L. Gandía, I. Mayorgas, P. Michelena, I. Cuchillo, R. de Pascual, F. Abad, et al., Human adrenal chromaffin cell calcium channels: drastic current facilitation in cell clusters, but not in isolated cells, Pflügers Archiv 436 (5) (1998) 696–704.

[10] S.E. Lee, S.H. Lee, Skin barrier and calcium, Annals of Dermatology 30 (3) (2018) 265–275.

[11] A. Hetzenauer, M. Sinnegger-Brauns, J. Striessnig, N. Singewald, Brain activation pattern induced by stimulation of L-type Ca2+-channels: contribution of Cav1.3 and Cav1.2 isoforms, Neuroscience 139 (3) (2006) 1005–1015.

[12] K.S. Pilch, K.H. Ramgoolam, A.C. Dolphin, Involvement of CaV2.2 channels and $\alpha2\delta$-1 in hippocampal homeostatic synaptic plasticity, bioRxiv (2022).

[13] A.A.S. Akha, N.J. Willmott, K. Brickley, A.C. Dolphin, A. Galione, S.V. Hunt, Anti-Ig-induced calcium influx in rat B lymphocytes mediated by cGMP through a dihydropyridine-sensitive channel, Journal of Biological Chemistry 271 (13) (1996) 7297–7300.

[14] K.L. Hoek, P. Antony, J. Lowe, N. Shinners, B. Sarmah, S.R. Wente, et al., Transitional B cell fate is associated with developmental stage-specific regulation of diacylglycerol and calcium signaling upon B cell receptor engagement, The Journal of Immunology 177 (8) (2006) 5405–5413.

[15] G. Grafton, L. Stokes, K.M. Toellner, J. Gordon, A non-voltage-gated calcium channel with L-type characteristics activated by B cell receptor ligation, Biochemical Pharmacology 66 (10) (2003) 2001–2009.

[16] L. Pelletier, M. Moreau, Cav1 channels is also a story of non excitable cells: application to calcium signalling in two different non related models, Biochimica Et Biophysica Acta. Molecular Cell Research 1868 (6) (2021) 118996.

[17] N. Rosa, E. Triffaux, V. Robert, M. Mars, M. Klein, G. Bouchaud, et al., The β and $\alpha2\delta$ auxiliary subunits of voltage-gated calcium channel 1 (Cav1) are required for TH2 lymphocyte function and acute allergic airway inflammation, Journal of Allergy and Clinical Immunology 142 (3) (2018) 892–903.

[18] I. Kadurin, L. Ferron, S.W. Rothwell, J.O. Meyer, L.R. Douglas, C.S. Bauer, et al., Proteolytic maturation of $\alpha2\delta$ represents a checkpoint for activation and neuronal trafficking of latent calcium channels, eLife (2016) 5:e21143.

[19] A. Davies, I. Kadurin, A. Alvarez-Laviada, L. Douglas, M. Nieto-Rostro, C.S. Bauer, et al., The $\alpha2\delta$ subunits of voltage-gated calcium channels form GPI-anchored proteins, a post-translational modification essential for function, Proceedings of the National Academy of Sciences 107 (4) (2010) 1654–1659.

[20] R.L. Cole, S.M. Lechner, M.E. Williams, P. Prodanovich, L. Bleicher, M.A. Varney, et al., Differential distribution of voltage-gated calcium channel alpha-2 delta ($\alpha2\delta$) subunit mRNA-containing cells in the rat central nervous system and the dorsal root ganglia, Journal of Comparative Neurology 491 (3) (2005) 246–269.

[21] C. Taylor, R. Garrido, Immunostaining of rat brain, spinal cord, sensory neurons and skeletal muscle for calcium channel alpha2-delta ($\alpha2$-δ) type 1 protein, Neuroscience 155 (2) (2008) 510–521.

[22] G.J. Obermair, G. Kugler, S. Baumgartner, P. Tuluc, M. Grabner, B.E. Flucher, The Ca2+ channel $\alpha2\delta$-1 subunit determines Ca2+ current kinetics in skeletal muscle but not targeting of α1S or excitation-contraction coupling, Journal of Biological Chemistry 280 (3) (2005) 2229–2237.

[23] V. Mastrolia, S.M. Flucher, G.J. Obermair, M. Drach, H. Hofer, E. Renström, et al., Loss of $\alpha2\delta$-1 calcium channel subunit function increases the susceptibility for diabetes, Diabetes 66 (4) (2017) 897–907.

[24] L. Pérez de Sevilla Müller, A. Sargoy, L. Fernández-Sánchez, A. Rodriguez, J. Liu, N. Cuenca, et al., Expression and cellular localization of the voltage-gated calcium channel $\alpha2\delta3$ in the rodent retina, Journal of Comparative Neurology 523 (10) (2015) 1443–1460.

[25] A. Klomp, R. Omichi, Y. Iwasa, R.J. Smith, Y.M. Usachev, A.F. Russo, et al., The voltage-gated Ca2+ channel subunit $\alpha2\delta$-4 regulates locomotor behavior and sensorimotor gating in mice, PLoS ONE 17 (3) (2022) e0263197.

[26] L. Ferron, S. Koshti, G.W. Zamponi, The life cycle of voltage-gated Ca2+ channels in neurons: an update on the trafficking of neuronal calcium channels, Neuronal Signaling 5 (1) (2021).

[27] J.S. Cassidy, L. Ferron, I. Kadurin, W.S. Pratt, A.C. Dolphin, Functional exofacially tagged N-type calcium channels elucidate the interaction with auxiliary $\alpha2\delta$-1 subunits, Proceedings of the National Academy of Sciences 111 (24) (2014) 8979–8984.

[28] M.B. Hoppa, B. Lana, W. Margas, A.C. Dolphin, T.A. Ryan, $\alpha2\delta$ expression sets presynaptic calcium channel abundance and release probability, Nature 486 (7401) (2012) 122–125.
[29] W.C. Risher, N. Kim, S. Koh, J.E. Choi, P. Mitev, E.F. Spence, et al., Thrombospondin receptor $\alpha2\delta$-1 promotes synaptogenesis and spinogenesis via postsynaptic Rac1, The Journal of Cell Biology 217 (10) (2018) 3747–3765.
[30] A. Tedeschi, S. Dupraz, C.J. Laskowski, J. Xue, T. Ulas, M. Beyer, et al., The calcium channel subunit Alpha2delta2 suppresses axon regeneration in the adult CNS, Neuron 92 (2) (2016) 419–434.
[31] C.L. Schöpf, C. Ablinger, S.M. Geisler, R.I. Stanika, M. Campiglio, W.A. Kaufmann, et al., Presynaptic $\alpha2\delta$ subunits are key organizers of glutamatergic synapses, Proceedings of the National Academy of Sciences 118 (14) (2021) e1920827118.
[32] Y. Wang, K.E. Fehlhaber, I. Sarria, Y. Cao, N.T. Ingram, D. Guerrero-Given, et al., The auxiliary calcium channel subunit $\alpha2\delta4$ is required for axonal elaboration, synaptic transmission, and wiring of rod photoreceptors, Neuron 93 (6) (2017) 1359–1374.
[33] I. Kadurin, A. Alvarez-Laviada, S.F.J. Ng, R. Walker-Gray, M. D'Arco, M.G. Fadel, et al., Calcium currents are enhanced by $\alpha2\delta$-1 lacking its membrane anchor, Journal of Biological Chemistry 287 (40) (2012) 33554–33566.
[34] G.M. Bernstein, O.T. Jones, Kinetics of internalization and degradation of N-type voltage-gated calcium channels: role of the $\alpha2/\delta$ subunit, Cell Calcium 41 (1) (2007) 27–40.
[35] J.S. Rougier, M. Albesa, N. Syam, G. Halet, H. Abriel, P. Viard, Ubiquitin-specific protease USP2-45 acts as a molecular switch to promote α 2 δ-1-induced downregulation of Cav 1.2 channels, Pflügers Archiv-European Journal of Physiology 467 (2015) 1919–1929.
[36] J. Chen, L. Li, S.R. Chen, H. Chen, J.D. Xie, R.E. Sirrieh, et al., The $\alpha2\delta$-1-NMDA receptor complex is critically involved in neuropathic pain development and gabapentin therapeutic actions, Cell Reports 22 (9) (2018) 2307–2321.
[37] J.J. Zhou, D.P. Li, S.R. Chen, Y. Luo, H.L. Pan, The $\alpha2\delta$-1–NMDA receptor coupling is essential for corticostriatal long-term potentiation and is involved in learning and memory, Journal of Biological Chemistry 293 (50) (2018) 19354–19364.
[38] N. Savalli, A. Pantazis, D. Sigg, J.N. Weiss, A. Neely, R. Olcese, The $\alpha2\delta$-1 subunit remodels CaV1.2 voltage sensors and allows Ca2+ influx at physiological membrane potentials, The Journal of General Physiology 148 (2) (2016) 147–159.
[39] P. Robinson, S. Etheridge, L. Song, P. Armenise, O.T. Jones, E.M. Fitzgerald, Formation of N-type (Cav2.2) voltage-gated calcium channel membrane microdomains: lipid raft association and clustering, Cell Calcium 48 (4) (2010) 183–194.
[40] A. Davies, L. Douglas, J. Hendrich, J. Wratten, A.T. Van Minh, I. Foucault, et al., The calcium channel $\alpha2\delta$-2 subunit partitions with CaV2.1 into lipid rafts in cerebellum: implications for localization and function, The Journal of Neuroscience 26 (34) (2006) 8748–8757.
[41] K. García, T. Nabhani, J. García, The calcium channel $\alpha2/\delta1$ subunit is involved in extracellular signalling, The Journal of Physiology 586 (3) (2008) 727–738.
[42] B. Fell, S. Eckrich, K. Blum, T. Eckrich, D. Hecker, G.J. Obermair, et al., $\alpha2\delta2$ controls the function and trans-synaptic coupling of Cav1.3 channels in mouse inner hair cells and is essential for normal hearing, The Journal of Neuroscience 36 (43) (2016) 11024–11036.
[43] C. Canti, M. Nieto-Rostro, I. Foucault, F. Heblich, J. Wratten, M. Richards, et al., The metal-ion-dependent adhesion site in the von Willebrand factor-A domain of $\alpha2\delta$ subunits is key to trafficking voltage-gated Ca2+ channels, Proceedings of the National Academy of Sciences 102 (32) (2005) 11230–11235.
[44] J. Brockhaus, M. Schreitmüller, D. Repetto, O. Klatt, C. Reissner, K. Elmslie, et al., α-Neurexins together with $\alpha2\delta$-1 auxiliary subunits regulate Ca2+ influx through Cav2.1 channels, The Journal of Neuroscience 38 (38) (2018) 8277–8294.
[45] R.C. Caylor, Y. Jin, B.D. Ackley, The Caenorhabditis elegans voltage-gated calcium channel subunits UNC-2 and UNC-36 and the calcium-dependent kinase UNC-43/CaMKII regulate neuromuscular junction morphology, Neural Development 8 (1) (2013) 1–13.

[46] P.T. Kurshan, A. Oztan, T.L. Schwarz, Presynaptic $\alpha2\delta$-3 is required for synaptic morphogenesis independent of its Ca2+-channel functions, Nature Neuroscience 12 (11) (2009) 1415–1423.
[47] T. Biederer, P.S. Kaeser, T.A. Blanpied, Transcellular nanoalignment of synaptic function, Neuron 96 (3) (2017) 680–696.
[48] E.H. Dennys, F.H. Norris, Amyotrophic lateral sclerosis: impairment of neuromuscular transmission, Archives of Neurology 36 (4) (1979) 202–205.
[49] R.A. Maselli, R.L. Wollman, C. Leung, B. Distad, S. Palombi, D.P. Richman, et al., Neuromuscular transmission in amyotrophic lateral sclerosis, Muscle & Nerve: Official Journal of the American Association of Electrodiagnostic Medicine 16 (11) (1993) 1193–1203.
[50] G. Bruneteau, S. Bauché, J.L. Gonzalez de Aguilar, G. Brochier, N. Mandjee, M.L. Tanguy, et al., Endplate denervation correlates with Nogo-A muscle expression in amyotrophic lateral sclerosis patients, Annals of Clinical and Translational Neurology 2 (4) (2015) 362–372.
[51] M. Dadon-Nachum, E. Melamed, D. Offen, The "dying-back" phenomenon of motor neurons in ALS, Journal of Molecular Neuroscience 43 (3) (2011) 470–477.
[52] J.P. Loeffler, G. Picchiarelli, L. Dupuis, J.L. Gonzalez De Aguilar, The role of skeletal muscle in amyotrophic lateral sclerosis, Brain Pathology 26 (2) (2016) 227–236.
[53] J. Penniston, A. Enyedi, Modulation of the plasma membrane Ca2+ pump, The Journal of Membrane Biology 165 (2) (1998) 101–109.
[54] G.J. Iacobucci, G.K. Popescu, Ca2+-dependent inactivation of GluN2A and GluN2B NMDA receptors occurs by a common kinetic mechanism, Biophysical Journal 118 (4) (2020) 798–812.
[55] M. Ben-Johny, D.T. Yue, Calmodulin regulation (calmodulation) of voltage-gated calcium channels, The Journal of General Physiology 143 (6) (2014) 679–692.
[56] H. Liang, C.D. DeMaria, M.G. Erickson, M.X. Mori, B.A. Alseikhan, D.T. Yue, Unified mechanisms of Ca2+ regulation across the Ca2+ channel family, Neuron 39 (6) (2003) 951–960.
[57] M.R. Tadross, R.W. Tsien, D.T. Yue, Ca2+ channel nanodomains boost local Ca2+ amplitude, Proceedings of the National Academy of Sciences 110 (39) (2013) 15794–15799.
[58] M. Heine, J. Heck, A. Ciuraszkiewicz, A. Bikbaev, Dynamic compartmentalization of calcium channel signalling in neurons, Neuropharmacology 169 (2020) 107556.
[59] P.A. Loehrer, L. Zieger, O.J. Simon, Update on paraneoplastic cerebellar degeneration, Brain Sciences 11 (11) (2021) 1414.
[60] O.D. Uchitel, S.H. Appel, F. Crawford, L. Sczcupak, Immunoglobulins from amyotrophic lateral sclerosis patients enhance spontaneous transmitter release from motor-nerve terminals, Proceedings of the National Academy of Sciences 85 (19) (1988) 7371–7374.
[61] O.D. Uchitel, F. Scornik, D. Protti, C. Fumberg, V. Alvarez, S.H. Appel, Long-term neuromuscular dysfunction produced by passive transfer of amyotrophic lateral sclerosis immunoglobulins, Neurology 42 (11) (1992) 2175.
[62] S.H. Appel, J.I. Engelhardt, J. Garcia, E. Stefani, Immunoglobulins from animal models of motor neuron disease and from human amyotrophic lateral sclerosis patients passively transfer physiological abnormalities to the neuromuscular junction, Proceedings of the National Academy of Sciences 88 (2) (1991) 647–651.
[63] E. Stefani, Calcium current and charge movement of mammalian muscle: action of amyotrophic lateral sclerosis immunoglobulins, The Journal of Physiology 444 (1) (1991) 723–742.
[64] R.G. Smith, S. Hamilton, F. Hofmann, T. Schneider, W. Nastainczyk, L. Birnbaumer, et al., Serum antibodies to L-type calcium channels in patients with amyotrophic lateral sclerosis, The New England Journal of Medicine 327 (24) (1992) 1721–1728.
[65] V. Magnelli, T. Sawada, O. Delbono, R.G. Smith, S.H. Appel, E. Stefani, The action of amyotrophic lateral sclerosis immunoglobulins on mammalian single skeletal muscle Ca2+ channels, The Journal of Physiology 461 (1) (1993) 103–118.

[66] O. Delbono, V. Magnelli, T. Sawada, R.G. Smith, S.H. Appel, E. Stefani, Fab fragments from amyotrophic lateral sclerosis IgG affect calcium channels of skeletal muscle, American Journal of Physiology. Cell Physiology 264 (3) (1993) C537–C543.
[67] R. Llinas, M. Sugimori, B. Cherksey, R.G. Smith, O. Delbono, E. Stefani, et al., IgG from amyotrophic lateral sclerosis patients increases current through P-type calcium channels in mammalian cerebellar Purkinje cells and in isolated channel protein in lipid bilayer, Proceedings of the National Academy of Sciences 90 (24) (1993) 11743–11747.
[68] R.G. Smith, M.E. Alexianu, G. Crawford, O. Nyormoi, E. Stefani, S.H. Appel, Cytotoxicity of immunoglobulins from amyotrophic lateral sclerosis patients on a hybrid motoneuron cell line, Proceedings of the National Academy of Sciences 91 (8) (1994) 3393–3397.
[69] A. Zhainazarov, P. Annunziata, S. Toneatto, E. Cherubini, A. Nistri, Serum fractions from amyotrophic lateral sclerosis patients depress voltage-activated Ca2+ currents of rat cerebellar granule cells in culture, Neuroscience Letters 172 (1–2) (1994) 111–114.
[70] F. Kimura, R.G. Smith, O. Delbono, O. Nyormoi, T. Schneider, W. Nastainczyk, et al., Amyotrophic lateral sclerosis patient antibodies label Ca2+ channel $\alpha 1$ subunit, Annals of Neurology: Official Journal of the American Neurological Association and the Child Neurology Society 35 (2) (1994) 164–171.
[71] D.R. Mosier, P. Baldelli, O. Delbono, R.G. Smith, M.E. Alexianu, S.H. Appel, et al., Amyotrophic lateral sclerosis immunoglobulins increase Ca2+ currents in a motoneuron cell line, Annals of Neurology: Official Journal of the American Neurological Association and the Child Neurology Society 37 (1) (1995) 102–109.
[72] J.I. Engelhardt, L. Siklós, L. Kőműves, R.G. Smith, S.H. Appel, Antibodies to calcium channels from ALS patients passively transferred to mice selectively increase intracellular calcium and induce ultrastructural changes in motoneurons, Synapse 20 (3) (1995) 185–199.
[73] V.A. Lennon, T.J. Kryzer, G.E. Griesmann, P.E. O'Suilleabhain, A.J. Windebank, A. Woppmann, et al., Calcium-channel antibodies in the Lambert–Eaton syndrome and other paraneoplastic syndromes, The New England Journal of Medicine 332 (22) (1995) 1467–1475.
[74] P.R. Andjus, L. Khiroug, A. Nistri, E. Cherubini, ALS IgGs suppress $Ca2+_i$ rise through P/Q-type calcium channels in central neurones in culture, NeuroReport 7 (12) (1996) 1914–1916.
[75] P.R. Andjus, Z. Stevic-Marinkovic, E. Cherubim, Immunoglobulins from motoneurone disease patients enhance glutamate release from rat hippocampal neurones in culture, The Journal of Physiology 504 (1) (1997) 103–112.
[76] H.D. Yan, W. Lim, K.W. Lee, J. Kim, Sera from amyotrophic lateral sclerosis patients reduce high-voltage activated Ca2+ currents in mice dorsal root ganglion neurons, Neuroscience Letters 235 (1–2) (1997) 69–72.
[77] L.V. Colom, M.E. Alexianu, D.R. Mosier, R.G. Smith, S.H. Appel, Amyotrophic lateral sclerosis immunoglobulins increase intracellular calcium in a motoneuron cell line, Experimental Neurology 146 (2) (1997) 354–360.
[78] V. La Bella, J.C. Goodman, S.H. Appel, Increased CSF glutamate following injection of ALS immunoglobulins, Neurology 48 (5) (1997) 1270–1272.
[79] D. Offen, S. Halevi, D. Orion, R. Mosberg, H. Stern-Goldberg, E. Melamed, et al., Antibodies from ALS patients inhibit dopamine release mediated by L-type calcium channels, Neurology 51 (4) (1998) 1100–1103.
[80] T.J. O'Shaughnessy, H. Yan, J. Kim, E.H. Middlekauff, K.W. Lee, L.H. Phillips, et al., Amyotrophic lateral sclerosis: serum factors enhance spontaneous and evoked transmitter release at the neuromuscular junction, Muscle & Nerve: Official Journal of the American Association of Electrodiagnostic Medicine 21 (1) (1998) 81–90.
[81] C. Grassi, M. Martire, D. Altobelli, G. Azzena, P. Preziosi, Characterization of Ca2+-channels responsible for K+-evoked [3H] noradrenaline release from rat brain cortex synaptosomes and their response to amyotrophic lateral sclerosis IgGs, Experimental Neurology 159 (2) (1999) 520–527.

[82] A. Pullen, P. Humphreys, Ultrastructural analysis of spinal motoneurones from mice treated with IgG from ALS patients, healthy individuals, or disease controls, Journal of the Neurological Sciences 180 (1–2) (2000) 35–45.
[83] S. Muchnik, A. Losavio, S. De Lorenzo, Effect of amyotrophic lateral sclerosis serum on calcium channels related to spontaneous acetylcholine release, Clinical Neurophysiology 113 (7) (2002) 1066–1071.
[84] S.A. Fratantoni, G. Weisz, A.M. Pardal, R.C. Reisin, O.D. Uchitel, Amyotrophic lateral sclerosis IgG-treated neuromuscular junctions develop sensitivity to L-type calcium channel blocker, Muscle & Nerve: Official Journal of the American Association of Electrodiagnostic Medicine 23 (4) (2000) 543–550.
[85] J.R. Carter, M. Mynlieff, Amyotrophic lateral sclerosis patient IgG alters voltage dependence of Ca2+ channels in dissociated rat motoneurons, Neuroscience Letters 353 (3) (2003) 221–225.
[86] A. Pullen, M. Demestre, R. Howard, R. Orrell, Passive transfer of purified IgG from patients with amyotrophic lateral sclerosis to mice results in degeneration of motor neurons accompanied by Ca2+ enhancement, Acta Neuropathologica 107 (1) (2004) 35–46.
[87] M. Demestre, R. Howard, R. Orrell, A. Pullen, Serine proteases purified from sera of patients with amyotrophic lateral sclerosis (ALS) induce contrasting cytopathology in murine motoneurones to IgG, Neuropathology and Applied Neurobiology 32 (2) (2006) 141–156.
[88] M.R. Pagani, R.C. Reisin, O.D. Uchitel, Calcium signaling pathways mediating synaptic potentiation triggered by amyotrophic lateral sclerosis IgG in motor nerve terminals, The Journal of Neuroscience 26 (10) (2006) 2661–2672.
[89] L.E. Gonzalez, M.L. Kotler, L.G. Vattino, E. Conti, R.C. Reisin, K.J. Mulatz, et al., Amyotrophic lateral sclerosis-immunoglobulins selectively interact with neuromuscular junctions expressing P/Q-type calcium channels, Journal of Neurochemistry 119 (4) (2011) 826–838.
[90] K. Vijayalakshmi, P.A. Alladi, S. Ghosh, V. Prasanna, B. Sagar, A. Nalini, et al., Evidence of endoplasmic reticular stress in the spinal motor neurons exposed to CSF from sporadic amyotrophic lateral sclerosis patients, Neurobiology of Disease 41 (3) (2011) 695–705.
[91] M. Milošević, M. Stenovec, M. Kreft, V. Petrušić, Z. Stević, S. Trkov, et al., Immunoglobulins G from patients with sporadic amyotrophic lateral sclerosis affects cytosolic Ca2+ homeostasis in cultured rat astrocytes, Cell Calcium 54 (1) (2013) 17–25.
[92] Y. Shi, K.S. Park, S.H. Kim, J. Yu, K. Zhao, L. Yu, et al., IgGs from patients with amyotrophic lateral sclerosis and diabetes target CaV$\alpha 2\delta 1$ subunits impairing islet cell function and survival, Proceedings of the National Academy of Sciences 116 (52) (2019) 26816–26822.
[93] I. Obál, B. Nógrádi, V. Meszlényi, R. Patai, G. Ricken, G.G. Kovacs, et al., Experimental motor neuron disease induced in mice with long-term repeated intraperitoneal injections of serum from ALS patients, International Journal of Molecular Sciences 20 (10) (2019) 2573.
[94] V. Meszlényi, R. Patai, T.F. Polgár, B. Nógrádi, L. Körmöczy, R. Kristóf, et al., Passive transfer of sera from ALS patients with identified mutations evokes an increased synaptic vesicle number and elevation of calcium levels in motor axon terminals, similar to sera from sporadic patients, International Journal of Molecular Sciences 21 (15) (2020) 5566.
[95] T.F. Polgár, V. Meszlényi, B. Nógrádi, L. Körmöczy, K. Spisák, K. Tripolszki, et al., Passive transfer of blood sera from ALS patients with identified mutations results in elevated motoneuronal calcium level and loss of motor neurons in the spinal cord of mice, International Journal of Molecular Sciences 22 (18) (2021) 9994.
[96] J. Engelhardt, J. Soós, I. Obál, L. Vigh, L. Siklós, Subcellular localization of IgG from the sera of ALS patients in the nervous system, Acta Neurologica Scandinavica 112 (2) (2005) 126–133.
[97] O. Nyormoi, Proteolytic activity in amyotrophic lateral sclerosis IgG preparations, Annals of Neurology: Official Journal of the American Neurological Association and the Child Neurology Society 40 (5) (1996) 701–706.
[98] L. Siklós, J. Engelhardt, Y. Harati, R.G. Smith, F. Joó, S.H. Appel, Ultrastructural evidence for altered calcium in motor nerve terminals in amyotrophc lateral sclerosis, Annals of Neurology 39 (2) (1996) 203–216.

[99] M. Bader, Tissue renin-angiotensin-aldosterone systems: targets for pharmacological therapy, Annual Review of Pharmacology and Toxicology 50 (2010) 439–465.

[100] R.M. Pfeiffer, B. Mayer, R.W. Kuncl, D.P. Check, E.K. Cahoon, D.R. Rivera, et al., Identifying potential targets for prevention and treatment of amyotrophic lateral sclerosis based on a screen of medicare prescription drugs, Amyotrophic Lateral Sclerosis and Frontotemporal Degeneration 21 (3–4) (2020) 235–245.

[101] N. Hu, H. Ji, Medications on hypertension, hyperlipidemia, diabetes, and risk of amyotrophic lateral sclerosis: a systematic review and meta-analysis, Neurological Sciences (2022) 1–11.

[102] F.C. Lin, C.P. Tsai, J.K.W. Lee, M.T. Wu, C.TC. Lee, Angiotensin-converting enzyme inhibitors and amyotrophic lateral sclerosis risk: a total population–based case-control study, JAMA Neurology 72 (1) (2015) 40–48.

[103] F. Bursch, N. Kalmbach, M. Naujock, S. Staege, R. Eggenschwiler, M. Abo-Rady, et al., Altered calcium dynamics and glutamate receptor properties in iPSC-derived motor neurons from ALS patients with C9orf72, FUS, SOD1 or TDP43 mutations, Human Molecular Genetics 28 (17) (2019) 2835–2850.

[104] K. Quinlan, J. Schuster, R. Fu, T. Siddique, C. Heckman, Altered postnatal maturation of electrical properties in spinal motoneurons in a mouse model of amyotrophic lateral sclerosis, The Journal of Physiology 589 (9) (2011) 2245–2260.

[105] G. Ringholz, S.H. Appel, M. Bradshaw, N. Cooke, D. Mosnik, P. Schulz, Prevalence and patterns of cognitive impairment in sporadic ALS, Neurology 65 (4) (2005) 586–590.

[106] P. McCombe, N. Wray, R. Henderson, Extra-motor abnormalities in amyotrophic lateral sclerosis: another layer of heterogeneity, Expert Review of Neurotherapeutics 17 (6) (2017) 561–577.

[107] P. Corcia, P.F. Pradat, F. Salachas, G. Bruneteau, N. le Forestier, D. Seilhean, et al., Causes of death in a post-mortem series of ALS patients, Amyotrophic Lateral Sclerosis: Official Publication of the World Federation of Neurology Research Group on Motor Neuron Diseases 9 (1) (2008) 59–62.

[108] A. Rosenbohm, B. Schmid, D. Buckert, W. Rottbauer, J. Kassubek, A.C. Ludolph, et al., Cardiac findings in amyotrophic lateral sclerosis: a magnetic resonance imaging study, Frontiers in Neurology 8 (2017) 479.

[109] H.C. Timmins, W. Saw, B.C. Cheah, C.S. Lin, S. Vucic, R.M. Ahmed, et al., Cardiometabolic health and risk of amyotrophic lateral sclerosis, Muscle & Nerve 56 (4) (2017) 721–725.

[110] L. Mach, T. Konecny, K. Helanova, A.S. Jaffe, E.J. Sorenson, V.K. Somers, et al., Elevation of cardiac troponin T in patients with amyotrophic lateral sclerosis, Acta Neurologica Belgica 116 (2016) 557–564.

[111] U. Kläppe, S. Chamoun, Q. Shen, A. Finn, B. Evertsson, H. Zetterberg, et al., Cardiac troponin T is elevated and increases longitudinally in ALS patients, Amyotrophic Lateral Sclerosis and Frontotemporal Degeneration 23 (1–2) (2022) 58–65.

[112] H. Gdynia, A. Kurt, S. Endruhn, A. Ludolph, A. Sperfeld, Cardiomyopathy in motor neuron diseases, Journal of Neurology, Neurosurgery and Psychiatry 77 (5) (2006) 671–673.

[113] J. Weis, I. Katona, G. Müller-Newen, C. Sommer, G. Necula, C. Hendrich, et al., Small-fiber neuropathy in patients with ALS, Neurology 76 (23) (2011) 2024–2029.

[114] E. Dalla Bella, R. Lombardi, C. Porretta-Serapiglia, C. Ciano, C. Gellera, V. Pensato, et al., Amyotrophic lateral sclerosis causes small fiber pathology, European Journal of Neurology 23 (2) (2016) 416–420.

[115] M. Nolano, V. Provitera, F. Manganelli, R. Iodice, G. Caporaso, A. Stancanelli, et al., Non-motor involvement in amyotrophic lateral sclerosis: new insight from nerve and vessel analysis in skin biopsy, Neuropathology and Applied Neurobiology 43 (2) (2017) 119–132.

[116] A. Chiò, G. Mora, G. Lauria, Pain in amyotrophic lateral sclerosis, The Lancet Neurology 16 (2) (2017) 144–157.

[117] A. Rappoport, Insulin in amyotrophic lateral sclerosis: impairment, tests and treatment, Neuroscience and Neurology (2023), https://doi.org/10.20944/preprints202212.0297.v3, https://www.preprints.org/manuscript/202212.0297/v3.

[118] K. Araki, A. Araki, D. Honda, T. Izumoto, A. Hashizume, Y. Hijikata, et al., TDP-43 regulates early-phase insulin secretion via CaV1.2-mediated exocytosis in islets, The Journal of Clinical Investigation 129 (9) (2019) 3578–3593.
[119] G. Coan, C.S. Mitchell, An assessment of possible neuropathology and clinical relationships in 46 sporadic amyotrophic lateral sclerosis patient autopsies, Neurodegenerative Diseases 15 (5) (2015) 301–312.
[120] L.C. Béland, A. Markovinovic, H. Jakovac, F. De Marchi, E. Bilic, L. Mazzini, et al., Immunity in amyotrophic lateral sclerosis: blurred lines between excessive inflammation and inefficient immune responses, Brain Communications 2 (2) (2020) fcaa124.
[121] D. Curti, A. Malaspina, G. Facchetti, C. Camana, L. Mazzini, P. Tosca, et al., Amyotrophic lateral sclerosis: oxidative energy metabolism and calcium homeostasis in peripheral blood lymphocytes, Neurology 47 (4) (1996) 1060–1064.
[122] A. Prasad, V. Bharathi, V. Sivalingam, A. Girdhar, B.K. Patel, Molecular mechanisms of TDP-43 misfolding and pathology in amyotrophic lateral sclerosis, Frontiers in Molecular Neuroscience 12 (2019) 25.
[123] S.C. Barber, P.J. Shaw, Oxidative stress in ALS: key role in motor neuron injury and therapeutic target, Free Radical Biology & Medicine 48 (5) (2010) 629–641.
[124] R.J. Ferrante, S.E. Browne, L.A. Shinobu, A.C. Bowling, M.J. Baik, U. MacGarvey, et al., Evidence of increased oxidative damage in both sporadic and familial amyotrophic lateral sclerosis, Journal of Neurochemistry 69 (5) (1997) 2064–2074.
[125] R.G. Smith, Y.K. Henry, M.P. Mattson, S.H. Appel, Presence of 4-hydroxynonenal in cerebrospinal fluid of patients with sporadic amyotrophic lateral sclerosis, Annals of Neurology: Official Journal of the American Neurological Association and the Child Neurology Society 44 (4) (1998) 696–699.
[126] W.A. Pedersen, W. Fu, J.N. Keller, W.R. Markesbery, S. Appel, R.G. Smith, et al., Protein modification by the lipid peroxidation product 4-hydroxynonenal in the spinal cords of amyotrophic lateral sclerosis patients, Annals of Neurology 44 (5) (1998) 819–824.
[127] H. Mitsumoto, R.M. Santella, X. Liu, M. Bogdanov, J. Zipprich, H.C. Wu, et al., Oxidative stress biomarkers in sporadic ALS, Amyotrophic Lateral Sclerosis 9 (3) (2008) 177–183.
[128] H. Blasco, C. Veyrat-Durebex, C. Bocca, F. Patin, P. Vourc'h, J. Kouassi Nzoughet, et al., Lipidomics reveals cerebrospinal-fluid signatures of ALS, Scientific Reports 7 (1) (2017) 1–10.
[129] E. Simpson, Y. Henry, J. Henkel, R. Smith, S.H. Appel, Increased lipid peroxidation in sera of ALS patients: a potential biomarker of disease burden, Neurology 62 (10) (2004) 1758–1765.
[130] T.M. Carrì, N. D'Ambrosi, M. Cozzolino, Pathways to mitochondrial dysfunction in ALS pathogenesis, Biochemical and Biophysical Research Communications 483 (4) (2017) 1187–1193.
[131] L. Dupuis, P.F. Pradat, A.C. Ludolph, J.P. Loeffler, Energy metabolism in amyotrophic lateral sclerosis, The Lancet Neurology 10 (1) (2011) 75–82.
[132] K. Mukund, S. Subramaniam, Skeletal muscle: a review of molecular structure and function, in health and disease, Wiley Interdisciplinary Reviews: Systems Biology and Medicine 12 (1) (2020) e1462.
[133] I.C. Smith, E. Bombardier, C. Vigna, A.R. Tupling, ATP consumption by sarcoplasmic reticulum Ca2+ pumps accounts for 40-50% of resting metabolic rate in mouse fast and slow twitch skeletal muscle, PLoS ONE 8 (7) (2013) e68924.
[134] M.E. Osler, J.R. Zierath, Minireview: adenosine 5'-monophosphate-activated protein kinase regulation of fatty acid oxidation in skeletal muscle, Endocrinology 149 (3) (2008) 935–941.
[135] Y.J. Liu, T.C. Ju, H.M. Chen, Y.S. Jang, L.M. Lee, H.L. Lai, et al., Activation of AMP-activated protein kinase $\alpha 1$ mediates mislocalization of TDP-43 in amyotrophic lateral sclerosis, Human Molecular Genetics 24 (3) (2015) 787–801.
[136] Y.J. Liu, L.M. Lee, H.L. Lai, Y. Chern, Aberrant activation of AMP-activated protein kinase contributes to the abnormal distribution of HuR in amyotrophic lateral sclerosis, FEBS Letters 589 (4) (2015) 432–439.

[137] N. Takeyama, S. Miki, A. Hirakawa, T. Tanaka, Role of the mitochondrial permeability transition and cytochrome C release in hydrogen peroxide-induced apoptosis, Experimental Cell Research 274 (1) (2002) 16–24.
[138] S. Marchi, V.A.M. Vitto, S. Patergnani, P. Pinton, High mitochondrial Ca2+ content increases cancer cell proliferation upon inhibition of mitochondrial permeability transition pore (mPTP), Cell Cycle 18 (8) (2019) 914–916.
[139] M.J. Hansson, R. Månsson, S. Morota, H. Uchino, T. Kallur, T. Sumi, et al., Calcium-induced generation of reactive oxygen species in brain mitochondria is mediated by permeability transition, Free Radical Biology & Medicine 45 (3) (2008) 284–294.
[140] H.K. Baumgartner, J.V. Gerasimenko, C. Thorne, P. Ferdek, T. Pozzan, A.V. Tepikin, et al., Calcium elevation in mitochondria is the main Ca2+ requirement for mitochondrial permeability transition pore (mPTP) opening, Journal of Biological Chemistry 284 (31) (2009) 20796–20803.
[141] M.R. Butler, H. Ma, F. Yang, J. Belcher, Y.Z. Le, K. Mikoshiba, et al., Endoplasmic reticulum (ER) Ca2+-channel activity contributes to ER stress and cone death in cyclic nucleotide-gated channel deficiency, Journal of Biological Chemistry 292 (27) (2017) 11189–11205.
[142] N.M. Connolly, J.H. Prehn, The metabolic response to excitotoxicity–lessons from single-cell imaging, Journal of Bioenergetics and Biomembranes 47 (1–2) (2015) 75–88.
[143] H.S. Marinho, C. Real, L. Cyrne, H. Soares, F. Antunes, Hydrogen peroxide sensing signaling and regulation of transcription factors, Redox Biology 2 (2014) 535–562.
[144] Y. Tan, T. Ichikawa, J. Li, Q. Si, H. Yang, X. Chen, et al., Diabetic downregulation of Nrf2 activity via ERK contributes to oxidative stress–induced insulin resistance in cardiac cells in vitro and in vivo, Diabetes 60 (2) (2011) 625–633.
[145] S.G. Ahn, D.J. Thiele, Redox regulation of mammalian heat shock factor 1 is essential for Hsp gene activation and protection from stress, Genes & Development 17 (4) (2003) 516–528.
[146] V. Ayala, A.B. Granado-Serrano, D. Cacabelos, A. Naudí, E.V. Ilieva, J. Boada, et al., Cell stress induces TDP-43 pathological changes associated with ERK1/2 dysfunction: implications in ALS, Acta Neuropathologica 122 (3) (2011) 259–270.
[147] T.J. Cohen, A.W. Hwang, T. Unger, J.Q. Trojanowski, V.M. Lee, Redox signalling directly regulates TDP-43 via cysteine oxidation and disulphide cross-linking, EMBO Journal 31 (5) (2012) 1241–1252.
[148] C. Colombrita, E. Zennaro, C. Fallini, M. Weber, A. Sommacal, E. Buratti, et al., TDP-43 is recruited to stress granules in conditions of oxidative insult, Journal of Neurochemistry 111 (4) (2009) 1051–1061.
[149] H.Y. Chang, S.C. Hou, T.D. Way, C.H. Wong, I.F. Wang, Heat-shock protein dysregulation is associated with functional and pathological TDP-43 aggregation, Nature Communications 4 (1) (2013) 1–11.
[150] X. Zuo, J. Zhou, Y. Li, K. Wu, Z. Chen, Z. Luo, et al., TDP-43 aggregation induced by oxidative stress causes global mitochondrial imbalance in ALS, Nature Structural & Molecular Biology 28 (2) (2021) 132–142.
[151] W.C. Xu, J.Z. Liang, C. Li, Z.X. He, H.Y. Yuan, B.Y. Huang, et al., Pathological hydrogen peroxide triggers the fibrillization of wild-type SOD1 via sulfenic acid modification of Cys-111, Cell Death & Disease 9 (2) (2018) 1–17.
[152] T. Arai, M. Hasegawa, H. Akiyama, K. Ikeda, T. Nonaka, H. Mori, et al., TDP-43 is a component of ubiquitin-positive tau-negative inclusions in frontotemporal lobar degeneration and amyotrophic lateral sclerosis, Biochemical and Biophysical Research Communications 351 (3) (2006) 602–611.
[153] M. Neumann, D.M. Sampathu, L.K. Kwong, A.C. Truax, M.C. Micsenyi, T.T. Chou, et al., Ubiquitinated TDP-43 in frontotemporal lobar degeneration and amyotrophic lateral sclerosis, Science 314 (5796) (2006) 130–133.
[154] C. Hetz, K. Zhang, R.J. Kaufman, Mechanisms regulation and functions of the unfolded protein response, Nature Reviews. Molecular Cell Biology 21 (8) (2020) 421–438.

[155] D. Kültz, Molecular and evolutionary basis of the cellular stress response, Annual Review of Physiology 67 (1) (2005) 225–257.
[156] F.L. Núñez-Santana, M.M. Oh, M.D. Antion, A. Lee, J.W. Hell, J.F. Disterhoft, Surface L-type Ca2+ channel expression levels are increased in aged hippocampus, Aging Cell 13 (1) (2014) 111–120.
[157] S.J. Moore, G.G. Murphy, The role of L-type calcium channels in neuronal excitability and aging, Neurobiology of Learning and Memory 173 (2020) 107230.
[158] A. Kumar, K. Bodhinathan, T.C. Foster, Susceptibility to calcium dysregulation during brain aging, Frontiers in Aging Neuroscience (2009) 2.
[159] A. Reiner, L. Medina, G. Figueredo-Cardenas, S. Anfinson, Brainstem motoneuron pools that are selectively resistant in amyotrophic lateral sclerosis are preferentially enriched in parvalbumin: evidence from monkey brainstem for a calcium-mediated mechanism in sporadic ALS, Experimental Neurology 131 (2) (1995) 239–250.
[160] B.K. Vanselow, B.U. Keller, Calcium dynamics and buffering in oculomotor neurones from mouse that are particularly resistant during amyotrophic lateral sclerosis (ALS)-related motoneurone disease, The Journal of Physiology 525 (Pt 2) (2000) 433.
[161] P. Laslo, J. Lipski, L.F. Nicholson, G.B. Miles, G.D. Funk, Calcium binding proteins in motoneurons at low and high risk for degeneration in ALS, NeuroReport 11 (15) (2000) 3305–3308.
[162] F. von Lewinski, B.U. Keller, Ca2+, mitochondria and selective motoneuron vulnerability: implications for ALS, Trends in Neurosciences 28 (9) (2005) 494–500.
[163] G.B. Miles, J. Lipski, A.R. Lorier, P. Laslo, G.D. Funk, Differential expression of voltage-activated calcium channels in III and XII motoneurones during development in the rat, European Journal of Neuroscience 20 (4) (2004) 903–913.
[164] C.A. Harwood, K. Westgate, S. Gunstone, S. Brage, N.J. Wareham, C.J. McDermott, et al., Long-term physical activity: an exogenous risk factor for sporadic amyotrophic lateral sclerosis?, Amyotrophic Lateral Sclerosis and Frontotemporal Degeneration 17 (5–6) (2016) 377–384.
[165] A.E. Visser, J.P. Rooney, F. D'Ovidio, H.J. Westeneng, R.C. Vermeulen, E. Beghi, et al., Multicentre, cross-cultural, population-based, case–control study of physical activity as risk factor for amyotrophic lateral sclerosis, Journal of Neurology, Neurosurgery and Psychiatry 89 (8) (2018) 797–803.
[166] T. Filippini, M. Fiore, M. Tesauro, C. Malagoli, M. Consonni, F. Violi, et al., Clinical and lifestyle factors and risk of amyotrophic lateral sclerosis: a population-based case-control study, International Journal of Environmental Research and Public Health 17 (3) (2020) 857.
[167] G.X. Chen, J. Douwes, L.H. van den Berg, B. Glass, D. McLean, A.M. 't Mannetje, Sports and trauma as risk factors for motor neurone disease: New Zealand case–control study, Acta Neurologica Scandinavica 145 (6) (2022) 770–785.
[168] D.H. Daneshvar, J. Mez, M.L. Alosco, Z.H. Baucom, I. Mahar, C.M. Baugh, et al., Incidence of and mortality from amyotrophic lateral sclerosis in national football league athletes, JAMA Network Open 4 (12) (2021) e2138801-1.
[169] F. Fang, U. Hållmarker, S. James, C. Ingre, K. Michaëlsson, A. Ahlbom, et al., Amyotrophic lateral sclerosis among cross-country skiers in Sweden, European Journal of Epidemiology 31 (3) (2016) 247–253.
[170] N. Scarmeas, T. Shih, Y. Stern, R. Ottman, L.P. Rowland, Premorbid weight, body mass, and varsity athletics in ALS, Neurology 59 (5) (2002) 773–775.
[171] S. Korner, J. Kammeyer, A. Zapf, M. Kuzma-Kozakiewicz, M. Piotrkiewicz, B. Kuraszkiewicz, et al., Influence of environment and lifestyle on incidence and progress of amyotrophic lateral sclerosis in a German ALS population, Aging and Disease 10 (2) (2019) 205.
[172] A. Rosenbohm, R. Peter, J. Dorst, J. Kassubek, D. Rothenbacher, G. Nagel, et al., Life course of physical activity and risk and prognosis of amyotrophic lateral sclerosis in a German ALS registry, Neurology 97 (19) (2021) e1955-63.

[173] S. Mamoor, Differential expression of CACNA2D1 in amyotrophic lateral sclerosis, https://doi.org/10.31219/osf.io/mnxup, https://osf.io/mnxup, 2022.

[174] F. D'Ovidio, A. d'Errico, E. Farina, A. Calvo, G. Costa, A. Chiò, Amyotrophic lateral sclerosis incidence and previous prescriptions of drugs for the nervous system, Neuroepidemiology 47 (1) (2016) 59–66.

[175] R. Miller, D. Gelinas, V. Dronsky, M. Mendoza, R. Barohn, W. Bryan, et al., Phase III randomized trial of gabapentin in patients with amyotrophic lateral sclerosis, Neurology 56 (7) (2001) 843–848.

[176] Recurrent Hypoventilation and Respiratory Failure During Gabapentin Therapy, Journal of the American Geriatrics Society 49 (4) (2001) 498.

[177] R.C. Pérez, M.G. Lechuga, M.M.L. Alvarez, A.A. Albisu, Gabapentin-induced central hypoventilation, Medicina Clinica 128 (13) (2007) 519.

[178] M. Tuccori, G. Lombardo, F. Lapi, A. Vannacci, C. Blandizzi, M.D. Tacca, Gabapentin-induced severe myopathy, The Annals of Pharmacotherapy 41 (7–8) (2007) 1301–1305.

[179] J. Lipson, S. Lavoie, D. Zimmerman, Gabapentin-induced myopathy in 2 patients on short daily hemodialysis, American Journal of Kidney Diseases 45 (6) (2005) e100-4.

[180] A. Siniscalchi, S. Mintzer, G. De Sarro, L. Gallelli, Myotoxicity induced by antiepileptic drugs: could be a rare but serious adverse event?, Psychopharmacology Bulletin 51 (4) (2021) 105–116.

[181] S. Ghosh, S. Villan, W. Al Yazeedi, Gabapentin-induced myositis in a patient with spinal cord injury–a case report, Qatar Medical Journal 2020 (2) (2020) 30.

[182] T.M. Coupal, D.R. Chang, K. Pennycooke, H.A. Ouellette, P.L. Munk, Radiologic findings in gabapentin-induced myositis, Journal of Radiology Case Reports 11 (4) (2017) 30.

[183] M.S. Choi, H. Jeon, H.S. Kim, B.H. Jang, Y.H. Lee, H.S. Park, et al., A case of gabapentin-induced rhabdomyolysis requiring renal replacement therapy, Hemodialysis International 21 (1) (2017) E4–E8.

[184] O. Bilgir, M. Çalan, F. Bilgir, L. Kebapçilar, A. Yüksel, Y. Yildiz, et al., Gabapentin-induced rhabdomyolysis in a patient with diabetic neuropathy, Internal Medicine 48 (12) (2009) 1085–1087.

[185] A. Desai, Y. Kherallah, C. Szabo, R. Marawar, Gabapentin or pregabalin induced myoclonus: a case series and literature review, Journal of Clinical Neuroscience 61 (2019) 225–234.

[186] K.R. Kaufman, A. Parikh, L. Chan, M. Bridgeman, M. Shah, Myoclonus in renal failure: two cases of gabapentin toxicity, Epilepsy & Behavior Case Reports 2 (2014) 8–10.

[187] Y.F. Shea, M.M.Y. Mok, R.S.K. Chang, Gabapentin-induced myoclonus in an elderly with end-stage renal failure, Journal of the Formosan Medical Association 113 (9) (2014) 660–661.

[188] A. Guddati, Z. Zafar, J. Cheng, S. Mohan, Treatment of gabapentin-induced myoclonus with continuous renal replacement therapy, Indian Journal of Nephrology 22 (1) (2012) 59.

[189] J.J. Verschuuren, J. Palace, H. Murai, M.R. Tannemaat, H.J. Kaminski, V. Bril, Advances and ongoing research in the treatment of autoimmune neuromuscular junction disorders, The Lancet Neurology 21 (2) (2022) 189–202.

[190] N. Boneva, T. Brenner, Z. Argov, Gabapentin may be hazardous in myasthenia gravis, Muscle & Nerve: Official Journal of the American Association of Electrodiagnostic Medicine 23 (8) (2000) 1204–1208.

[191] J. Barclay, N. Balaguero, M. Mione, S.L. Ackerman, V.A. Letts, J. Brodbeck, et al., Ducky mouse phenotype of epilepsy and ataxia is associated with mutations in the Cacna2d2 gene and decreased calcium channel current in cerebellar Purkinje cells, The Journal of Neuroscience 21 (16) (2001) 6095–6104.

[192] G.A. Fuller-Bicer, G. Varadi, S.E. Koch, M. Ishii, I. Bodi, N. Kadeer, et al., Targeted disruption of the voltage-dependent calcium channel $\alpha 2/\delta$-1-subunit, American Journal of Physiology. Heart and Circulatory Physiology 297 (1) (2009) H117–H124.

[193] J. Jankovic, J. Mazziotta, S. Pomeroy, N. Newman, Bradley and Daroff's Neurology in Clinical Practice, 8th edition, Elsevier, 2021.

[194] S.J. Guillot, M. Bolborea, L. Dupuis, Dysregulation of energy homeostasis in amyotrophic lateral sclerosis, Current Opinion in Neurology 34 (5) (2021) 773–780.
[195] E. D'Amico, G. Grosso, J.W. Nieves, A. Zanghì, P. Factor-Litvak, H. Mitsumoto, Metabolic abnormalities, dietary risk factors and nutritional management in amyotrophic lateral sclerosis, Nutrients 13 (7) (2021) 2273.
[196] C. Toth, V. Hebert, C. Gougeon, H. Virtanen, J.K. Mah, D. Pacaud, Motor unit number estimations are smaller in children with type 1 diabetes mellitus: a case–cohort study, Muscle & Nerve 50 (4) (2014) 593–598.
[197] K. Maratova, O. Soucek, J. Matyskova, Z. Hlavka, L. Petruzelkova, B. Obermannova, et al., Muscle functions and bone strength are impaired in adolescents with type 1 diabetes, Bone 106 (2018) 22–27.
[198] K. Muramatsu, M. Niwa, T. Tamaki, M. Ikutomo, Y. Masu, T. Hasegawa, et al., Effect of streptozotocin-induced diabetes on motoneurons and muscle spindles in rats, Neuroscience Research 115 (2017) 21–28.
[199] S. Oveisgharan, A.W. Capuano, S. Nag, S. Agrawal, L.L. Barnes, D.A. Bennett, et al., Association of hemoglobin A1C with TDP-43 pathology in community-based elders, Neurology 96 (22) (2021) e2694-703.
[200] M. Illario, S. Monaco, A.L. Cavallo, I. Esposito, P. Formisano, L. D'Andrea, et al., Calcium-calmodulin-dependent kinase II (CaMKII) mediates insulin-stimulated proliferation and glucose uptake, Cellular Signalling 21 (5) (2009) 786–792.
[201] S. Monaco, M. Illario, M.R. Rusciano, G. Gragnaniello, G. Di Spigna, E. Leggiero, et al., Insulin stimulates fibroblast proliferation through calcium-calmodulin-dependent kinase II, Cell Cycle 8 (13) (2009) 2024–2030.
[202] D. Wright, C. Fick, J. Olesen, K. Lim, B. Barnes, B. Craig, A role for calcium/calmodulin kinase in insulin stimulated glucose transport, Life Sciences 74 (7) (2004) 815–825.
[203] R. Suzuki, K. Lee, E. Jing, S.B. Biddinger, J.G. McDonald, T.J. Montine, et al., Diabetes and insulin in regulation of brain cholesterol metabolism, Cell Metabolism 12 (6) (2010) 567–579.
[204] H. Shimano, R. Sato, SREBP-regulated lipid metabolism: convergent physiology–divergent pathophysiology, Nature Reviews Endocrinology 13 (12) (2017) 710.
[205] R. Willmann, S. Pun, L. Stallmach, G. Sadasivam, A.F. Santos, P. Caroni, et al., Cholesterol and lipid microdomains stabilize the postsynapse at the neuromuscular junction, EMBO Journal 25 (17) (2006) 4050–4060.
[206] J.E. Baenziger, J.A. Domville, J.D. Therien, The Role of Cholesterol in the Activation of Nicotinic Acetylcholine Receptors, Current Topics in Membranes, vol. 80, Elsevier, 2017, pp. 95–137.
[207] B.P. Head, H.H. Patel, P.A. Insel, Interaction of membrane/lipid rafts with the cytoskeleton: impact on signaling and function: membrane/lipid rafts, mediators of cytoskeletal arrangement and cell signaling, Biochimica Et Biophysica Acta. Biomembranes 1838 (2) (2014) 532–545.
[208] S.N. Whitehead, S. Gangaraju, A. Aylsworth, S.T. Hou, Membrane raft disruption results in neuritic retraction prior to neuronal death in cortical neurons, BioScience Trends 6 (4) (2012) 183–191.
[209] A. Wuolikainen, J. Acimovic, A. Lövgren-Sandblom, P. Parini, P.M. Andersen, I. Björkhem, Cholesterol, oxysterol, triglyceride, and coenzyme Q homeostasis in ALS. Evidence against the hypothesis that elevated 27-hydroxycholesterol is a pathogenic factor, PLoS ONE 9 (11) (2014) e113619.
[210] J.C. Dodge, E.H. Jensen, J. Yu, S.P. Sardi, A.R. Bialas, T.V. Taksir, et al., Neutral lipid cacostasis contributes to disease pathogenesis in amyotrophic lateral sclerosis, The Journal of Neuroscience 40 (47) (2020) 9137–9147.
[211] J. Schumacher, R. Peter, G. Nagel, D. Rothenbacher, A. Rosenbohm, A. Ludolph, et al., Statins, diabetes mellitus and prognosis of amyotrophic lateral sclerosis: data from 501 patients of a population-based registry in southwest Germany, European Journal of Neurology 27 (8) (2020) 1405–1414.

[212] S. Apostolski, J. Nikolić, C. Bugarski-Prokopljević, V. Miletić, S. Pavlović, S. Filipović, Serum and CSF immunological findings in ALS, Acta Neurologica Scandinavica 83 (2) (1991) 96–98.
[213] M. Oldstone, L. Perrin, C. Wilson, F. Norris Jr, Evidence for immune-complex formation in patients with amyotrophic lateral sclerosis, The Lancet 308 (7978) (1976) 169–172.
[214] I.A. Saleh, T. Zesiewicz, Y. Xie, K.L. Sullivan, A.M. Miller, N. Kuzmin-Nichols, et al., Evaluation of humoral immune response in adaptive immunity in ALS patients during disease progression, Journal of Neuroimmunology 215 (1–2) (2009) 96–101.
[215] J.I. Engelhardt, J. Tajti, S.H. Appel, Lymphocytic infiltrates in the spinal cord in amyotrophic lateral sclerosis, Archives of Neurology 50 (1) (1993) 30–36.
[216] D.R. Beers, W. Zhao, J. Wang, X. Zhang, S. Wen, D. Neal, et al., ALS patients' regulatory T lymphocytes are dysfunctional, and correlate with disease progression rate and severity, JCI Insight 2 (5) (2017).
[217] R.K. Sheean, F.C. McKay, E. Cretney, C.R. Bye, N.D. Perera, D. Tomas, et al., Association of regulatory T-cell expansion with progression of amyotrophic lateral sclerosis: a study of humans and a transgenic mouse model, JAMA Neurology 75 (6) (2018) 681–689.
[218] S. Garbuzova-Davis, D.G. Hernandez-Ontiveros, M.C. Rodrigues, E. Haller, A. Frisina-Deyo, S. Mirtyl, et al., Impaired blood–brain/spinal cord barrier in ALS patients, Brain Research 1469 (2012) 114–128.
[219] D.R. Beers, S.H. Appel, Immune dysregulation in amyotrophic lateral sclerosis: mechanisms and emerging therapies, The Lancet Neurology 18 (2) (2019) 211–220.
[220] N. Feddermann-Demont, A. Junge, K.P. Weber, M. Weller, J. Dvořák, A.A. Tarnutzer, Prevalence of potential sports-associated risk factors in Swiss amyotrophic lateral sclerosis patients, Brain and Behavior 7 (4) (2017) e00630.
[221] M. Kanmogne, R.S. Klein, Neuroprotective versus neuroinflammatory roles of complement: from development to disease, Trends in Neurosciences 44 (2) (2021) 97–109.
[222] G. Morgan, R. Levinsky, Clinical significance of IgG subclass deficiency, Archives of Disease in Childhood 63 (7) (1988) 771.
[223] X. Sui, J.H. Geng, Y.H. Li, G.Y. Zhu, W.H. Wang, Calcium channel $\alpha 2\delta 1$ subunit (CACNA2D1) enhances radioresistance in cancer stem-like cells in non-small cell lung cancer cell lines, Cancer Management and Research 10 (2018) 5009.
[224] T. Kawamata, H. Akiyama, T. Yamada, P. McGeer, Immunologic reactions in amyotrophic lateral sclerosis brain and spinal cord tissue, The American Journal of Pathology 140 (3) (1992) 691.
[225] X. Chen, W. Feng, R. Huang, X. Guo, Y. Chen, Z. Zheng, et al., Evidence for peripheral immune activation in amyotrophic lateral sclerosis, Journal of the Neurological Sciences 347 (1–2) (2014) 90–95.
[226] M. Wang, Z. Liu, J. Du, Y. Yuan, B. Jiao, X. Zhang, et al., Evaluation of peripheral immune activation in amyotrophic lateral sclerosis, Frontiers in Neurology (2021) 1028.
[227] A.L. Kjældgaard, K. Pilely, K.S. Olsen, A.Ø. Lauritsen, S.W. Pedersen, K. Svenstrup, et al., Complement profiles in patients with amyotrophic lateral sclerosis: a prospective observational cohort study, Journal of Inflammation Research 14 (2021) 1043.
[228] H. Donnenfeld, R. Kascsak, H. Bartfeld, Deposits of IgG and C3 in the spinal cord and motor cortex of ALS patients, Journal of Neuroimmunology 6 (1) (1984) 51–57.
[229] M. Sta, R. Sylva-Steenland, M. Casula, J. De Jong, D. Troost, E. Aronica, et al., Innate and adaptive immunity in amyotrophic lateral sclerosis: evidence of complement activation, Neurobiology of Disease 42 (3) (2011) 211–220.
[230] El. Bahia, N. Idrissi, S. Bosch, V. Ramaglia, E. Aronica, F. Baas, D. Troost, Complement activation at the motor end-plates in amyotrophic lateral sclerosis, Journal of Neuroinflammation 13 (1) (2016) 1–12.
[231] M.R. Turner, R. Goldacre, S. Ramagopalan, K. Talbot, M.J. Goldacre, Autoimmune disease preceding amyotrophic lateral sclerosis: an epidemiologic study, Neurology 81 (14) (2013) 1222–1225.

[232] C. Cui, E. Longinetti, H. Larsson, J. Andersson, Y. Pawitan, F. Piehl, et al., Associations between autoimmune diseases and amyotrophic lateral sclerosis: a register-based study, Amyotrophic Lateral Sclerosis and Frontotemporal Degeneration 22 (3–4) (2021) 211–219.
[233] M. Seelen, P.T. van Doormaal, A.E. Visser, M.H. Huisman, M.H. Roozekrans, S.W. de Jong, et al., Prior medical conditions and the risk of amyotrophic lateral sclerosis, Journal of Neurology 261 (10) (2014) 1949–1956.
[234] A. Gaimari, M. Fusaroli, E. Raschi, E. Baldin, L. Vignatelli, F. Nonino, et al., Amyotrophic lateral sclerosis as an adverse drug reaction: a disproportionality analysis of the food and drug administration adverse event reporting system, Drug Safety (2022) 1–11.
[235] H.T. Gotaas, G.O. Skeie, N.E. Gilhus, Myasthenia gravis and amyotrophic lateral sclerosis: a pathogenic overlap, Neuromuscular Disorders 26 (6) (2016) 337–341.
[236] M. del Mar Amador, N. Vandenberghe, N. Berhoune, J.P. Camdessanché, S. Gronier, E. Delmont, et al., Unusual association of amyotrophic lateral sclerosis and myasthenia gravis: a dysregulation of the adaptive immune system?, Neuromuscular Disorders 26 (6) (2016) 342–346.
[237] S. de Pasqua, F. Cavallieri, R. D'Angelo, F. Salvi, N. Fini, R. D'Alessandro, et al., Amyotrophic lateral sclerosis and myasthenia gravis: association or chance occurrence?, Neurological Sciences 38 (2017) 441–444.
[238] R.K. Hajela, K.M. Huntoon, W.D. Atchison, Lambert–Eaton syndrome antibodies target multiple subunits of voltage-gated Ca2+ channels, Muscle & Nerve 51 (2) (2015) 176–184.
[239] R. Zhou, R.R. Caspi, Ocular immune privilege, F1000 biology reports (2010) 2.
[240] A. Badou, M.K. Jha, D. Matza, R.A. Flavell, Emerging roles of L-type voltage-gated and other calcium channels in T lymphocytes, Frontiers in Immunology 4 (2013) 243.
[241] J.E. McRory, J. Hamid, C.J. Doering, E. Garcia, R. Parker, K. Hamming, et al., The CACNA1F gene encodes an L-type calcium channel with unique biophysical properties and tissue distribution, The Journal of Neuroscience 24 (7) (2004) 1707–1718.
[242] B. Davenport, Y. Li, J.W. Heizer, C. Schmitz, A.L. Perraud, Signature channels of excitability no more: L-type channels in immune cells, Frontiers in Immunology 6 (2015) 375.
[243] J.Y. Zhang, P.P. Zhang, W.P. Zhou, J.Y. Yu, Z.H. Yao, J.F. Chu, et al., L-type Cav1.2 calcium channel-α-1C regulates response to rituximab in diffuse large B-cell lymphoma, Clinical Cancer Research 25 (13) (2019) 4168–4178.
[244] P. Hemon, Y. Renaudineau, M. Debant, N. Le Goux, S. Mukherjee, W. Brooks, et al., Calcium signaling: from normal B cell development to tolerance breakdown and autoimmunity, Clinical Reviews in Allergy & Immunology 53 (2017) 141–165.
[245] R. Zhang, R. Gascon, R.G. Miller, D.F. Gelinas, J. Mass, K. Hadlock, et al., Evidence for systemic immune system alterations in sporadic amyotrophic lateral sclerosis (sALS), Journal of Neuroimmunology 159 (1–2) (2005) 215–224.
[246] D. Troost, J. Van den Oord, J.V.D. Jong, Immunohistochemical characterization of the inflammatory infiltrate in amyotrophic lateral sclerosis, Neuropathology and Applied Neurobiology 16 (5) (1990) 401–410.
[247] L. Provinciali, M. Laurenzi, L. Vesprini, A. Giovagnoli, C. Bartocci, M. Montroni, et al., Immunity assessment in the early stages of amyotrophic lateral sclerosis: a study of virus antibodies and lymphocyte subsets, Acta Neurologica Scandinavica 78 (6) (1988) 449–454.
[248] J.R. Burrell, M.C. Kiernan, S. Vucic, J.R. Hodges, Motor neuron dysfunction in frontotemporal dementia, Brain 134 (9) (2011) 2582–2594.
[249] C. Lomen-Hoerth, J. Murphy, S. Langmore, J. Kramer, R. Olney, B. Miller, Are amyotrophic lateral sclerosis patients cognitively normal?, Neurology 60 (7) (2003) 1094–1097.
[250] L. Liu-Yesucevitz, A. Bilgutay, Y.J. Zhang, T. Vanderwyde, A. Citro, T. Mehta, et al., Tar DNA binding protein-43 (TDP-43) associates with stress granules: analysis of cultured cells and pathological brain tissue, PLoS ONE 5 (10) (2010) e13250.
[251] K. Rascovsky, J.R. Hodges, D. Knopman, M.F. Mendez, J.H. Kramer, J. Neuhaus, et al., Sensitivity of revised diagnostic criteria for the behavioural variant of frontotemporal dementia, Brain 134 (9) (2011) 2456–2477.

[252] M.L. Schroeter, B. Vogt, S. Frisch, G. Becker, A. Seese, H. Barthel, et al., Dissociating behavioral disorders in early dementia-an FDG-PET study, Psychiatry Research: Neuroimaging 194 (3) (2011) 235–244.
[253] W.W. Seeley, D.A. Carlin, J.M. Allman, M.N. Macedo, C. Bush, B.L. Miller, et al., Early frontotemporal dementia targets neurons unique to apes and humans, Annals of Neurology: Official Journal of the American Neurological Association and the Child Neurology Society 60 (6) (2006) 660–667.
[254] E.J. Kim, M. Sidhu, S.E. Gaus, E.J. Huang, P.R. Hof, B.L. Miller, et al., Selective frontoinsular von economo neuron and fork cell loss in early behavioral variant frontotemporal dementia, Cerebral Cortex 22 (2) (2012) 251–259.
[255] S.S. Pineda, H. Lee, B.E. Fitzwalter, S. Mohammadi, L.J. Pregent, M.E. Gardashli, et al., Single-cell profiling of the human primary motor cortex in ALS and FTLD, bioRxiv 2021.
[256] E.A. Nimchinsky, B.A. Vogt, J.H. Morrison, P.R. Hof, Spindle neurons of the human anterior cingulate cortex, Journal of Comparative Neurology 355 (1) (1995) 27–37.
[257] X. Gu, Z. Gao, X. Wang, X. Liu, R.T. Knight, P.R. Hof, et al., Anterior insular cortex is necessary for empathetic pain perception, Brain 135 (9) (2012) 2726–2735.
[258] M. Rutgen, E.M. Seidel, G. Silani, I. Riecansky, A. Hummer, C. Windischberger, et al., Placebo analgesia and its opioidergic regulation suggest that empathy for pain is grounded in self pain, Proceedings of the National Academy of Sciences 112 (41) (2015) E5638–E5646.
[259] P.D. Fletcher, L.E. Downey, H.L. Golden, C.N. Clark, C.F. Slattery, R.W. Paterson, et al., Pain and temperature processing in dementia: a clinical and neuroanatomical analysis, Brain 138 (11) (2015) 3360–3372.
[260] C.R. Marshall, C.J. Hardy, M. Allen, L.L. Russell, C.N. Clark, R.L. Bond, et al., Cardiac responses to viewing facial emotion differentiate frontotemporal dementias, Annals of Clinical and Translational Neurology 5 (6) (2018) 687–696.
[261] M.T. Gailliot, R.F. Baumeister, The physiology of willpower: linking blood glucose to self-control, Personality and Social Psychology Review 11 (4) (2007) 303–327.
[262] D. Adlersberg, H. Dolger, Medico-legal problems of hypoglycemic reactions in diabetes, Annals of Internal Medicine 12 (11) (1939) 1804–1815.
[263] O. Piguet, Å. Petersén, B. Yin Ka Lam, S. Gabery, K. Murphy, J.R. Hodges, et al., Eating and hypothalamus changes in behavioral-variant frontotemporal dementia, Annals of neurology. 69 (2) (2011) 312–319.
[264] M. Bocchetta, E. Gordon, E. Manning, J. Barnes, D.M. Cash, M. Espak, et al., Detailed volumetric analysis of the hypothalamus in behavioral variant frontotemporal dementia, Journal of Neurology 262 (12) (2015) 2635–2642.
[265] F. Kumfor, J.L. Hazelton, J.A. Rushby, J.R. Hodges, O. Piguet, Facial expressiveness and physiological arousal in frontotemporal dementia: phenotypic clinical profiles and neural correlates, Cognitive, Affective & Behavioral Neuroscience 19 (2019) 197–210.
[266] I. Im, J.P. Jun, S. Hwang, M.H. Ko, Swallowing outcomes in patients with subcortical stroke associated with lesions of the caudate nucleus and insula, Journal of International Medical Research 46 (9) (2018) 3552–3562.
[267] S. Morbelli, M. Ferrara, F. Fiz, B. Dessi, D. Arnaldi, A. Picco, et al., Mapping brain morphological and functional conversion patterns in predementia late-onset bvFTD, European Journal of Nuclear Medicine and Molecular Imaging 43 (7) (2016) 1337–1347.
[268] M. Fukai, T. Hirosawa, M. Kikuchi, S. Hino, T. Kitamura, Y. Ouchi, et al., Different patterns of glucose hypometabolism underlie functional decline in frontotemporal dementia and Alzheimer's disease: FDG-PET study, Neuropsychiatry 8 (2) (2018) 441–447.
[269] R.M. Ahmed, M. MacMillan, L. Bartley, G.M. Halliday, M.C. Kiernan, J.R. Hodges, et al., Systemic metabolism in frontotemporal dementia, Neurology 83 (20) (2014) 1812–1818.
[270] A. Golimstok, N. Cámpora, J.I. Rojas, M.C. Fernandez, C. Elizondo, E. Soriano, et al., Cardiovascular risk factors and frontotemporal dementia: a case–control study, Translational Neurodegeneration 3 (1) (2014) 1–6.

[271] R. Zanardini, L. Benussi, S. Fostinelli, C. Saraceno, M. Ciani, B. Borroni, et al., Serum C-peptide, visfatin, resistin, and ghrelin are altered in sporadic and GRN-associated frontotemporal lobar degeneration, Journal of Alzheimer's Disease 61 (3) (2018) 1053–1060.
[272] C. Yoon, M. Kang, H. Shin, S. Jeon, J.J. Yang, S. Kim, et al., Higher C-peptide levels are associated with regional cortical thinning in 1093 cognitively normal subjects, European Journal of Neurology 21 (10) (2014) 1318.
[273] J.D. Woolley, B.K. Khan, A. Natesan, A. Karydas, M. Dallman, P. Havel, et al., Satiety-related hormonal dysregulation in behavioral variant frontotemporal dementia, Neurology 82 (6) (2014) 512–520.
[274] C.S. Jensen, H.S. Gleerup, C.S. Musaeus, S.G. Hasselbalch, P. Høgh, G. Waldemar, et al., Cerebrospinal fluid glucose is not altered in patients with dementia, Clinical Biochemistry 112 (2023) 1–5.
[275] I. Ferrer, T. Tuñón, M. Serrano, R. Casas, S. Alcantara, M. Zujar, et al., Calbindin D-28k and parvalbumin immunoreactivity in the frontal cortex in patients with frontal lobe dementia of non-Alzheimer type associated with amyotrophic lateral sclerosis, Journal of Neurology, Neurosurgery and Psychiatry 56 (3) (1993) 257–261.
[276] A. Spalloni, S. Caioli, E. Bonomi, C. Zona, E. Buratti, A. Alberici, et al., Cerebrospinal fluid from frontotemporal dementia patients is toxic to neurons, Biochimica Et Biophysica Acta. Molecular Basis of Disease 1867 (6) (2021) 166122.
[277] J.S. Katzeff, F. Bright, K. Lo, J.J. Kril, A. Connolly, B. Crossett, et al., Altered serum protein levels in frontotemporal dementia and amyotrophic lateral sclerosis indicate calcium and immunity dysregulation, Scientific Reports 10 (1) (2020) 1–12.
[278] K. Phan, Y. He, R. Pickford, S. Bhatia, J.S. Katzeff, J.R. Hodges, et al., Uncovering pathophysiological changes in frontotemporal dementia using serum lipids, Scientific Reports 10 (1) (2020) 1–13.
[279] K. Imamura, N. Sahara, N.M. Kanaan, K. Tsukita, T. Kondo, Y. Kutoku, et al., Calcium dysregulation contributes to neurodegeneration in FTLD patient iPSC-derived neurons, Scientific Reports 6 (1) (2016) 1–10.
[280] F. Palluzzi, R. Ferrari, F. Graziano, V. Novelli, G. Rossi, D. Galimberti, et al., A novel network analysis approach reveals DNA damage, oxidative stress and calcium/cAMP homeostasis-associated biomarkers in frontotemporal dementia, PLoS ONE 12 (10) (2017) e0185797.
[281] K. Younes, L.A. Lepow, C. Estrada, P.E. Schulz, Auto-antibodies against P/Q- and N-type voltage-dependent calcium channels mimicking frontotemporal dementia, SAGE Open Medical Case Reports 6 (2018) 2050313X17750928.
[282] F. Arshad, F. Varghese, A. Paplikar, Y. Gangadhar, S. Ramakrishnan, J.R. Chaudhuri, et al., Role of autoantibodies in neurodegenerative dementia: an emerging association, Dementia and Geriatric Cognitive Disorders 50 (2) (2021) 153–160.
[283] B. Borroni, J. Stanic, C. Verpelli, M. Mellone, E. Bonomi, A. Alberici, et al., Anti-AMPA GluA3 antibodies in frontotemporal dementia: a new molecular target, Scientific Reports 7 (1) (2017) 1–10.
[284] J.Y. Li, Z.Y. Cai, X.H. Sun, D.C. Shen, X.Z. Yang, M.S. Liu, et al., Blood–brain barrier dysfunction and myelin basic protein in survival of amyotrophic lateral sclerosis with or without frontotemporal dementia, Neurological Sciences 43 (2022) 3201–3210.
[285] K. Katisko, E. Solje, A.M. Koivisto, J. Krüger, T. Kinnunen, P. Hartikainen, et al., Prevalence of immunological diseases in a Finnish frontotemporal lobar degeneration cohort with the C9orf72 repeat expansion carriers and non-carriers, Journal of Neuroimmunology 321 (2018) 29–35.
[286] P. Gami-Patel, M. Scarioni, F.H. Bouwman, B.D. Boon, J.C. van Swieten, N. Brain Bank, et al., The severity of behavioural symptoms in FTD is linked to the loss of GABRQ-expressing VENs and pyramidal neurons, Neuropathology and Applied Neurobiology 48 (4) (2022) e12798.

[287] A.L. Nana, M. Sidhu, S.E. Gaus, J.H.L. Hwang, L. Li, Y. Park, et al., Neurons selectively targeted in frontotemporal dementia reveal early stage TDP-43 pathobiology, Acta Neuropathologica 137 (1) (2019) 27–46.
[288] M. Boccardi, F. Sabattoli, M.P. Laakso, C. Testa, R. Rossi, A. Beltramello, et al., Frontotemporal dementia as a neural system disease, Neurobiology of Aging 26 (1) (2005) 37–44.
[289] W.W. Seeley, R. Crawford, K. Rascovsky, J.H. Kramer, M. Weiner, B.L. Miller, et al., Frontal paralimbic network atrophy in very mild behavioral variant frontotemporal dementia, Archives of Neurology 65 (2) (2008) 249–255.
[290] Y. Wang, D. Shen, B. Hou, X. Sun, X. Yang, J. Gao, et al., Brain structural and perfusion changes in amyotrophic lateral sclerosis-frontotemporal dementia patients with cognitive and motor onset: a preliminary study, Brain Imaging and Behavior (2022) 1–11.
[291] Z. Képes, F. Nagy, Á. Budai, S. Barna, R. Esze, S. Somodi, et al., Age, BMI and diabetes as independent predictors of brain hypoperfusion, Nuclear Medicine Review 24 (1) (2021) 11–15.
[292] K. Yaffe, C.M. Falvey, N. Hamilton, T.B. Harris, E.M. Simonsick, E.S. Strotmeyer, et al., Association between hypoglycemia and dementia in a biracial cohort of older adults with diabetes mellitus, JAMA Internal Medicine 173 (14) (2013) 1300–1306.
[293] S.H. Appel, D. Beers, L. Siklos, J.I. Engelhardt, D.R. Mosier, Calcium: the darth vader of ALS, Amyotrophic Lateral Sclerosis and Other Motor Neuron Disorders 2 (1) (2001) 47–54.
[294] R. Patai, B. Nógrádi, J.I. Engelhardt, L. Siklós, Calcium in the pathomechanism of amyotrophic lateral sclerosis–taking center stage?, Biochemical and Biophysical Research Communications 483 (4) (2017) 1031–1039.
[295] A. Mackensen, F. Müller, D. Mougiakakos, S. Böltz, A. Wilhelm, M. Aigner, et al., Anti-CD19 CAR T cell therapy for refractory systemic lupus erythematosus, Nature Medicine (2022) 1–9.
[296] J. Hendrich, A.T. Van Minh, F. Heblich, M. Nieto-Rostro, K. Watschinger, J. Striessnig, et al., Pharmacological disruption of calcium channel trafficking by the $\alpha 2\delta$ ligand gabapentin, Proceedings of the National Academy of Sciences 105 (9) (2008) 3628–3633.

Chapter 10

A galactose theory of Parkinson's disease

10.1 Introduction

Parkinson's disease (PD) is the main movement disorder [1,2]. Movement symptoms result from the degeneration of brain dopamine (DA) neurons, mainly in the substantia nigra pars compacta (SNc). Locus coeruelus (LC) norepinephrine (NEP) neurons also degenerate early [3]. The cognitive impairment shown by many PD patients can be explained by reduced NEP [4] and DA. Although substantial empirical data has been gathered about PD during the last decades, there is still no complete theory explaining the disease. In particular, a theory of PD must explain why gut symptoms such as constipation precede onset by more than a decade [5], and the specific vulnerability of DA and NEP neurons [3].

Here I present a complete theory of PD (T*PD). It is complete in the sense that it explains its etiology, symptoms, pathophysiology, and treatment. The theory is supported by strong evidence, and points to novel optimal treatment directions.

Theory overview. PD patients have a higher gut abundance of mucin-degrading bacteria (e.g., Akkermansia Muciniphila (akkm)), which can be due to (epi)genetic reasons (e.g., higher mucin production), maternal transfer during birth, diet (e.g., milk consumption), infections, pollution, antibiotics treatment, etc. Since galactose is a major component of mucin and competes with glucose for transport and uptake, this results in higher than normal brain galactose uptake, and lower than normal brain glucose uptake. Galactose undergoes oxidative metabolism like glucose, but it is a less efficient substrate for glycolysis. As a result, glutathione (GSH) production, which depends on glycolysis and the pentose phosphate pathway (PPP), is decreased. GSH is the main anti-oxidant that counters the oxidative damage induced by iron, and its deficiency leads to cell death by ferroptosis [6].

Neuromelanin (NM) is a pigment produced via iron-mediated oxidation of catecholamines [7], protecting cells from iron-induced oxidative stress (oxis) [8]. SNc DA neurons and LC NEP neurons have a substantially higher NM expression than other brain cells [7], indicating that they have the highest sensitivity to iron toxicity. Hence, they are the first to suffer the results of decreased GSH. These neurons manage to protect themselves for many years (e.g., via alpha-synuclein (aSyn) and NM), but this protection eventually collapses, due

The Science of the Brain. https://doi.org/10.1016/B978-0-44-345008-2.00016-3

to the general aging-related decrease in the efficiency of cellular processes and to aSyn and NM accumulation.

Glycolysis-oxphos imbalance in PD can also be caused or enhanced by mutations in genes involved in mitochondrial oxphos and iron metabolism.

10.2 T*PD theory of PD

T*PD explains PD as follows.

1. PD involves an imbalance between galactose and glucose in favor of the former. This yields reduced glycolysis.
2. The main source for this imbalance is a higher abundance of mucin-degrading bacteria in the gut microbiome (GMB).
3. The imbalance yields GSH deficiency, exposing cells to oxidative iron toxicity. The cells that are most sensitive to this are those that continuously secrete catecholamines and express neuromelanin.
4. The phenomenon is a small-scale one, and the main damage occurs with the deterioration of cellular defenses with aging, and with the accumulation of NM and alpha-synuclein (aSyn).
5. Some genetic mutations can enhance these processes.

Here I elaborate on each of these points.

Galactose. Galactose is a monosaccharide found in milk products (as lactose, containing one galactose molecule and one glucose molecule), fruits and vegetables [9]. It is absorbed by intestinal endothelial cells via the sodium-glucose linked transporter type I (SGLT1), and released into the circulation via glucose transporter type 2 (GLUT2). Normally, most of the ingested galactose remains in the liver, with a small amount entering the brain (via GLUT3 and GLUT4) and other organs [10]. However, a higher load reduces liver clearance [11], and following an intraperitoneal galactose load, brain uptake is higher than the livers', retaining galactose for a longer duration than the liver and that of brain glucose [10].

The main metabolic pathway of galactose is the Leloir pathway, where it is converted to UDP-Gal and UDP-Glc. Through these, galactose can be used for glycogen synthesis, glycolysis, and glycosylation. However, it fuels glycolysis at a much slower rate than glucose does [9,12,13]. As a result, its contribution to the PPP, which is essential for GSH synthesis, is smaller, it induces higher oxidative stress and oxphos gene transcription than glucose [14], and reduces glycogen synthesis.

Two additional metabolic pathways, used in case of excess, are the galactonate pathway and galactitol. Galactitol does not diffuse across the cell membranes, and when it accumulates, it leads to depletion of NADPH, decreased glutathione reductase activity, and increased oxis. Galactitol accumulation exerts negative feedback on the first step of the Leloir pathway, increasing its accumulation [9].

Thus, galactose decreases anabolic processes and increases oxidative stress. Indeed, there is a rodent model of aging in which chronic subcutaneous galactose injections induce mitochondrial dysfunction, oxidative stress, inflammation, apoptosis, and decreased neurotrophic factors [13]. These effects are ameliorated by alpha-lipoic acid, an iron chelator [15].

The galactose aging model also shows increased GSK3b, which suppresses glycogen synthesis [16]. Note that (i) glycogenolysis is required for the astrocyte Na^+/K^+-ATPase [17], (ii) the glutamate-glutamine cycle depends on K^+ and Na^+ gradients, and (iii) glutamate is used for GSH production. These data imply that glutamate uptake may be impaired in PD, leading to excitotoxicity.

Mucin-degrading gut bacteria. The human gut microbiome (GMB) is comprised of a large number of species and sub-species. Several of these can degrade mucin, the protective mucus layer of the gut and the respiratory tract [18,19]. Galactose is a fundamental component of mucin. The main mucin-degrading bacterium is akkm (the only member of verrucomicrobia present in humans), which clearly plays an important part in PD and has all of the prototypical properties needed for explaining it. Other species include bacteroidetes, bifidobacteria, firmicutes, and lactobacteria.

Unlike some mucin-degrading bacteria, akkm liberates mucin but does not use it [20]. In parallel, akkm increases the thickness of the gut mocus layer [21], and upregulates genes involved in maintaining the intestinal barrier [22]. These effects increase galactose absorption and decrease glucose absorption [23].

High GMB akkm may be secondary to increased mucin production due to (epi)genetic reasons, diet effects (e.g., consumption of particular milk products), and other inherited or acquired alterations of the GMB. For example, akkm is increased in the galactose-induced aging mouse model [24]. Importantly, mucin production is enhanced by gut infections [25]. Since akkm is highly heritable [26], a family or personal history of infections can trigger PD in many people.

Neuromelanin, iron. One clearly unique aspect of brain DA and NEP cells is that they are the only ones with substantial expression of neuromelanin (NM). NM is a pigment resulting from the oxidation of catecholamines by iron(III) to o-quinones, which yield NM [7]. NM is not degradable and it is insoluble, accumulating in cells. Thus, the expression of NM indicates a state with a high reactive iron potential. Indeed, SNc DA neurons have higher basal oxphos and oxis than ventral tegmental area (VTA) DA neurons, which are less sensitive in PD [27].

Ferroptosis is an iron-dependent, caspase-independent cell death pathway whose key features are GSH depletion and lipid peroxidation [6]. The PPP, which depends on glycolysis, is essential for the production of GSH [28]. GSH binding to iron prevents the oxidation of iron(II), maintaining iron solubility and preventing the generation of the hydroxyl radical from hydrogen peroxide (the fenton reaction) [6]. Hydroxyl radicals are highly potent agents of lipid peroxidation. GSH depletion allows iron to yield hydroxyl radicals, lipid peroxidation, and ferroptosis.

Thus, the following picture emerges. When GSH production is sufficient, it prevents the formation of iron(III) and lipid peroxidation. When GSH diminishes (e.g., with aging), iron(III) is formed and drives the formation of NM, which neutralizes iron toxicity, including the production of toxic catecholamine metabolites and of the hydroxyl radical [29]. Indeed, reactive iron is not present in NM-containing neurons, while neurons without NM have reactive iron deposits [7]. With severe GSH deficiency, as in PD, there is lipid peroxidation and eventually ferroptosis.

Aging. Age is the leading risk factor for PD. In over 75% of patients, the age of onset is older than 65 years, and in 90-95% it is older than 50 years [30]. Aging involves a general decrease in the efficiency of brain cellular processes, inducing an increase in relevant harmful processes such as lipid peroxidation, mitochondrial dysfunction, and dysregulated metabolism [31]. Moreover, the specific causal processes discussed above are also affected by aging. The capacity of the liver for galactose elimination decreases with aging, starting around 63 years [32]. The galactose-based aging model shows many of the characteristics of normal aging [13]. GSH synthesis significantly decreases with aging [33]. Both oxidative iron [34] and NM [7] increase with aging. Lipid peroxidation is increased 2-fold in SNc DA neurons vs. the basal ganglia and prefrontal cortex in aging [35].

Alpha-synuclein (aSyn). PD has been traditionally strongly associated with aggregates of aSyn in the degenerating neurons. However, it is now recognized that such aggregates are also present in many other neurons and tissues [30]. aSyn is recruited by increased oxis [36] and iron (via an iron-responsive DNA element) [37]. There is higher aSyn accumulation in NM cells [38]. Monomeric (but not fibrillar) aSyn prevents lipid peroxidation [39], and knockout neurons are more vulerable to oxis [40]. aSyn converts large spherical vesicles into very small ones with higher curvature [41], inhibits membrane fusion, and induces mitochondria fragmentation [42]. It is present in mitochondria-associated endoplasmic reticulum membranes, streamlinining Ca^{2+} transfer [43]. Finally, it promotes glucose uptake and glycolysis [44,45].

Thus, the role of aSyn seems to be to protect cells from excessive oxphos- and iron-induced oxis. It is easily activated in basically all cell types (in fact, the kinases promoting its Ser129 phosphorylation are constitutively active [46]), indicating that it is the first line of defense against such toxicity. As explained above, cells that continuously secrete catecholamines are more vulnerable than other cells, and need further defenses in the form of NM. In PD, higher chronic oxis induces chronic aSyn recruitment, misfolding, and phosphorylation, which eventually lead to its aggregation. This further impairs mitoch function and promotes degeneration.

Genetic mutations. In a minority of patients, PD is associated with gene mutations (in parkin (park2), DJ1 (park7), pink1, LRRK2). All of these genes are essential for mitochondria function, specifically with respect to oxis [47]. For example, parkin overexpression decreases oxis, protects from DA- or 6-OHDA-induced apoptosis, and mutants are associated with increased lipid peroxidation [47]. DJ1 is protective against H2O2, 6-OHDA, rotenone, and MPTP (widely used animal models of PD). DJ1 also enhances GSH levels [47].

Another associated gene is GBA, which shows decreased activity in sporadic PD [48]. GBA breaks down glucosylceramide to glucose and ceramide. Decreased activity implies decreased glucose around membranes, exacerbating the imbalance problem in PD.

It is not clear whether these mutations require higher mucin-degrading bacteria to cause the disease. They may be able to do so on their own, or alternatively, it is possible that they do require a basic galactose problem, and their presence only accelerates disease onset.

Animal models. There are several animal models for PD, based on rotenone, paraquat, 6-OHDA, MPTP/MPP+, etc. [1]. These models mimic the oxis and mitochondria aspects of PD, but not the galactose aspect.

10.3 Evidence

T*PD is supported by strong evidence.

10.3.1 Gut bacteria, mucin

Mucin-degrading bacteria. Increased abundance of mucin-degrading bacteria, mainly akkm, is consistently reported in PD [49,50]. Other relevant bacteria include some bifidobacterium, bacteroides, lactobacillus, and christensenellaceae species.

Constipation. PD patients show gut-related prodromal symptoms, mainly constipation, which precede movement symptoms by decades. Akkm and high gut mucin are associated with constipation [51,52].

Olfaction. PD patients also show very early prodromal olfactory symptoms [1]. Mucin is expressed at the respiratory tract, including the nasal cavity, which hosts mucin-degrading bacteria [53].

aSyn. Patients show aSyn pathology in the gut and olfactory mucosa [54].

Pneumonia. Respiratory diseases are very common in PD [55], and have been reported to be the leading cause of death [56,57]. Usually explained via swallowing difficulties, it is possibly better explained via respiratory mucin expression.

HPL infection. Helicobacter pylori (HPL) is a gut bacterium, associated with increased PD risk [55]. HPL degrades mucin and liberates galactose [58].

Pollution. Exposure to air pollution increases risk (but not in all studies) [59]. Environmental pollution and pesticides enhance oxis burden in the respiratory tracts and increase gut mucus [60].

10.3.2 Galactose

Milk. Consumption of dairy products, mainly milk, is a PD risk factor [61]. Milk increases the amount of gut galactose. Many mucin-degrading bacteria, including akkm, bacteroides, and bifidobacteria can degrade human milk oligosaccharides [62].

Galactitol. There is some direct evidence for excessive galactose in PD. CSF galactitol, whose production indicates excessive galactose, is increased by 1.26x in PD [63]. Galactitol is increased 3.1x in most brain areas in PD with cognitive decline [64]. In preonset PD, plasma galactitol is decreased [65] (with a similar trend reported as well [66]). This may show higher brain intracellular accumulation.

Glycosylation. Abnormally high glycosylation and glycation are common [67].

Galactosemia. Galactosemia is a disease that involves accumulation of galactose due to reduced function of an enzyme that breaks it down. A high percentage of patients show motor problems, mainly tremor and dystonia [68], and progressive worsening is common [68,69]. Striatal dopamine denervation has been reported in one case report, and L-dopa improved tremor in another [70,71].

Both galactosemia [72] and PD patients [73] show decreased bone mass and bone problems.

10.3.3 Glucose

Reduced glucose. Patient CSF shows decreased glucose and lactate [74,75]. Lower blood glucose elevation following food intake is associated with increased PD risk [76]. This supports lower glucose gut absorption.

Glycolysis. G6PD and 6PGD (PPP-supporting enzymes) are decreased in the putamen in early PD stages [77]. Patient SNc DA cells show decreased glycolysis [78]. Plasma PPP and glycolysis are dysregulated compared to essential tremor patients [79].

Glycogen. GSK3b, which suppresses glycogen synthesis, is found in patient Lewy bodies in midbrain and pons neurons [80]. Glycogen synthesis rate is decreased in patient visual cortex [81].

Glycolysis medication. Glycolysis-enhancing drugs decrease PD risk [82].

Uptake. PET imaging studies consistently report reduced glucose uptake in non-degenerating brain areas [83–85]. This supports excess of ATP in brain cells (in T*PD, due to galactose), since ATP excess is the main factor that downregulates glucose receptors.

Reduced glucose uptake in olfaction pathways is correlated with olfactory dysfunction in patients [86].

Diet. Patients eat significantly more carbohydrates preonset [87], and show sweet craving [88,89], showing that the brain does not receive sufficient amounts of glucose.

Diabetes. People with type 2 diabetes (DM2) have a higher PD risk, but PD patients have a lower risk of DM2 [90]. T*PD explains this as follows. In DM2, there is reduced cellular uptake of glucose, and a higher PD risk indicates that this might be part of the problem in PD. In PD, there is lower blood glucose (due to competition with galactose for gut absorption), which reduces DM2 risk.

Note that gut bacteria such as akkm are usually viewed as beneficial in DM2 and inflammatory bowel disease, because they reduce blood glucose and enhance barrier function. In T*PD, such bacteria are the main culprits.

BMI. PD patients are commonly underweight, with a significant proportion fulfilling criteria for malnutrition [91]. Conversely, being underweight (prodromally) increases risk [92]. Mucin reduces gut absorption of nutrients used for fat storage, and galactose poorly supports growth processes.

10.3.4 Oxidative stress

Mitochondria. There is overwhelming evidence showing mitochondria (especially complex I) damage in PD [2]. Factors that impair mitochondria function (e.g., pesticides) are associated with increased PD risk [61]. Higher mitochondria oxis is also present in patient skin fibroblasts [93].

Chronic systemic complex I inhibition by rotenone causes highly selective SNc DA degeneration, associated with hypokinesia and ridigity [94].

GSH. The data with respect to GSH in PD overwhelmingly points to a decrease, in the SNc [95–97], including preonset [98,99], in other brain areas [100], in CSF [101], and in blood [102–104].

Iron. There is excessive total iron and iron(III) accumulation in the SNc in PD [100,105–107], including preonset [108].

Lipid peroxidation. Patient brains show high lipid peroxidation [109–112].

Neuromelanin. Virtually all patients exhibit substantial loss of neuromelanin-containing LC NEP neurons [7]. (See also cancer below.) Lateral SNc neuromelanin positively correlates with posterior putamen DA functionality in patients [113].

10.3.5 Sympathetic nervous system

Early sympathetic degeneration. Early sympathetic nervous system (SNS) symptoms (daytime sleepiness, decreased lipolysis, cardiac SNS dysfunction) are very common in PD [114], showing that SNS cells degenerate early.

PD risk is higher with decreased serum triglycerides [115] and long chain fatty acids [116]. Note that this seemingly contradicts the datum stated earlier of being underweight increasing risk. That datum was due to GMB, and the one here to SNS function (lipolysis).

REM sleep behavior disorder (RBD). RBD involves large movements during the rapid eye movement (REM) phase of sleep ("acting out dreams"). RBD is often one of the prodromal signs of PD [30]. Muscle atonia during REM sleep is normally mediated by projections from the sublateral dorsal nucleus (SLD), located just below the LC. SLD neurons contain NM, and are affected in PD to about the same extent as the LC [117]. This yields prodromal symtpoms like the other sympathetic prodromal symptoms in PD.

10.3.6 Risk & protective factors

Alcohol. Mild alcohol consumption is associated with decreased PD risk [118]. Alcohol depletes akkm, firmicutes, and lactobacteria [119].

Smoking. Smoking is associated with decreased PD risk [120]. Smoking depletes gut mucin-degrading bacteria (akkm, bifidobacteria, bifidobacteria, firmicutes) [119].

Caffeine. Caffeine decreases PD risk [61]. Caffeine has been shown to oppose galactose-induced oxis [121]. Akkm is negatively associated with caffeine consumption [52].

Traumatic brain injury (TBI). TBI increases PD risk [61]. TBI induces iron and reactive oxygen species accumulation, dysfunctional iron metabolism, and upregulates ferroptosis genes and neural degeneration [122].

Infections. Infections increase PD risk [55]. Infections increase gut mucin production [25].

Ibuprofen. Chronic ibuprofen (and to a lesser extent, also other NSAIDs) treatment reduces PD risk [123]. Such treatment is known to increase gut permeability, allowing nutrient entry.

Exercise. Moderate to intense exercise is associated with decreased risk [124]. This either occurs because the capacity of exercising shows an unimpaired SNS (reverse causality), or because exercise is actively helpful, e.g., by enhancing glycolysis.

Cancer. All cancer types are decreased in PD [125], except melanoma, which is increased [126]. The decrease occurs because cancer utilizes aerobic glycolysis, which is reduced in PD due to galactose. Melanoma is increased because melanocytes are specifically sensitive to oxis, as attested by their high melanin expression (however, the precise mechanisms of melanoma are not fully understood).

10.4 Treatment

Current drug-based treatments attempt to increase brain DA. While these drugs may help movement symptoms (at least for some time), they do not address the real cause of the disease, and are associated with several negative adverse effects.

According to T*PD, the optimal treatment for PD is to reduce galactose load while enhancing glucose metabolism. This needs to be done early, before neurons have been irrevocably damaged. Fortunately, gut symptoms can be easily detected, allowing early screening.

Fecal tests for the relative abundance of mucin-degrading bacteria, blood levels of galactose and its metabolites, and GSH levels in all tissues (including blood and skin cells and fibroblasts) constitute promising biomarkers.

Galactose load can be theoretically reduced via a galactose restricted diet. This is currently the only treatment for galactosemia. In practice, this approach is very difficult, due to the large number of food items that contain galactose. Nonetheless, most milk products should be avoided (high-fat yogurts and some high-fat cheese are low in galactose and can be consumed).

One treatment approach is to remove or reduce gut mucin-degrading bacteria, especially akkm. This can be done via fecal transplants, or via antibiotics or other drugs that have this effect. Common antibiotics decrease relative akkm abundance, but they also increase other mucin-degrading bacteria. Thus, akkm-specific drugs should be developed. Nonetheless, even common antibiotics may improve PD state, because these other species may not over-enhance gut barrier in the way that akkm does.

It is not clear whether complete eradication of gut bacteria (via non-selective antibiotics) is beneficial, but it can be attempted in the absence of other treatments.

A promising approach is to develop drugs that reduce gut mucin levels by targeting mucin production genes (MUC2, MUC5AC, others). Reducing mucin levels has three benefits. First, it would directly relieve galactose load. Second, it would reduce the relative abundance of mucin-degrading bacteria, depriving them of their main nutrients. Finally, it would address olfaction and respiration problems.

Exercise reduces PD risk. However, as explained above, this could be via reverse causality.

Adrenergic receptor agonists relieve the pressure off the SNS, and prodromal beta2-AR is indeed protective in a 1.76M Israeli cohort [127]. Similarly, propranolol (a beta blocker) increases risk 2.6-fold.

10.5 Discussion

I presented the first complete theory of PD. T*PD is complete in the sense that it explains the etiology, symptoms, pathology, and risk factors of the disease.

A complete theory can be wrong (partially or fully), but being complete is the minimal requirement from a theory.

In T*PD, PD occurs following a particular composition of the GMB, with an increased abundance of mucin-degrading bacteria. This in turn can result from many events, including infections, diet, inheritance, etc. Mechanistically, this particular composition yields higher levels of galactose and lower levels of glucose in the brain, which increases oxis and decreases glycolysis and GSH production, leaving the cell more exposed to ferroptosis. SNc and LC cells are the brain cells most sensitive to this, as indicated by their uniquely high expression of neuromelanin.

This account unifies the two most important questions about the disease: the gut and olfactory connection (with prodromal symptoms that precede diagnosis by over a decade), and the specific vulnerability of SNc and LC neurons.

Evidence. T*PD is supported by diverse and wide evidence, relating to the GMB, galactose, glucose (glycolysis, diabetes, BMI, imaging), oxis (mitochondria, GSH, iron, lipid peroxidation), the SNS, and risk and protective factors (smoking, alcohol, caffeine, exercise, ibuprofen, traumatic brain injury, infections, and melanoma). One piece of evidence that is relatively small is direct evidence for higher galactose levels in patient blood.

Other theories. A recent large multi-author review of PD did not mention the gut or GMB at all [1]. The idea that PD is an energy disease has been raised but without mechanistic gut and brain details [128]. The idea that the increased risk with milk consumption is due to galactose has been phrased [129,130], again without mechanisms and without linking it to other phenomena. A GMB hypothesis has been formulated, with an emphasis only on aSyn, inflammation, and brain fatty acids [131]. A brain-side hypothesis was raised in which PD involves a toxic feedback loop between iron, oxis, aSyn, and NM [8]. Thus, no existing theory is close to T*PD.

aSyn propagation. One of the established ideas in PD research is that the disease starts in the periphery (gut, olfactory tract) and spreads upwards to the brain [1]. However, this is based on Lewy pathology, whose distribution is not consistent with the disease [132]. As far as I know, the idea that the harmful agents are metabolic agents that spread from the gut through the blood has never been raised.

Treatment. An encouraging aspect of T*PD is that it implies several possible ways of treating the disease, some of which are relatively not difficult to implement. Precise modifications of the GMB are difficult to achieve, but a reduction of mucin degradation is probably possible. This treatment should start before DA and NEP neurons have accumulated too much damage, but fortunately, the presence of prodromal symptoms allows us to identify the risk years in advance.

List of abbreviations

akkm: Akkermansia Muciniphila.
aSyn: alpha-synuclein.
GMB: gut microbiome.
GSH: glutathione.
HPL: helicobacter pylori.
LC: locus coeruelus.
NEP: norepinephrine.
NM: neuromelanin.
PD: Parkinson's disease.
PPP: pentose phosphate pathway.
RBD: REM sleep behavior disorder.
SNc: substantia nigra pars compacta.
SNS: sympathetic nervous system.
TBI: traumatic brain injury.
T*PD: the theory of PD presented in this paper.

Acknowledgments

I thank Naama Rappoport-Levin, M.D., for discussions on the theory presented here.

References

[1] J. Obeso, C. Goetz, A. Lang, D. Weintraub, E. Bezard, et al., Past, present, and future of Parkinson's disease: a special essay on the 200th Anniversary of the Shaking Palsy, Movement Disorders 32 (9) (2017) 1264–1310.
[2] H.R. Morris, M.G. Spillantini, C.M. Sue, C.H. Williams-Gray, The pathogenesis of Parkinson's disease, The Lancet 403 (10423) (2024) 293–304.
[3] D.J. Surmeier, J.A. Obeso, G.M. Halliday, Selective neuronal vulnerability in Parkinson disease, Nature Reviews. Neuroscience 18 (2) (2017) 101.
[4] S.J. Sara, The locus coeruleus and noradrenergic modulation of cognition, Nature Reviews. Neuroscience 10 (3) (2009) 211–223.
[5] K.L. Adams-Carr, J.P. Bestwick, S. Shribman, A. Lees, A. Schrag, A.J. Noyce, Constipation preceding Parkinson's disease: a systematic review and meta-analysis, Journal of Neurology, Neurosurgery and Psychiatry 87 (7) (2016) 710–716.
[6] S.J. Guiney, P.A. Adlard, A.I. Bush, D.I. Finkelstein, S. Ayton, Ferroptosis and cell death mechanisms in Parkinson's disease, Neurochemistry International 104 (2017) 34–48.
[7] F.A. Zucca, J. Segura-Aguilar, E. Ferrari, P. Muñoz, I. Paris, D. Sulzer, et al., Interactions of iron, dopamine and neuromelanin pathways in brain aging and Parkinson's disease, Progress in Neurobiology 155 (2017) 96–119.
[8] Z. Jansen van Rensburg, S. Abrahams, S. Bardien, C. Kenyon, Toxic feedback loop involving iron, reactive oxygen species, α-synuclein and neuromelanin in Parkinson's disease and intervention with turmeric, Molecular Neurobiology 58 (11) (2021) 5920–5936.
[9] F. Conte, N. van Buuringen, N.C. Voermans, D.J. Lefeber, Galactose in human metabolism, glycosylation and congenital metabolic diseases: time for a closer look, Biochimica et Biophysica Acta. G, General Subjects 1865 (8) (2021) 129898.

[10] M. Roser, D. Josic, M. Kontou, K. Mosetter, P. Maurer, W. Reutter, Metabolism of galactose in the brain and liver of rats and its conversion into glutamate and other amino acids, Journal of Neural Transmission 116 (2009) 121–129.
[11] J.M. Henderson, M.H. Kutner, R.P. Bain, First-order clearance of plasma galactose: the effect of liver disease, Gastroenterology 83 (5) (1982) 1090–1096.
[12] C. Aguer, D. Gambarotta, R.J. Mailloux, C. Moffat, R. Dent, R. McPherson, et al., Galactose enhances oxidative metabolism and reveals mitochondrial dysfunction in human primary muscle cells, PLoS ONE 6 (12) (2011) e28536.
[13] T. Shwe, W. Pratchayasakul, N. Chattipakorn, S.C. Chattipakorn, Role of D-galactose-induced brain aging and its potential used for therapeutic interventions, Experimental Gerontology 101 (2018) 13–36.
[14] R. Rossignol, R. Gilkerson, R. Aggeler, K. Yamagata, S.J. Remington, R.A. Capaldi, Energy substrate modulates mitochondrial structure and oxidative capacity in cancer cells, Cancer Research 64 (3) (2004) 985–993.
[15] X. Cui, P. Zuo, Q. Zhang, X. Li, Y. Hu, J. Long, et al., Chronic systemic D-galactose exposure induces memory loss, neurodegeneration, and oxidative damage in mice: protective effects of R-α-lipoic acid, Journal of Neuroscience Research 83 (8) (2006) 1584–1590.
[16] M.Y. Xia, X.Y. Zhao, Q.L. Huang, H.Y. Sun, C. Sun, J. Yuan, et al., Activation of Wnt/β-catenin signaling by lithium chloride attenuates d-galactose-induced neurodegeneration in the auditory cortex of a rat model of aging, FEBS Open Bio 7 (6) (2017) 759–776.
[17] M.E. Gibbs, D.S. Hutchinson, R.J. Summers, Role of β-adrenoceptors in memory consolidation: β3-adrenoceptors act on glucose uptake and β2-adrenoceptors on glycogenolysis, Neuropsychopharmacology 33 (10) (2008) 2384–2397.
[18] I. Brockhausen, H. Schachter, P. Stanley, O-GalNAc glycans, in: Essentials of Glycobiology, 2nd edition, 2009.
[19] M. Yamaguchi, K. Yamamoto, Mucin glycans and their degradation by gut microbiota, Glycoconjugate Journal 40 (4) (2023) 493–512.
[20] M. Derrien, E.E. Vaughan, C.M. Plugge, W.M. de Vos, Akkermansia muciniphila gen. nov., sp. nov., a human intestinal mucin-degrading bacterium., I nternational journal of systematic and evolutionary microbiology 54 (5) (2004) 1469–1476.
[21] A. Everard, C. Belzer, L. Geurts, J.P. Ouwerkerk, C. Druart, L.B. Bindels, et al., Cross-talk between Akkermansia muciniphila and intestinal epithelium controls diet-induced obesity, Proceedings of the National Academy of Sciences 110 (22) (2013) 9066–9071.
[22] C. Martin-Gallausiaux, D. Garcia-Weber, A. Lashermes, P. Larraufie, L. Marinelli, V. Teixeira, et al., Akkermansia muciniphila upregulates genes involved in maintaining the intestinal barrier function via ADP-heptose-dependent activation of the ALPK1/TIFA pathway, Gut Microbes 14 (1) (2022) 2110639.
[23] C. Depommier, M. Van Hul, A. Everard, N.M. Delzenne, W.M. De Vos, P.D. Cani, Pasteurized Akkermansia muciniphila increases whole-body energy expenditure and fecal energy excretion in diet-induced obese mice, Gut Microbes 11 (5) (2020) 1231–1245.
[24] Y. Xu, Y. Yang, B. Li, Y. Xie, Y. Shi, G. Le, Dietary methionine restriction improves gut microbiota composition and prevents cognitive impairment in D-galactose-induced aging mice, Food & Function 13 (24) (2022) 12896–12914.
[25] J.J. Kim, W.I. Khan, Goblet cells and mucins: role in innate defense in enteric infections, Pathogens 2 (1) (2013) 55–70.
[26] L. Chen, V. Collij, S. Hu, et al., Environmental factors shaping the gut microbiome in a Dutch population, Nature 604 (7907) (2022) 732–739.
[27] C. Pacelli, N. Giguère, M.J. Bourque, M. Lévesque, R.S. Slack, L.É. Trudeau, Elevated mitochondrial bioenergetics and axonal arborization size are key contributors to the vulnerability of dopamine neurons, Current Biology 25 (18) (2015) 2349–2360.
[28] A. Stincone, A. Prigione, T. Cramer, M.M. Wamelink, K. Campbell, E. Cheung, et al., The return of metabolism: biochemistry and physiology of the pentose phosphate pathway, Biological Reviews 90 (3) (2015) 927–963.

[29] L. Zecca, L. Casella, A. Albertini, C. Bellei, F.A. Zucca, M. Engelen, et al., Neuromelanin can protect against iron-mediated oxidative damage in system modeling iron overload of brain aging and Parkinson's disease, Journal of Neurochemistry 106 (4) (2008) 1866–1875.
[30] B.R. Bloem, M.S. Okun, C. Klein, Parkinson's disease, The Lancet 397 (10291) (2021) 2284–2303.
[31] M.P. Mattson, T.V. Arumugam, Hallmarks of brain aging: adaptive and pathological modification by metabolic states, Cell Metabolism 27 (6) (2018) 1176–1199.
[32] M. Schnegg, B.H. Lauterburg, Quantitative liver function in the elderly assessed by galactose elimination capacity, aminopyrine demethylation and caffeine clearance, Journal of Hepatology 3 (2) (1986) 164–171.
[33] J.H. Suh, S.V. Shenvi, B.M. Dixon, H. Liu, A.K. Jaiswal, R.M. Liu, et al., Decline in transcriptional activity of Nrf2 causes age-related loss of glutathione synthesis, which is reversible with lipoic acid, Proceedings of the National Academy of Sciences 101 (10) (2004) 3381–3386.
[34] G. Hebbrecht, W. Maenhaut, J. De Reuck, Brain trace elements and aging, Nuclear Instruments & Methods in Physics Research. Section B, Beam Interactions With Materials and Atoms 150 (1-4) (1999) 208–213.
[35] E. Floor, M.G. Wetzel, Increased protein oxidation in human substantia nigra pars compacta in comparison with basal ganglia and prefrontal cortex measured with an improved dinitrophenylhydrazine assay, Journal of Neurochemistry 70 (1) (1998) 268–275.
[36] M. Hashimoto, A. Takeda, L.J. Hsu, T. Takenouchi, E. Masliah, Role of cytochrome c as a stimulator of α-synuclein aggregation in Lewy body disease, Journal of Biological Chemistry 274 (41) (1999) 28849–28852.
[37] B. Chen, X. Wen, H. Jiang, J. Wang, N. Song, J. Xie, Interactions between iron and α-synuclein pathology in Parkinson's disease, Free Radical Biology & Medicine 141 (2019) 253–260.
[38] Q. Xuan, S.L. Xu, D.H. Lu, S. Yu, M. Zhou, K. Uéda, et al., Increase expression of α-synuclein in aged human brain associated with neuromelanin accumulation, Journal of Neural Transmission 118 (2011) 1575–1583.
[39] M. Zhu, Z.J. Qin, D. Hu, L.A. Munishkina, A.L. Fink, α-synuclein can function as an antioxidant preventing oxidation of unsaturated lipid in vesicles, Biochemistry 45 (26) (2006) 8135–8142.
[40] R.E. Musgrove, A.E. King, T.C. Dickson, α-Synuclein protects neurons from apoptosis downstream of free-radical production through modulation of the MAPK signalling pathway, Neurotoxicity Research 23 (2013) 358–369.
[41] N. Mizuno, J. Varkey, N.C. Kegulian, B.G. Hegde, N. Cheng, R. Langen, et al., Remodeling of lipid vesicles into cylindrical micelles by α-synuclein in an extended α-helical conformation, Journal of Biological Chemistry 287 (35) (2012) 29301–29311.
[42] F. Kamp, N. Exner, A.K. Lutz, N. Wender, J. Hegermann, B. Brunner, et al., Inhibition of mitochondrial fusion by α-synuclein is rescued by PINK1, Parkin and DJ-1, EMBO Journal 29 (20) (2010) 3571–3589.
[43] S. Paillusson, P. Gomez-Suaga, R. Stoica, D. Little, P. Gissen, M.J. Devine, et al., α-Synuclein binds to the ER–mitochondria tethering protein VAPB to disrupt Ca2+ homeostasis and mitochondrial ATP production, Acta Neuropathologica 134 (2017) 129–149.
[44] G. Rodriguez-Araujo, H. Nakagami, H. Hayashi, M. Mori, T. Shiuchi, Y. Minokoshi, et al., Alpha-synuclein elicits glucose uptake and utilization in adipocytes through the Gab1/PI3K/Akt transduction pathway, Cellular and Molecular Life Sciences 70 (2013) 1123–1133.
[45] H. Qiao, X. He, Q. Zhang, H. Yuan, D. Wang, L. Li, et al., Alpha-synuclein induces microglial migration via PKM2-dependent glycolysis, International Journal of Biological Macromolecules 129 (2019) 601–607.
[46] K.Y. Chau, H.L. Ching, A.H. Schapira, J.M. Cooper, Relationship between alpha synuclein phosphorylation, proteasomal inhibition and cell death: relevance to Parkinson's disease pathogenesis, Journal of Neurochemistry 110 (3) (2009) 1005–1013.

[47] V. Dias, E. Junn, M.M. Mouradian, The role of oxidative stress in Parkinson's disease, Journal of Parkinson's Disease 3 (4) (2013) 461–491.
[48] M.E. Gegg, A.H. Schapira, The role of glucocerebrosidase in Parkinson disease pathogenesis, The FEBS Journal 285 (19) (2018) 3591–3603.
[49] E.M. Hill-Burns, J.W. Debelius, J.T. Morton, W.T. Wissemann, M.R. Lewis, Z.D. Wallen, et al., Parkinson's disease and Parkinson's disease medications have distinct signatures of the gut microbiome, Movement Disorders 32 (5) (2017) 739–749.
[50] S. Romano, G.M. Savva, J.R. Bedarf, I.G. Charles, F. Hildebrand, A. Narbad, Meta-analysis of the Parkinson's disease gut microbiome suggests alterations linked to intestinal inflammation, npj Parkinson's Disease 7 (1) (2021) 27.
[51] F. Scheperjans, V. Aho, P.A. Pereira, K. Koskinen, L. Paulin, E. Pekkonen, et al., Gut microbiota are related to Parkinson's disease and clinical phenotype, Movement Disorders 30 (3) (2015) 350–358.
[52] K. Murakami, H. Okubo, S. Sasaki, Dietary intake in relation to self-reported constipation among Japanese women aged 18–20 years, European Journal of Clinical Nutrition 60 (5) (2006) 650–657.
[53] L.A. Adolf, S. Heilbronner, Nutritional interactions between bacterial species colonising the human nasal cavity: current knowledge and future prospects, Metabolites 12 (6) (2022) 489.
[54] L.Y. Ma, G.L. Liu, D.X. Wang, M.M. Zhang, W.Y. Kou, T. Feng, Alpha-synuclein in peripheral tissues in Parkinson's disease, ACS Chemical Neuroscience 10 (2) (2019) 812–823.
[55] H. Wang, X. Liu, C. Tan, W. Zhou, J. Jiang, W. Peng, et al., Bacterial, viral, and fungal infection-related risk of Parkinson's disease: meta-analysis of cohort and case–control studies, Brain and Behavior 10 (3) (2020) e01549.
[56] L. Morgante, G. Salemi, F. Meneghini, A.E. Di Rosa, A. Epifanio, F. Grigoletto, et al., Parkinson disease survival: a population-based study, Archives of Neurology 57 (4) (2000) 507–512.
[57] D.W. Ryu, K. Han, A.H. Cho, Mortality and causes of death in patients with Parkinson's disease: a nationwide population-based cohort study, Frontiers in Neurology 14 (2023) 1236296.
[58] B. Slomiany, V. Murty, J. Piotrowski, Y. Liau, P. Sundaram, A. Slomiany, Glycosulfatase activity of Helicobacter pylori toward gastric mucin, Biochemical and Biophysical Research Communications 183 (2) (1992) 506–513.
[59] H. Murata, L.M. Barnhill, J.M. Bronstein, Air pollution and the risk of Parkinson's disease: a review, Movement Disorders 37 (5) (2022) 894–904.
[60] K. Gillois, M. Lévêque, V. Théodorou, H. Robert, M. Mercier-Bonin, Mucus: an underestimated gut target for environmental pollutants and food additives, Microorganisms 6 (2) (2018) 53.
[61] A. Ascherio, M.A. Schwarzschild, The epidemiology of Parkinson's disease: risk factors and prevention, The Lancet Neurology 15 (12) (2016) 1257–1272.
[62] E. Luna, S.G. Parkar, N. Kirmiz, S. Hartel, E. Hearn, M. Hossine, et al., Utilization efficiency of human milk oligosaccharides by human-associated Akkermansia is strain dependent, Applied and Environmental Microbiology 88 (1) (2022) e01487-21.
[63] A. Wuolikainen, P. Jonsson, M. Ahnlund, H. Antti, S.L. Marklund, T. Moritz, et al., Multiplatform mass spectrometry analysis of the CSF and plasma metabolomes of rigorously matched amyotrophic lateral sclerosis, Parkinson's disease and control subjects, Molecular BioSystems 12 (4) (2016) 1287–1298.
[64] M. Scholefield, S.J. Church, G. Taylor, D. Knight, R.D. Unwin, G.J. Cooper, Multi-regional alterations in glucose and purine metabolic pathways in the Parkinson's disease dementia brain, npj Parkinson's Disease 9 (1) (2023) 66.
[65] S.S. Ahmed, W. Santosh, S. Kumar, H.T.T. Christlet, Metabolic profiling of Parkinson's disease: evidence of biomarker from gene expression analysis and rapid neural network detection, Journal of Biomedical Science 16 (1) (2009) 1–12.
[66] M. Konjevod, J. Sáiz, C. Barbas, A. Bergareche, E. Ardanaz, J.M. Huerta, et al., A set of reliable samples for the study of biomarkers for the early diagnosis of Parkinson's disease, Frontiers in Neurology 13 (2022) 844841.

[67] P.A. Videira, M. Castro-Caldas, Linking glycation and glycosylation with inflammation and mitochondrial dysfunction in Parkinson's disease, Frontiers in Neuroscience 12 (2018) 381.
[68] B. Panis, A.M. Bosch, A. Burlina, D.J. Coman, M.L. Couce, A.M. Das, et al., Brain function in classic galactosemia, a galactosemia network (GalNet) members review, Frontiers in Genetics 15 (2024) 1355962.
[69] I. Rubio-Agusti, M. Carecchio, K.P. Bhatia, M. Kojovic, I. Parees, H.S. Chandrashekar, et al., Movement disorders in adult patients with classical galactosemia, Movement Disorders 28 (6) (2013) 804–810.
[70] A. Poisson, E. Roze, C. Demily, S. Thobois, Evidence for dopaminergic denervation in classical galactosemia, Movement Disorders: Official Journal of the Movement Disorder Society 32 (6) (2017) 940–942.
[71] M. Boca, A. Whone, Letter to the editor on "Evidence for dopaminergic denervation in classical galactosemia". Movement disorders, Official Journal of the Movement Disorder Society 32 (12) (2017) 1797.
[72] B. van Erven, M.M. Römers, M.E. Rubio-Gozalbo, Revised Proposal for the Prevention of Low Bone Mass in Patients with Classic Galactosemia, JIMD Reports, vol. 17, Springer, 2014, pp. 41–46.
[73] K.M. Torsney, A.J. Noyce, K.M. Doherty, J.P. Bestwick, R. Dobson, A.J. Lees, Bone health in Parkinson's disease: a systematic review and meta-analysis, Journal of Neurology, Neurosurgery and Psychiatry 85 (10) (2014) 1159–1166.
[74] P.A. LeWitt, J. Li, M. Lu, T.G. Beach, C.H. Adler, L. Guo, et al., 3-hydroxykynurenine and other Parkinson's disease biomarkers discovered by metabolomic analysis, Movement Disorders 28 (12) (2013) 1653–1660.
[75] A. Öhman, L. Forsgren, NMR metabonomics of cerebrospinal fluid distinguishes between Parkinson's disease and controls, Neuroscience Letters 594 (2015) 36–39.
[76] K. Murakami, Y. Miyake, S. Sasaki, K. Tanaka, W. Fukushima, C. Kiyohara, et al., Dietary glycemic index is inversely associated with the risk of Parkinson's disease: a case–control study in Japan, Nutrition 26 (5) (2010) 515–521.
[77] L. Dunn, G.F. Allen, A. Mamais, H. Ling, A. Li, K.E. Duberley, et al., Dysregulation of glucose metabolism is an early event in sporadic Parkinson's disease, Neurobiology of Aging 35 (5) (2014) 1111–1115.
[78] M. Elstner, C.M. Morris, K. Heim, A. Bender, D. Mehta, E. Jaros, et al., Expression analysis of dopaminergic neurons in Parkinson's disease and aging links transcriptional dysregulation of energy metabolism to cell death, Acta Neuropathologica 122 (2011) 75–86.
[79] E.A. Ostrakhovitch, E.S. Song, J.K. Macedo, M.S. Gentry, J.E. Quintero, C. van Horne, et al., Analysis of circulating metabolites to differentiate Parkinson's disease and essential tremor, Neuroscience Letters 769 (2022) 136428.
[80] M. Nagao, H. Hayashi, Glycogen synthase kinase-3beta is associated with Parkinson's disease, Neuroscience Letters 449 (2) (2009) 103–107.
[81] M. Rango, C. Bonifati, N. Bresolin, Parkinson's disease and brain mitochondrial dysfunction: a functional phosphorus magnetic resonance spectroscopy study, Journal of Cerebral Blood Flow and Metabolism 26 (2) (2006) 283–290.
[82] J.E. Simmering, M.J. Welsh, L. Liu, N.S. Narayanan, A. Pottegård, Association of glycolysis-enhancing α-1 blockers with risk of developing Parkinson disease, JAMA Neurology 78 (4) (2021) 407–413.
[83] J.L. Eberling, B.C. Richardson, B.R. Reed, N. Wolfe, W.J. Jagust, Cortical glucose metabolism in Parkinson's disease without dementia, Neurobiology of Aging 15 (3) (1994) 329–335.
[84] Y. Hosokai, Y. Nishio, K. Hirayama, A. Takeda, T. Ishioka, Y. Sawada, et al., Distinct patterns of regional cerebral glucose metabolism in Parkinson's disease with and without mild cognitive impairment, Movement Disorders: Official Journal of the Movement Disorder Society 24 (6) (2009) 854–862.

[85] Y. Xu, X. Wei, X. Liu, J. Liao, J. Lin, C. Zhu, et al., Low cerebral glucose metabolism: a potential predictor for the severity of vascular parkinsonism and Parkinson's disease, Aging and Disease 6 (6) (2015) 426.
[86] T. Baba, A. Takeda, A. Kikuchi, Y. Nishio, Y. Hosokai, K. Hirayama, et al., Association of olfactory dysfunction and brain metabolism in Parkinson's disease, Movement Disorders 26 (4) (2011) 621–628.
[87] E. Ådén, M. Carlsson, E. Poortvliet, H. Stenlund, J. Linder, M. Edström, et al., Dietary intake and olfactory function in patients with newly diagnosed Parkinson's disease: a case-control study, Nutritional Neuroscience 14 (1) (2011) 25–31.
[88] W. Hellenbrand, A. Seidler, H. Boeing, B.P. Robra, P. Vieregge, P. Nischan, et al., Diet and Parkinson's disease I: a possible role for the past intake of specific foods and food groups: results from a self-administered food-frequency questionnaire in a case-control study, Neurology 47 (3) (1996) 636–643.
[89] E. Cassani, M. Barichella, V. Ferri, G. Pinelli, L. Iorio, C. Bolliri, et al., Dietary habits in Parkinson's disease: adherence to Mediterranean diet, Parkinsonism & Related Disorders 42 (2017) 40–46.
[90] F. Camargo Maluf, D. Feder, A. Alves de Siqueira Carvalho, et al., Analysis of the relationship between type II diabetes mellitus and Parkinson's disease: a systematic review, in: Parkinson's Disease, 2019.
[91] J.M. Sheard, S. Ash, P.A. Silburn, G.K. Kerr, Prevalence of malnutrition in Parkinson's disease: a systematic review, Nutrition Reviews 69 (9) (2011) 520–532.
[92] W.P. Cheshire Jr., Z.K. Wszolek, Body mass index is reduced early in Parkinson's disease, Parkinsonism & Related Disorders 11 (1) (2005) 35–38.
[93] C.M. Deus, S.P. Pereira, T. Cunha-Oliveira, F.B. Pereira, N. Raimundo, P.J. Oliveira, Mitochondrial remodeling in human skin fibroblasts from sporadic male Parkinson's disease patients uncovers metabolic and mitochondrial bioenergetic defects, Biochimica et Biophysica Acta. Molecular Basis of Disease 1866 (3) (2020) 165615.
[94] R. Betarbet, T.B. Sherer, G. MacKenzie, M. Garcia-Osuna, A.V. Panov, J.T. Greenamyre, Chronic systemic pesticide exposure reproduces features of Parkinson's disease, Nature Neuroscience 3 (12) (2000) 1301–1306.
[95] J. Sian, D.T. Dexter, A.J. Lees, S. Daniel, Y. Agid, F. Javoy-Agid, et al., Alterations in glutathione levels in Parkinson's disease and other neurodegenerative disorders affecting basal ganglia, Annals of Neurology: Official Journal of the American Neurological Association and the Child Neurology Society 36 (3) (1994) 348–355.
[96] S.J. Kish, C. Morito, O. Hornykiewicz, Glutathione peroxidase activity in Parkinson's disease brain, Neuroscience Letters 58 (3) (1985) 343–346.
[97] E. Sofic, K. Jellinger, Reduced and oxidized glutathione in the substantia nigra of patients with Parkinson's disease, Neuroscience Letters 142 (2) (1992) 128–130.
[98] P. Jenner, D. Dexter, J. Sian, A. Schapira, C. Marsden, Oxidative stress as a cause of nigral cell death in Parkinson's disease and incidental Lewy body disease, Annals of Neurology: Official Journal of the American Neurological Association and the Child Neurology Society 32 (S1) (1992) S82–S87.
[99] R. Pearce, A. Owen, S. Daniel, P. Jenner, C. Marsden, Alterations in the distribution of glutathione in the substantia nigra in Parkinson's disease, Journal of Neural Transmission 104 (1997) 661–677.
[100] P. Riederer, E. Sofic, W.D. Rausch, B. Schmidt, G.P. Reynolds, K. Jellinger, et al., Transition metals, ferritin, glutathione, and ascorbic acid in parkinsonian brains, Journal of Neurochemistry 52 (2) (1989) 515–520.
[101] W. Maetzler, S.P. Schmid, I. Wurster, I. Liepelt, A. Gaenslen, T. Gasser, et al., Reduced but not oxidized cerebrospinal fluid glutathione levels are lowered in Lewy body diseases, Movement Disorders 26 (1) (2011) 176–181.
[102] D.O. Cristalli, N. Arnal, F.A. Marra, M.J. de Alaniz, C.A. Marra, Peripheral markers in neurodegenerative patients and their first-degree relatives, Journal of the Neurological Sciences 314 (1–2) (2012) 48–56.

[103] S. Charisis, E. Ntanasi, M. Stamelou, G. Xiromerisiou, M. Maraki, A.S. Veskoukis, et al., Plasma glutathione and prodromal Parkinson's disease probability, Movement Disorders 37 (1) (2022) 200–205.

[104] Q. He, Z. Zhang, B. Fu, J. Chen, J. Liu, Changes in serum uric acid, glutathione, and amyloid-β1-42 levels in Parkinson's disease patients and their association with disease progression and cognitive decline, Current Medical Research and Opinion (2024) 105–113.

[105] E. Sofic, P. Riederer, H. Heinsen, H. Beckmann, G. Reynolds, G. Hebenstreit, et al., Increased iron (III) and total iron content in post mortem substantia nigra of parkinsonian brain, Journal of Neural Transmission 74 (1988) 199–205.

[106] D. Dexter, F. Wells, A. Lee, F. Agid, Y. Agid, P. Jenner, et al., Increased nigral iron content and alterations in other metal ions occurring in brain in Parkinson's disease, Journal of Neurochemistry 52 (6) (1989) 1830–1836.

[107] B.F.G. Popescu, M.J. George, U. Bergmann, A.V. Garachtchenko, M.E. Kelly, R.P. McCrea, et al., Mapping metals in Parkinson's and normal brain using rapid-scanning x-ray fluorescence, Physics in Medicine and Biology 54 (3) (2009) 651.

[108] W.W. Martin, M. Wieler, M. Gee, Midbrain iron content in early Parkinson disease: a potential biomarker of disease status, Neurology 70 (16 Part 2) (2008) 1411–1417.

[109] A. Yoritaka, N. Hattori, K. Uchida, M. Tanaka, E.R. Stadtman, Y. Mizuno, Immunohistochemical detection of 4-hydroxynonenal protein adducts in Parkinson disease, in: Proceedings of the National Academy of Science, vol. 93, 1996, pp. 2696–2701.

[110] M.L. Selley, (E)-4-hydroxy-2-nonenal may be involved in the pathogenesis of Parkinson's disease, Free Radical Biology & Medicine 25 (2) (1998) 169–174.

[111] R.J. Castellani, G. Perry, S.L. Siedlak, A. Nunomura, S. Shimohama, J. Zhang, et al., Hydroxynonenal adducts indicate a role for lipid peroxidation in neocortical and brainstem Lewy bodies in humans, Neuroscience Letters 319 (1) (2002) 25–28.

[112] E. Dalfó, I. Ferrer, Early α-synuclein lipoxidation in neocortex in Lewy body diseases, Neurobiology of Aging 29 (3) (2008) 408–417.

[113] F. Depierreux, E. Parmentier, L. Mackels, K. Baquero, C. Degueldre, E. Balteau, et al., Parkinson's disease multimodal imaging: F-DOPA PET, neuromelanin-sensitive and quantitative iron-sensitive MRI, npj Parkinson's Disease 7 (1) (2021) 57.

[114] D. Berg, R.B. Postuma, C.H. Adler, B.R. Bloem, P. Chan, B. Dubois, et al., MDS research criteria for prodromal Parkinson's disease, Movement Disorders 30 (12) (2015) 1600–1611.

[115] K. Sääksjärvi, P. Knekt, S. Männistö, J. Lyytinen, M. Heliövaara, Prospective study on the components of metabolic syndrome and the incidence of Parkinson's disease, Parkinsonism & Related Disorders 21 (10) (2015) 1148–1155.

[116] M. Trupp, P. Jonsson, A. Öhrfelt, H. Zetterberg, O. Obudulu, L. Malm, et al., Metabolite and peptide levels in plasma and CSF differentiating healthy controls from patients with newly diagnosed Parkinson's disease, Journal of Parkinson's Disease 4 (3) (2014) 549–560.

[117] D. García-Lorenzo, C. Longo-Dos Santos, C. Ewenczyk, S. Leu-Semenescu, C. Gallea, G. Quattrocchi, et al., The coeruleus/subcoeruleus complex in rapid eye movement sleep behaviour disorders in Parkinson's disease, Brain 136 (7) (2013) 2120–2129.

[118] D. Zhang, H. Jiang, J. Xie, Alcohol intake and risk of Parkinson's disease: a meta-analysis of observational studies, Movement Disorders 29 (6) (2014) 819–822.

[119] G. Capurso, E. Lahner, The interaction between smoking, alcohol and the gut microbiome, Best Practice & Research Clinical Gastroenterology 31 (5) (2017) 579–588.

[120] C.B. Breckenridge, C. Berry, E.T. Chang, R.L. Sielken Jr., J.S. Mandel, Association between Parkinson's disease and cigarette smoking, rural living, well-water consumption, farming and pesticide use: systematic review and meta-analysis, PLoS ONE 11 (4) (2016) e0151841.

[121] F. Ullah, T. Ali, N. Ullah, M.O. Kim, Caffeine prevents d-galactose-induced cognitive deficits, oxidative stress, neuroinflammation and neurodegeneration in the adult rat brain, Neurochemistry International 90 (2015) 114–124.

[122] B.S. Xie, Y.Q. Wang, Y. Lin, Q. Mao, J.F. Feng, G.Y. Gao, et al., Inhibition of ferroptosis attenuates tissue damage and improves long-term outcomes after traumatic brain injury in mice, CNS Neuroscience & Therapeutics 25 (4) (2019) 465–475.

[123] A. Samii, M. Etminan, M.O. Wiens, S. Jafari, NSAID use and the risk of Parkinson's disease: systematic review and meta-analysis of observational studies, Drugs & Aging 26 (2009) 769–779.
[124] K.C. Paul, Y.H. Chuang, I.F. Shih, A. Keener, Y. Bordelon, J.M. Bronstein, et al., The association between lifestyle factors and Parkinson's disease progression and mortality, Movement Disorders 34 (1) (2019) 58–66.
[125] A. Bajaj, J.A. Driver, E.S. Schernhammer, Parkinson's disease and cancer risk: a systematic review and meta-analysis, Cancer Causes & Control 21 (2010) 697–707.
[126] A. Bose, G.A. Petsko, D. Eliezer, Parkinson's disease and melanoma: co-occurrence and mechanisms, Journal of Parkinson's Disease 8 (3) (2018) 385–398.
[127] N. Gronich, D.R. Abernethy, E. Auriel, I. Lavi, G. Rennert, W. Saliba, β2-adrenoceptor agonists and antagonists and risk of Parkinson's disease, Movement Disorders 33 (9) (2018) 1465–1471.
[128] S. Amano, D. Kegelmeyer, S.L. Hong, Rethinking energy in parkinsonian motor symptoms: a potential role for neural metabolic deficits, Frontiers in Systems Neuroscience 8 (2015) 242.
[129] A.R. Sarni, L. Baroni, Milk and Parkinson disease: could galactose be the missing link, Mediterranean Journal of Nutrition and Metabolism 12 (1) (2019) 91–118.
[130] J.D. Adams, Possible causes of Parkinson's disease, Frontiers in Bioscience-Landmark 26 (8) (2021) 387–394.
[131] M.F. Munoz-Pinto, N. Empadinhas, S.M. Cardoso, The neuromicrobiology of Parkinson's disease: a unifying theory, Ageing Research Reviews 70 (2021) 101396.
[132] S. Engelender, O. Isacson, The threshold theory for Parkinson's disease, Trends in Neurosciences 40 (1) (2017) 4–14.

Chapter 11

A lipid-raft theory of Alzheimer's disease

11.1 Introduction

Alzheimer's disease (AD) is the main type of dementia, affecting dozens of millions of people [1]. Despite extensive research (215,000 papers indexed in PubMed, 1.9 million in Google Scholar) and many hypotheses [2], there is at present no coherent theory of AD. The dominant explanation is the amyloid β (Aβ) hypothesis, but it is not a complete theory and is widely criticized [3].

The minimal requirement for any theory of AD is to explain the following major facts. The main AD symptom is memory impairment, starting with anterograde memory and progressing to retrograde memory. Other cognitive deficits are also present [1]. Olfaction and hearing problems occur very early, as do retinal abnormalities [4]. There are two disease variants, sporadic and familial autosomal dominant (FAD), with the former appearing only in relatively old age. The defining AD pathologies are intracellular neurofibrillary tangles (NFTs), which are associated with hyperphosphorylated tau (hyper p-tau), and extracellular plaques containing Aβ [1]. Tau pathology shows good spatial and temporal correlation with symptoms [5], but plaques are also commonly present in nondemented people during aging, and not all demented people exhibit them [3]. Several basic cellular components show dysfunctions that often precede NFTs and plaques, including in mitochondria and in lipid (especially cholesterol) and calcium homeostasis [6]. AD involves early synaptic damage and loss, followed by severe neurodegeneration [7]. Carrying the apolipoprotein (Apo) E4 isoform is strongly associated with AD, while ApoE2 is almost completely protective. There are other risk factors (female sex, viral infection, brain injury, insulin resistance (IR), inflammation, damaged brain blood vessels, and stress), and protective factors (education). Obesity and being underweight increase risk, but being overweight is protective.

This article presents a new theory of AD, the lipid-raft theory of AD (T*AD), which explains all of these facts. To do so, it first presents a new theory of brain plasticity; the theory of adaptive response plasticity (T*PL), which explains how neural activity yields memory formation; and the physiological roles of the main AD agents. The focus on plasticity is motivated by the fact that initial memory symptoms involve anterograde amnesia of benign everyday events [1]. This points to an early impairment in normal memory formation processes, i.e., in

The Science of the Brain. https://doi.org/10.1016/B978-0-44-345008-2.00017-5

brain plasticity. Current descriptions of brain plasticity are incomplete and do not address AD agents, prompting the development of a new theory.

T*PL and T*AD address the major established facts known about brain plasticity and AD, methodically identified via a thorough examination of the scientific literature (hundreds of thousands of papers) done over more than 10 years. Both theories are supported by very strong evidence.

11.1.1 Overview of the theory of adaptive response plasticity

In T*PL, the organism can be in one of three states. The steady state involving neurons, their interconnections (synapses), and glia is supported by stable receptors and channels, the cytoskeleton, adhesion and scaffolding molecules, trans-synaptic nanodomains, extracellular matrix (ECM), myelin, and various constitutively active enzymes. Novelty-induced neural activity initiates a plasticity process consisting of two stages. First, a candidate generation (Cgen) stage involves the formation of elements competing for long-term enhancement. Candidates include existing synapses, new synapses, new neurite branches, and (sometimes) new neurons. This stage involves destabilization of the steady state, immediate potentiation of neurotransmission, and structural changes, and it is what underlies short-term memory (STM) (Fig. 11.1). Second, competition resolution (Cres) consists of the enhancement of winning candidates, the elimination of losers, and restabilization (Fig. 11.2). Winner enhancement starts early but involves a relatively long process in which the evoked changes undergo consolidation to establish a new steady state (Fig. 11.3).

Crucially, the switch from Cgen to Cres depends on the formation of plasma-membrane (PM) lipid rafts (LRs), ordered lipid nanodomains enriched in cholesterol, sphingomyelin (SPM), and phospholipids, which are essential for connecting the membrane to the cytoskeleton, the ECM, and synaptic partners and hence for receptor trafficking and signaling, winner enhancement, and stabilization. The role of tau is to promote cytoskeleton growth and stability in winning synapses. It is activated in a PM LR–dependent manner via dephosphorylation during early winner enhancement and inactivated during Cgen and loser removal. The role of amyloid precursor protein (APP) is to manage cholesterol during plasticity. APP has two mutually exclusive cleavage products, soluble APP α (sAPPα) and Aβ. sAPPα is a major Cgen agent promoting cholesterol synthesis and transport. The incorporation of sufficient amounts of cholesterol in LRs triggers the production of Aβ, which terminates Cgen and removes losing candidates.

11.1.2 Overview of the lipid-raft theory of Alzheimer's disease

Once plasticity in health is understood, we can see what goes wrong in AD. T*AD provides a complete mechanistic account of AD symptoms, pathology, and risk factors. The central thesis is that AD is caused by impaired formation of PM LRs, mainly due to insufficient neural uptake of cholesterol, which is normally produced by astrocytes and transported to neurons via ApoE.

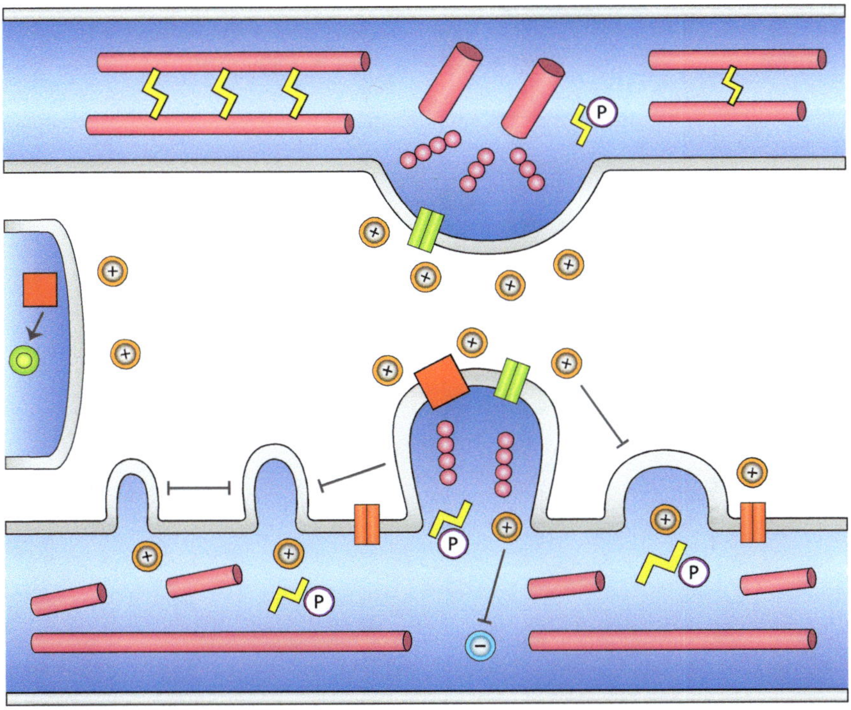

FIGURE 11.1 Candidate generation (Cgen). Candidate generation (Cgen). Neural activity triggers the release and activation of Cgen agents [e.g., tissue plasminogen activator, matrix metallopeptidase 9, brain-derived neurotrophic factor; circled plus symbols]. (a) These agents induce phosphorylation (P) of tau (yellow shapes), which destabilizes cytoskeleton microtubules (pink cylinders) to allow candidate generation; (b) induce the formation of competing candidates [four postsynaptic dendritic spines, one presynaptic axon bouton, and calcium-permeable glutamate receptors (red cylinders)] supported by dynamic actin (pink circles); (c) suppress competition-resolution agents (circled minus symbols); and (d) promote candidate growth. sAPPα (red square) is located outside lipid rafts (green cylinders) and promotes Cgen. In astrocytes, sAPPα promotes synthesis of cholesterol (green circle). The presynaptic neuron is shown at the top, and the postsynaptic neuron is shown at the bottom; an astrocyte is shown on the left. Abbreviation: sAPPα, soluble amyloid precursor protein α.

Reduced formation of PM LRs prolongs Cgen and prevents Cres (Fig. 11.4), with three major consequences. First, STM is not converted to long-term memory (LTM), explaining AD anterograde amnesia. Second, the cytoskeleton is not linked to the membrane properly, leading to excessive p-tau, mitochondrial problems, impairment in all signaling triggered by PM receptors (including growth factor signaling), and eventual neurodegeneration. Tau phosphorylation is a direct consequence of the core mechanism of the disease, explaining the correlation between tau pathology and symptom severity.

A third consequence of impaired PM LRs is increased cholesterol production by neurons. In many cases, this is not sufficient to produce PM LRs and

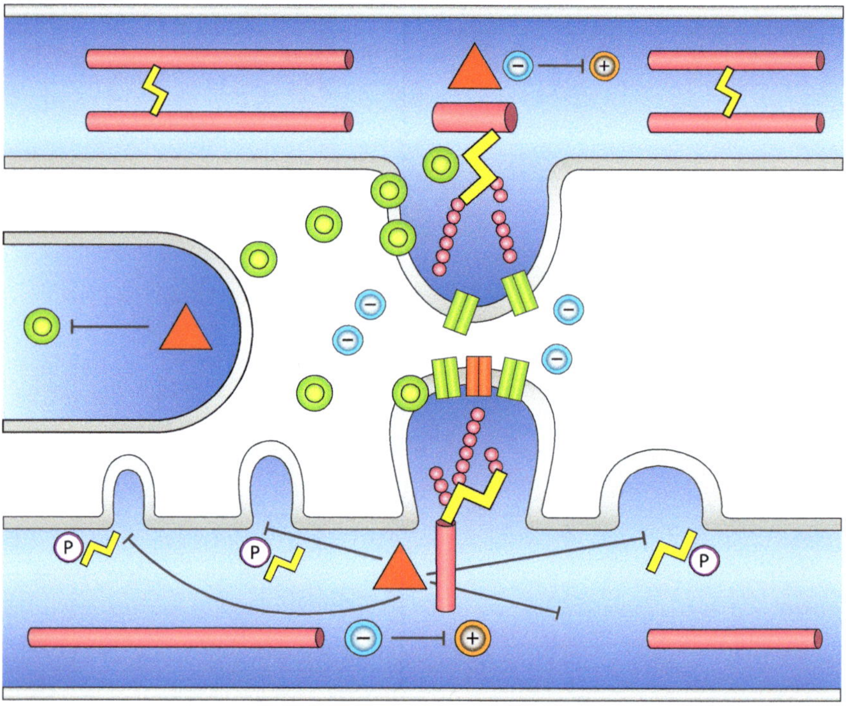

FIGURE 11.2 Competition resolution (Cres). Astrocyte-produced cholesterol (green circles) transported by apolipoprotein E triggers the switch to Cres (circled minus symbols represent Cres agents), which includes production of amyloid β (Aβ) (red triangle) and formation of lipid rafts (green cylinders). Winning candidates are enhanced; active tau (yellow shapes; P indicates phosphorylation) supports growth by linking microtubules (pink cylinders) and active actin (pink circles); calcium-permeable glutamate receptors (red cylinders) translocate to synapses; and Aβ suppresses losing candidates, cholesterol, and candidate-generation agents (circled plus symbols). The presynaptic neuron is shown at the top, and the postsynaptic neuron is shown at the bottom; an astrocyte is shown on the left.

stimulates chronic Aβ production, leading to membrane Aβ cation channels that induce calcium toxicity and to Aβ aggregation. In other cases, neural cholesterol production does manage to establish PM LRs, with intact plasticity accompanied by excessive Aβ. This explains why Aβ plaques are associated only weakly with AD symptoms and why cognitively healthy people can exhibit them. They are neither causal nor essential for the disease.

Neurodegeneration is exacerbated by the fact that many plasticity agents obey a double-edged plasticity (DEP) principle, whereby an agent can support both Cgen and Cres, depending on the amount or cleavage. Crucially, Ca^{2+} is a DEP agent, with high Ca^{2+} marking winners and low Ca^{2+} inducing loser elimination. Since the LR impairment leads to chronic plasticity processes that involve relatively small calcium amounts, AD involves chronic loser elimination processes that yield degeneration.

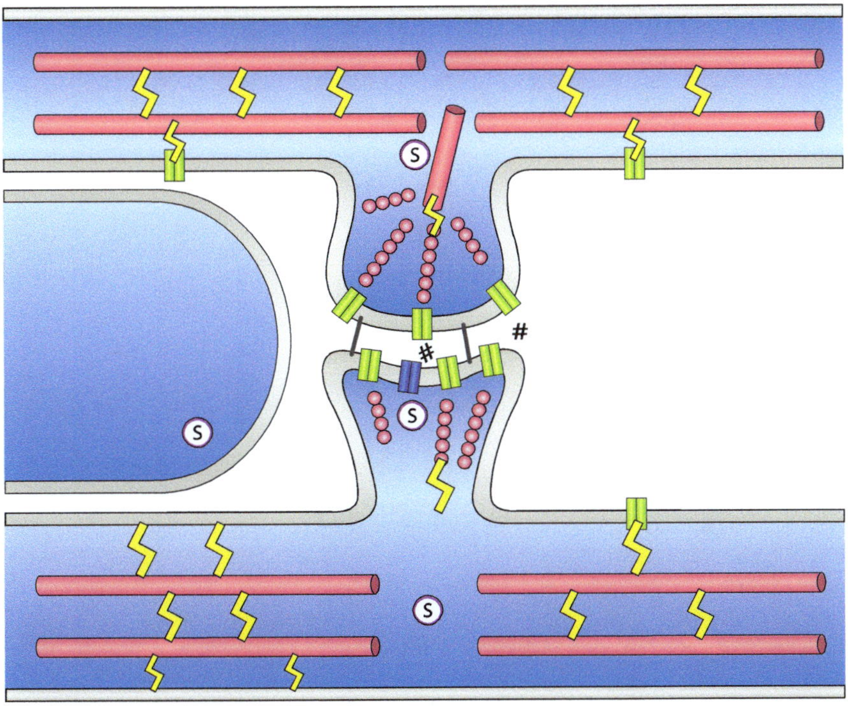

FIGURE 11.3 **The stable state**. Presynaptic and postsynaptic winners and the astrocyte processes supporting the new synapse complete their growth. Stability agents (S) maintain the stable state. Protein phosphatase 2A (PP2A) dephosphorylates tau (yellow shapes) to allow it to support structural elements. Lipid rafts (green cylinders) cooperate with the cytoskeleton (pink cylinders represent microtubules, and pink circles represent dynamic actin) to support receptor anchoring. Synaptic glutamate receptors are switched to be calcium impermeable (blue cylinders). Adhesion molecules (black lines) connect the two sides of the new synapse and form nanodomains, with protection from the extracellular matrix (hash symbols). The presynaptic neuron is shown at the top, and the postsynaptic neuron is shown at the bottom; an astrocyte is shown on the left.

Impaired formation of PM LRs can stem from several causes. In general, it occurs due to an accumulation of risk factors, the strongest of which is aging. Other risk factors include ApoE4, infection by viruses that target LRs, brain IR (which impairs cholesterol synthesis), damaged brain vasculature, brain injury, stress, and chronic neuroinflammation.

The following sections detail T*PL, T*AD, the evidence for these theories, and AD risk factors.

11.2 The theory of adaptive response plasticity

Brain responses with any element of novelty trigger plasticity processes that alter the paths involved in response execution to facilitate the activation of this response in similar future situations. Plasticity can modify, create, or remove

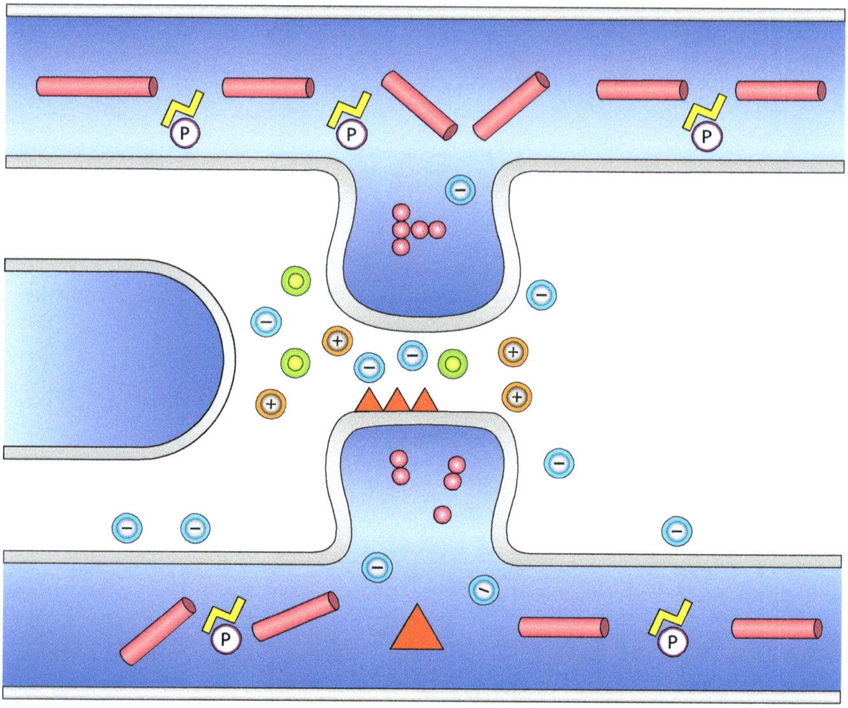

FIGURE 11.4 Chronic plasticity and impaired competition resolution (Cres) in Alzheimer's disease (AD). In AD, cholesterol (green circles) is not incorporated sufficiently into plasma membrane lipid rafts (LRs) (e.g., due to reduced transport by apolipoprotein E4). As a result, synapse formation is not completed, manifesting as anterograde amnesia. LR deficiency impairs the switch from candidate generation (Cgen) to Cres (circled minus symbols indicate Cres agents) and results in a state of chronicity in which Cgen agents (circled plus symbols) remain present. Although chronicity starts with Cgen agents, the resulting state is biased toward Cres functionality due to the double-edged plasticity (DEP) principle. This yields hyper p-tau (yellow shapes; P indicates phosphorylation), neurite retraction, cytoskeleton collapse (pink cylinders represent microtubules, and pink circles represent dynamic actin), and eventually cell death, which manifest as retrograde amnesia. Chronic cholesterol production induces amyloid β (Aβ) (red triangles) plaques, and Aβ forms toxic cation pores. The presynaptic neuron is shown at the top, and the postsynaptic neuron is shown at the bottom; an astrocyte is shown on the left. Intracellular cholesterol and endosomal problems are not shown.

synapses, neurite branches, neurons, glia, and glial processes. The fundamental plasticity task is to identify or create the existing or new elements to be modified, perform the modification, and integrate the changes into the existing network. T*PL explains how this is done.

During the stable steady state, the brain uses a variety of mechanisms to achieve execution efficiency via structural and molecular stability. When plasticity is required, a two-stage process is initiated. The first stage, candidate generation (Cgen), involves destabilization of the steady state to allow modifications and generation of potential elements to be modified. These include synapses to be potentiated, new neurite branches, new boutons and spines, and new neurons. Candidates are generated in all areas in which there is novelty-related execution, as indicated by high calcium influx. A single neuron normally contains many synapse candidates, to provide a variety of options for optimal plasticity. The changes done at this stage promote high calcium influx via membrane insertion of calcium-permeable (CP) receptors.

Candidates compete for long-term persistence, the winners being those who have managed to gain sustained support from intracellular calcium. Competition occurs in a race-like manner, not directly, although candidates do compete indirectly over limited cellular resources.

In the second stage, competition resolution (Cres), winning candidates are enhanced, losing ones are eliminated, and the relevant structures are stabilized. Winner enhancement optimizes neurotransmission in terms of time and energy by creating spatially and temporally focused signaling and by replacing the CP receptors added during Cgen with receptors that allow the passage of less or no calcium. Winning spines are structurally supported via the formation of an actin cytoskeleton, which requires tau-mediated connectivity to cytoskeleton microtubules (MTBs) and the formation of trans-synaptic nanodomains. Losing spines and branches are retracted and removed, with appropriate modifications to the cytoskeleton. There is a relatively long consolidation process, much of it occurring during sleep, that involves protein synthesis to reestablish membranes, cytoskeletons, and the ECM.

There is overwhelming evidence that neural activity changes neurotransmission and induces new synapses, dendritic spines, axonal boutons, branching points, and (sometimes) neurons; that the neurons and neurites connected by new synapses participate in the inducing responses; that these changes undergo stabilization and consolidation; and that this process underlies memory [8]. There is also strong direct evidence for interspine competition [9]. Further evidence is given in Section 11.4.

The switch from Cgen to Cres is triggered by the formation of PM LRs, which are essential for connecting the membrane to the cytoskeleton, the ECM, and synaptic partners and thus for trafficking and anchoring receptors and scaffold proteins to winning candidates and for linking presynaptic and postsynaptic cells. The most sensitive element in LR formation is cholesterol, because it is produced by astrocytes and transported to neurons. Unlike other astrocyte-produced agents (e.g., glutamine, lactate), cholesterol has a large hydrophobic domain, and its transport requires relatively heavy machinery (ApoE). APP is a central plasticity protein whose major physiological role is to manage cholesterol during plasticity, with sAPPα promoting its synthesis and Aβ terminating it.

T*PL is a general theory in which plasticity consists of a single, well-defined process evoked in all plasticity-inducing contexts, including neonatal development, adult learning, and recovery after injury. It also operates in the same manner across all body tissues. These aspects are not detailed here due to my focus on the brain and AD.

11.2.1 Double-edged plasticity

The brain does not know in advance which candidates will win and which will lose, so both winners and losers are stimulated by the same agents. To distinguish between winners and losers, biology uses a mechanism that I call double-edged plasticity (DEP). In DEP, different agent amounts, rates, or cleavages can induce opposite effects. To induce amount-dependent effects, the agent binds different receptors or domains with different affinities. Usually, winners and losers use low and high affinities (high and low amounts), respectively. Brain agents are chemical and propagate through media, so only a focused execution path receives a high amount, defining where the winners are located.

Many important agents directly obey DEP. Calcium activates Ca^{2+}calmodulin-dependent protein kinase II (CaMKII) and protein phosphatase 2B (PP2B), promoting Cgen or Cres (see Section 11.2.6). Dopamine has two receptor families, the low-affinity D1R family that supports vigorous activity [via the G protein–coupled receptors (GPCRs) Gs and Gq] and the high-affinity D2R family that opposes it (via Gi/o) [10]. Similarly, high- and low-affinity serotonin 5-HT1 and 5-HT2 receptors suppress and promote effortful activity, respectively [11].

Another mechanism that supports DEP is different cleavages of a protein. To induce cleavage effects, the precleavage and various postcleavage agents activate different signaling pathways. This is the case with APP (see Section 11.2.4) and growth factors [brain-derived neurotrophic factor (BDNF) and neural growth factor (NGF)], whose mature forms support candidate and winner growth while their proforms support loser removal (see Section 11.2.6).

11.2.2 Long-term potentiation and long-term depression

The notions of long-term potentiation (LTP) and long-term depression (LTD), which are ubiquitously used in relation to plasticity, are not used in T*PL. LTP occurs in both Cgen (all over) and Cres (in winners), and LTD occurs in Cres in both winners and losers. These terms are suitable for describing the local effects of specific experimental conditions but not for the high-level theory.

The following sections detail the steady state, Cgen, cholesterol and LRs, and Cres, with an emphasis on the T*PL aspects that are most relevant to AD.

11.2.3 The steady state

The main relevant components of the steady state are the cytoskeleton, adhesion and scaffold proteins, the ECM, myelin, and constitutive enzyme activity.

Cytoskeleton. The cytoskeleton supports intracellular trafficking, including that of mitochondria and growth factors; exocytosis; and endocytosis and is crucial for neurotransmission and plasticity [12]. It has three main ingredients, MTBs, located mainly in axons but also in dendritic spines; intermediate filaments; and F-actin, located in spines. MTB and actin stability are mainly supported by Map1b and cofilin, respectively. Tau is discussed in Section 11.2.6.

Adhesion. A variety of synaptic adhesion proteins (e.g., neuroligin, neurexin, LRRTM) connect pre- and postsynaptic sites to improve physical stability and signaling [13]. An important role of these proteins is to establish trans-synaptic nanocolumns and cytoskeleton-connected synaptic nanodomains that restrict the spatial propagation of neurotransmitters to provide rapid and efficient activation of downstream signaling [13]. Stable localization of receptors at the PM is assisted by scaffold proteins such as PSD95 and GRIP1 [14].

Extracellular matrix. The brain's ECM is mainly arranged in perineuronal nets and the perinodal ECM [15]. It is synthesized following neural activity and provides stability. It closes the critical period of plasticity during development, opposes the lateral diffusion of some synaptic proteins to extrasynaptic sites, and augments synaptic adhesion [15]. Integrins are a family of cell surface ECM adhesion molecules that support cytoskeleton-based bidirectional trafficking [16]. Thus, the steady state includes a global skeleton that connects all cells to each other via cytoskeletons, adhesion molecules, and ECM.

Myelin. Oligodendrocyte (OLG) processes enwrap neural axons in a myelin sheath mainly made of OLG-produced cholesterol. Myelin protects axons and improves neurotransmission.

Constitutive activity. There are many proteins that are constitutively active to support the steady state. The ones most relevant here are CaMKII, protein kinase M zeta (PKMzeta), and glycogen synthase kinase 3 (GSK3β) (see Section 11.2.6).

11.2.4 Candidate generation

Cgen is triggered in acute states involving protein kinase A (PKA) activation and strong Ca^{2+} influx, depolarizing the cell and inducing action potentials. This is rapidly followed by the release of the growth factor proforms proBDNF and proNGF [17] (both pre- and postsynaptically); tissue plasminogen activator (tPA), which cleaves proforms to their mature forms, BDNF and NGF [18]; and matrix metallopeptidase 9 (MMP9), which digests ECM and adhesion molecules [19]. Cell detachment from the ECM activates integrin signaling and yields the endocytosis of LR components such as caveolin1, destabilizing the steady state [16].

PKA, MARK2, and high levels of Ca^{2+}activated CaMKII phosphorylate tau at S262, S356, and S214, and ERK phosphorylates tau at S199 and S202 [20]. Phosphorylation of tau inactivates it to destabilize the existing MTB–actin cytoskeleton and is essential for neurite formation. ERK also destabilizes myelin [21]. Thus, Cgen destabilizes both extracellular and intracellular stabilization mechanisms.

A central T*PL tenet is that Cgen is a state of cholesterol deficiency. In support, statins, which decrease cholesterol synthesis, increase expression of tPA and p11 (another agent that facilitates growth factor maturation) and BDNF maturation activity [22], and cholesterol deficiency induces hyperphosphorylation of tau, axonal degeneration, and MTB depolymerization (breakdown) [23]. NGF is a plasticity agent supporting winners. It cooperates with the Akt axis (see Section 11.2.6) to promote cholesterol synthesis and rapid axonal growth [24].

Silent synapses contain N-methyl-d-aspartic acid receptors (NMDARs; mainly the GluN2B subunit) but not α-amino-3-hydroxy-5-methyl-4-isoxazolepropionic acid receptors (AMPARs) [25]. BDNF acts via tropomyosin receptor kinase B (TrkB) and enhances GluN2B currents to promote neurite branching [26] and trafficking of AMPARs (mainly the GluA1 subunit) to silent synapses, unsilencing them [25]. These unsilenced synapses are branching candidates. CaMKII binding to GluN2B is needed for spinogenesis [27]. Wnt protein, which promotes growth during development, also promotes axonal branching during Cgen [28].

GluA2-lacking AMPARs are calcium permeable. CP-AMPARs are located at extrasynaptic or synaptic sites, and mark synaptic candidates. During Cgen, PKA and CaMKII stimulate GluA1 surface expression via phosphorylation at S845 and S831 [29], with ERK promoting GluA1 trafficking to synapses [30]. Existing synapses are not degraded but are destabilized via the digestion of adhesion molecules, and their excitatory currents are enhanced by switching AMPARs to be calcium permeable via GluA2 endocytosis promoted by protein kinase C (PKC) phosphorylation at S880 [31].

Most PKC isoforms are activated by calcium. In addition to GluA2 endocytosis, PKC promotes membrane incorporation of GluA1 via pS181 [32] and activation of the Rho GTPase Rac1, which promotes spinogenesis via the actin cytoskeleton [33].

Reelin is an agent that promotes neural migration and growth during development, after which its expression diminishes. In the adult brain, it is expressed by excitatory neurons in entorhinal cortex (ETRC) layer 2 projecting into the hippocampus, GABAergic neurons in cortical layers 1/2, and retrosplenial cortex-projecting GABAergic hippocampus neurons [34]. All of these neurons have axons in long-distance pathways. Reelin is a Cgen agent promoting APPα cleavage [35] and neurite branching [36]. In T*PL, its role is to promote the integration of new neurons and events into the network.

Amyloid precursor protein and soluble amyloid precursor protein α. Amyloid precursor protein (APP) is a transmembrane protein cleaved by α-secretase to yield sAPPα, with the remaining part later cleaved by γ-secretase, or by β-secretase (BACE1) followed by γ-secretase to generate Aβ. Despite extensive research on Aβ and APP [37], to my knowledge there is no coherent account of their physiological roles. T*PL provides such an explanation, in which sAPPα and Aβ are Cgen and Cres agents, respectively. A specific role of APP is to manage cholesterol, with sAPPα promoting its synthesis and transport and Aβ terminating its synthesis and promoting extrusion.

APP transcription is mainly promoted by Cgen agents, including BDNF [38] and ERK [39]. α cleavage (i.e., sAPPα production) is promoted by Cgen agents, including BDNF [40], NGF [41], tPA [42], MMP9 [43], and PKC [44]. Supporting the T*PL thesis that Cgen is a state in which membrane cholesterol is needed, α cleavage is stimulated by reduced membrane cholesterol [45] and occurs in non-LR domains [46]. sAPPα promotes cholesterol synthesis. The intracellular part created by sAPPα cleavage increases SREBP2, the main agent inducing cholesterol synthesis, in cells with low cholesterol, including human astrocytes [47]. sAPPα directly binds to and activates insulin receptors [48], which activate SREBP2 via the PI3K–Akt–mTOR axis and increase α-secretase expression [49].

sAPPα is a major Cgen agent. It rapidly increases surface extrasynaptic GluA1, decreases GluA2 and GluA3 and de novo GluA2 synthesis [50], and promotes neurite growth, branching, spine density, and spine volume [51]. It is an adhesion molecule that promotes axonal outgrowth and synaptogenesis [52].

Cgen directly opposes Cres by suppressing BACE1 via several Cgen agents, including sAPPα [53], NGF, TrkA [43], and BDNF (via SORLA) [54]. Cgen does not end until winners can stably grow, which requires PM LRs.

Short-term memory. Cgen is what supports STM. In particular, it has been repeatedly shown that GluA1 is essential for STM, with knockout animals showing normal spatial reference memory but markedly impaired spatial working memory and STM [55].

11.2.5 Cholesterol, apolipoprotein E, and lipid rafts

Cgen is a cholesterol-deficient state, and the incorporation of cholesterol in LRs switches the cell from Cgen to Cres. Cholesterol is a vital element in all body tissues [56]. The brain is the most cholesterol-rich organ, containing over 20% of body cholesterol. Cholesterol is a major ingredient of LRs and myelin. It is also the precursor of steroids, which are major plasticity agents. Cholesterol does not cross the blood–brain barrier. Brain cholesterol is produced in astrocytes, transported to neurons in ApoE particles, and taken up via ApoE receptors [mainly the low-density lipoprotein receptor (LDLR) and LDLR-related protein 1 (LRP1)]. ApoE transcription is promoted in growth situations via growth factors (BDNF and NGF) and estrogen [57–59]. It is normally produced by neurons only in small amounts, with production increasing in conditions of stress, injury, and resource deficiency [60].

Cholesterol synthesis is mainly stimulated by SREBPs [61], which also promote LDLR expression. SREBPs are activated by lack of PM cholesterol and by ERK and insulin–Akt signaling (see Section 11.2.6). The brain-specific cholesterol metabolite 24S-hydroxycholesterol (and its non-brain oxysterol counterpart 27-hydroxycholesterol) and intracellular cholesterol excess suppress SREBP and activate nuclear liver X receptors (LXRs), which promote ApoE and the transporters ABCA1 and ABCG1. These extrude cholesterol by lipidating ApoE and transporting it across the membrane.

Apolipoprotein E isoforms. Humans have three ApoE isoforms that differ in amount produced and transport capacity: ApoE2, ApoE3, and ApoE4, in order from greatest to lowest production and transport capacity [62]. ApoE4 has the highest receptor affinity, saturating receptors faster. These properties can have both positive and negative consequences. ApoE4 is more efficient in terms of speed and resources, explaining its various positive effects [e.g., improving cognition during youth [63]]. However, the fact that the neurons of ApoE4 carriers receive less cholesterol makes them vulnerable in aging, as discussed in this article.

Lipid rafts. LRs are dynamic membrane nanodomains enriched in cholesterol; sphin-golipids, mainly SPM; and glycerophospholipids such as gangliosides [64]. LRs were originally controversial due to technical difficulties but are now fully accepted. LRs increase local membrane rigidity and serve to anchor proteins and link the membrane to the cytoskeleton and the ECM, thereby supporting the connection between the intracellular and extracellular environments, specifically extracellular induced signaling [16,65]. They are a major site of membrane proteins and are central cytoskeleton trafficking targets, interfacing with the actin cytoskeleton [64]. MTB proteins, mainly tau, associate with LRs, and impairing this association yields axonal retraction [65,66].

Palmitoylation targets proteins to LRs and is required for stable membrane anchoring of many proteins, including synaptic density proteins, glutamate receptors and their recycling proteins, steroid receptors, GPCRs, and actin-regulating proteins required for spine growth [67]. Caveolae are LRs that contain caveolin1 and show as membrane invaginations. They are essential for membrane anchoring and trafficking of tyrosine kinase receptors such as TrkA (the NGF receptor) and the insulin receptor [68]. LRs and cholesterol are required for the activation of nicotinic receptors [69].

LRs are essential for plasticity. Synaptogenesis requires astrocyte-derived cholesterol [70]. Depletion of cholesterol or sphingolipids leads to gradual loss of hippocampus dendritic spines and synapses and to surface AMPAR instability [71]. Cholesterol depletion blocks winner enhancement in hippocampus CA1 [72], an area that shows specific vulnerability in AD (see Section 11.4.6).

LRs are present in intracellular membranes as well, including in mitochondria-associated endoplasmic reticulum membranes (MAMs), which are essential for mitochondria function [73], and in the trans-Golgi network and recycling endosomes [74].

11.2.6 Competition resolution: winners and losers

Cgen induces indiscriminate destabilization, candidate generation, and cellular calcium influx in the vicinity of active sites. Cholesterol induces a switch from Cgen to Cres in two ways. It allows winner enhancement through LRs and it stimulates the production of Aβ, which is the main loser-removal agent.

Cres has four main components. First, calcium influx is reduced in both winners and losers. Calcium must be restrained because it can be toxic. Most relevantly here, calcium activates calmodulin, whose continued binding to PSD95 rapidly (within 15 minutes) decreases its palmitoylation and synaptic location and increases AMPAR endocytosis, rendering synapses unusable [75]. This time frame is consistent with the duration of STM. Calcium is restrained by switching GluN2B to the GluN2A subunit [76], replacing CP-AMPARs with CI-AMPARs by adding GluA2 [77], and endocytosis of GluA1 via PP2B [78].

Second, the cytoskeleton is linked to the PM in winners to support trafficking, with tau being a major player (see Section 2.6.2). Third, winning synapses are stabilized, including through the formation of nanodomains for efficient neurotransmission [79]. Finally, the membrane is returned to a stable condition by removing losing candidates (see Section 2.6.3).

Winner determination. Ca^{2+} is a DEP agent, with large amounts (or rates) activating kinases (mainly CaMKII) that promote winners, and small amounts activating phosphatases (mainly PP2B) to eliminate losers [80]. It is not possible to restrain calcium before some persistent enhancement of winners occurs, because strong, focused, persistent calcium is what determines winner status. Once LRs are incorporated into the PM, Cres can enhance winning candidates and remove losing ones to establish a new steady state.

There are two main agents involved in winner enhancement, CaMKII and PKC. Both start their activity during Cgen (because winners need to be generated first (see Section 11.2.4) and continue during Cres.

CaMKII is activated by high calcium concentrations [27] during Cgen. It binds GluN2B, translocates with it to synapses, and promotes GluA1 channel conductance via phosphorylation at S831 [27]. It also induces spine growth via Rac1 [81]. When Cres starts, CaMKII undergoes autophosphorylation at T286, which allows it to continue activation without calcium. In this way, it can support synapse consolidation during Cres and possibly even the maintenance of synapses in the steady state. It promotes synapse stabilization and the formation of nanodomains via segregation of AMPARs and NLG from GluN2B [79] and the switch from GluN2B to GluN2A [76].

PKC is activated by sustained calcium release from intracellular stores. During Cgen, it promotes GluA1 synaptic delivery via S818 phosphorylation [32], structural growth via Rac1 [33], production of sAPPα over Aβ [44], and GluA2 endocytosis [14]. During Cres, it promotes the switch from GluN2B to GluN2A [76] and prevents winner damage due to Aβ (endocytosed APP undergoes β cleavage, unless this is opposed by PKC). At plasticity termination, its constitutively active form, PKMzeta, supports LTM [82].

Candidate synapses that become large enough allow the invasion of MTBs and tau [83], an important factor in winner determination.

Tau. Tau binds cytoskeleton MTBs and was initially thought to support MTB stability. However, its detachment from MTBs does not destabilize them or impair axonal transport [84]. It is now viewed as a cross-linker of the MTB and actin cytoskeletons that promotes dynamic changes including axonal elongation, synapse formation, and stabilization of growing neurites [85].

During Cgen, tau is inactivated via phosphorylation (see Section 11.2.4) to oppose its stabilization effect. During Cres, it is activated in winners to promote their structural stabilization and cytoskeleton linking and inactivated in losers to allow their removal. Activation in winners is done by phosphatases, mainly PP2A [86]. Methylated (stronger) PP2A is enriched in LRs and decreases p-tau [87]. Inactivation in losers is mainly done by GSK3b and cyclin dependent kinase 5 (Cdk5), assisted by p75 [88].

As noted in section 2.5.2, active tau requires LRs to achieve its effects [65,66]. Reducing cholesterol (which induces a loser-like, non-LR state) yields hyperphosphorylation of tau at the GSK3 and PKA sites [89]. Excess tau is secreted via direct translocation through the PM, and this action is supported by cholesterol and SPM [90]. Thus, extracellular tau is a normal by-product of plasticity-inducing activity.

Amyloid β. Aβ is a major Cres agent whose main role is to remove losers. The switch from α to β cleavage of APP, and thus initiation of Aβ production, occurs when LRs have been formed. Cholesterol clearly stimulates Aβ production and is needed for it, as its depletion inhibits BACE1 and γ-secretase additively [91,92]. In turn, Aβ provides negative feedback on cholesterol synthesis [93], supporting the T*PL view that cholesterol synthesis occurs in Cgen but not Cres.

BACE1 operates in intracellular compartments (endosomes and Golgi), so Aβ can be produced without the formation of PM LRs [94] (as described in Section 11.3.3, this has important implications in AD). PM LRs are a feature of winners, while the main role of Aβ is to remove losers, which are spatially segregated from winners.

Aβ production is also promoted by the Cres agents p75 and JNK [95,96]. Aβ promotes Cres by enhancing GSK3β [48,88], PP2B [78,97], proNGF [98], p75 [88], PTEN [99], JNK [96], and RhoA (which opposes Rac1) [100]. Aβ's loser removal functionality is obtained via three main mechanisms, involving RhoA; p-tau, via GSK3b, JNK; and p75, which is a high-affinity receptor for proBDNF and proNGF and a low-affinity receptor for NGF. p75 stops neurite growth and induces apoptosis [26]; with Aβ, p75 activates sphingomyelinase to remove SPM from the PM [93], thereby cleaning losing candidates from LR components and restoring membrane integrity.

Aβ opposes Cgen through these agents (e.g., GSK3β opposes Akt and thus insulin signaling, PP2B opposes BDNF, and PTEN opposes mTOR) and other mechanisms [e.g., it inhibits NGF [48] and nicotinic acetylcholine receptors (nAChRs), mainly the CP α-7 subunit [101]].

The ECM, which promotes the stable postplasticity state, contains several agents (e.g., heparan sulfate proteoglycan) that are contained in LRs and bind and take up Aβ [102].

Aβ is a DEP agent, possibly to prevent it from impairing winners. Aβ oligomers readily insert in membranes to form cation-selective pores [101,103]. At low (picomolar) concentrations, the resulting calcium influx promotes the function of the α7 subunit of nAChRs [101], explaining the positive effect that low Aβ concentrations can have on LTP and growth [104]. At higher (nanomolar) concentrations, Aβ inhibits nAChRs and decreases plasticity [101,104].

In summary, Aβ terminates Cgen, promotes Cres, especially loser removal, and terminates cholesterol synthesis. The common view of Aβ as a negative agent stems from the fact that loser removal involves reduced spine density and LTD. However, loser removal is essential for cellular health, and Aβ has a crucial healthy role in plasticity. Indeed, Aβ disruption prevents the consolidation and stabilization of memory [105].

Consolidation. This stage takes place after activity termination and involves protein synthesis and trafficking to the winning candidates, completion of loser removal, cytoskeleton stabilization, ECM and myelin production, and other actions needed to establish a stable steady state. Consolidation is one of the major processes taking place during sleep [106].

11.2.7 Summary

Brain plasticity starts with destabilization of the stable state, coupled with indiscriminate increases in neural excitability and the generation of structural candidates competing for enhancement. Winners are determined by sustained calcium signaling. Incorporation of cholesterol in PM LRs triggers a switch to restabilization, which involves winner enhancement and loser removal. The major agents in these processes are the AD-associated agents tau, APP, and cholesterol (with other lipids). sAPPα promotes the initial Cgen stage. Cholesterol induces a switch to the production of Aβ, which promotes loser removal. The formation of PM LRs allows activated tau to extend the cytoskeleton and link it to the enhanced winning synapses. Both Aβ and tau phosphorylation are crucial for normal, healthy plasticity.

11.3 The lipid-raft theory of Alzheimer's disease

Provided with a theory of brain plasticity that explains the roles of the main AD agents, it is now possible to understand what goes wrong in AD. This section presents the LR theory of AD (T*AD) and shows how it accounts for AD symptoms and pathology. Risk factors, protective factors, and strong evidence supporting the theory are given in subsequent sections. Unless explicitly noted, the discussion is about sporadic AD, not FAD.

11.3.1 Mechanisms underlying symptoms and pathology

My starting point for explaining AD consists of the following three clues. First, the strongest genetic risk factor in AD, carrying ApoE4, points to reduced transport, neural uptake, or neural trafficking of cholesterol. Second, the characteristic symptom of AD, impaired anterograde memory with functioning STM, points to a problem in the initiation of Cres or in winner enhancement. Third, the main AD pathologies, hyperphosphorylated tau and Aβ, point to chronic Cgen or excessive loser removal. Neurodegeneration is a natural consequence of these pathologies and of chronic loser removal.

The main role of cholesterol in short-term plasticity is in LRs. Thus, the first clue leads to the hypothesis of impaired LR formation. Impaired LR formation impairs the switch from STM to LTM and from Cgen to Cres, explaining memory symptoms (the second clue). LRs and Cres are essential for tau dephosphorylation, explaining the tau part of the third clue (see Section 11.3.3 for the Aβ part). Neurons can produce cholesterol in response to stress to support Aβ production, but they cannot supplant astrocyte-derived cholesterol for PM LRs [70]. Thus, we reach the following hypothesis: AD symptoms and pathology are caused by impaired formation of PM LRs, which is in turn caused by reduced neural uptake or trafficking of astrocyte-produced cholesterol.

11.3.2 Chronicity

The formation of PM LRs triggers the switch from Cgen to Cres. When this process is impaired, we can expect both Cgen and Cres to be active at the same time but with smaller agent amounts than those involved in healthy plasticity and with a prolonged duration. I use the term chronicity to refer to this state throughout this article (Fig. 11.4). In early disease stages, chronicity should yield an increase in both Cgen and Cres agents. With disease progression, brain resources get depleted, so Cres should increase and Cgen decrease. This is exactly what the evidence shows (see Section 11.4.4).

Many plasticity agents obey DEP and are present in smaller amounts during chronicity. As a result, their effects are tilted toward Cres. Specifically, chronic calcium presence induces loser removal and neurodegeneration. Thus, the continued activation of Cgen, which could compensate for cholesterol deficiency by promoting its synthesis, actually exacerbates the situation. Moreover, because biological systems extensively rely on negative feedback, chronicity desensitizes receptors and pathways, impairing many cellular signaling pathways.

11.3.3 Cholesterol and amyloid β

A straightforward explanation for reduced PM LRs is that cholesterol synthesis is decreased. Indeed, there are data indicating that ApoE4 is associated with reduced cholesterol synthesis capacity [107], and there is evidence for reduced cholesterol in AD (see Section 11.4.2). However, chronic synthesis is at least as likely, since cholesterol synthesis continues as long as it does not get incorporated properly in the PM. Thus, AD can involve both cholesterol deficiency (in PM LRs) and excess. Chronic synthesis happens in both astrocytes and neurons, which increase cholesterol production under stress. Neural production may be able to counter membrane damage incurred by injury [60], but it generally does not compensate for cholesterol deficiency during plasticity [70,108].

Cholesterol stimulates Aβ production, yielding two types of neurons associated with chronic cholesterol in AD. In the first type, chronic neural cholesterol production eventually manages to form PM LRs. Such neurons form synapses and do not show tau pathology but do show excessive Aβ production, causing Aβ secretion and aggregation. This explains why Aβ is common in aging and why Aβ plaques are not strongly correlated with AD symptoms and tau pathology. In the second type, chronic cholesterol production does not compensate for reduced PM LRs, and these neurons show plasticity impairment and both tau and Aβ pathology. Since Aβ binds cholesterol [103], Aβ plaques are expected to contain cholesterol in both neural types, as is indeed the case [109].

11.3.4 Tau

LRs are crucial for cytoskeleton-PM linking, neurite growth, and neurite stabilization, and tau has a major role in these functions [65,66]. LRs promote the switch to Cres and allow tau dephosphorylation in winners. LR impairment promotes the cytosolic localization of tau and p-tau, and tau–membrane disconnect may facilitate the helical tau conformation found in NFTs [110]. Propagating p-tau is hypothesized to spread AD pathology [5], and tau is indeed secreted as a normal consequence of neural activity [90] (see Section 2.6.2). T*PL explains this tau secretion as a way of clearing excessive inactive tau generated during Cgen, but it is possible that it occurs in AD, which involves excessive inactive tau. Nonetheless, gradual spreading is not well supported by the evidence [111].

11.3.5 Core cause

The mechanisms of AD can be explained by impaired PM LRs, and these can be explained by reduced uptake or trafficking of cholesterol. Why does this happen? Although the link with ApoE4 is very strong, there are people carrying this isoform (even homozygotes) who do not get the disease. In addition, there are ApoE3 carriers with AD.

The parsimonious answer to this question is that cholesterol metabolism, and specifically LRs, are normally reduced in aging [56,83] (which incidentally explains why memory is reduced in normal aging), and a variety of risk factors can push this reduction beyond the damage threshold. Some viruses enter cells via LRs and impair lipid metabolism (this includes COVID-19, which might explain its long-lasting cognitive symptoms). IR and impaired vasculature affect all plasticity stages and can specifically induce cholesterol deficiency. Sleep problems, chronic inflammation, and chronic stress promote a state similar to chronic destabilization. Brain injury involves acute destabilization that can become chronic. Polyunsaturated fatty acids (PUFAs) are also present in LRs and reduced in aging. These risk factors are expanded upon in Section 11.5. In addition, lipid metabolism is supported by many genes, providing ample opportunity for small gene changes to predispose a person to less efficient metabolism, especially in aging. Such changes can manifest as sporadic AD even in ApoE3 carriers.

Gonadal steroids are major plasticity agents and are reduced abruptly and relatively early in women (versus a gradual loss in men), explaining why women have an increased AD risk at younger ages and a faster cognitive decline after diagnosis [112].

11.3.6 Autosomal dominant Alzheimer's disease

The core cause of autosomal dominant AD (which approximately overlaps with FAD) is different from that of sporadic AD, and involves decrease-of-function mutations in the PSEN1 gene, whose protein (presenilin 1) is a major component of γ-secretase, or mutations in the γ-secretase APP cleavage site [113]. Such mutations affect both sAPPα and Aβ, which are central plasticity agents. Hence, these mutations can seriously damage plasticity, explaining the earlier age of onset of the disease. The reason that the brain manages to support plasticity until middle age is probably the large functional redundancy between the various Cgen and Cres agents.

11.4 Evidence

In addition to the salient evidence regarding tau, Aβ, and ApoE4, many other lines of evidence provide support for T*AD, including evidence concerning LRs, cholesterol, PUFAs, plasticity agents, synapse issues, the brain areas of earliest damage, genetics, and other diseases. These lines of evidence are presented in this section. Risk factors also provide support for the theory and are discussed in Section 11.5.

11.4.1 Lipid rafts

LRs are reported to be reduced or abnormal in AD. In mixed ApoE3/ApoE4 carriers, membrane cholesterol was decreased by 36%, with abnormal LRs [114]. Neuronal LRs are strongly altered in frontal cortex and ETRC from the earliest stages of the disease (before NFTs) [115]. The changes include lower cholesterol, SPM, and PUFAs [115]. Thcsc ncurons show increased sterol esters, which may indicate excessive cholesterol synthesis with impaired incorporation into LRs. Patient temporal cortex contains significantly lower numbers of LRs, with those remaining being depleted of cholesterol [116]. Frontal and temporal cortex LRs contain significantly higher levels of the gangliosides GM1 and GM2 [116]. Flotillin and gangliosides, strong LR markers, show marked abnormalities in patient brain, cerebrospinal fluid (CSF), and serum [117–119]. In most cases, these abnormalities also occur in patients with mild cognitive impairment, showing that it is an early event in the disease. Flotillin accumulates in lysosomes in NFT-positive neurons, showing the link between LRs and tau pathology [120]. A recent review summarized strong evidence that Aβ plaques contain cholesterol and gangliosides [109].

11.4.2 Cholesterol

Dysregulated lipid metabolism, especially accumulation of lipids in glia, was noted as a third major AD pathology right from the start, over 100 years ago [121]. Cholesterol and lipid dysregulation is a strong characteristic of AD [121]. As predicted by T*AD, both lower and higher cholesterol are reported. Lower cholesterol is reported in temporal cortex [122] and CSF [123,124], especially in patients with severe disease [125]. Seladin1, an enzyme that mediates the conversion of desmosterol to cholesterol, is reduced in AD, specifically in vulnerable regions [126]. ETRC and hippocampus show lower cholesterol synthesis, which is significantly associated with AD pathology (however, cholesterol levels themselves were normal, which might indicate chronicity) [127].

Most of the evidence points to chronically increased cholesterol synthesis. Neurons with NFT tau show higher levels of unesterified cholesterol [128]. Cholesterol and ceramides accumulate in AD brain in a vulnerable region (frontal cortex) but not the cerebellum [129]. ETRC shows elevated cholesterol esters, SPM, and ganglioside GM3 [130]. Patients with AD show higher brain cholesterol levels and decreased levels of LXR (cholesterol extrusion) [131]. Increased ABCA1 (sterol extrusion) expression correlates strongly with dementia severity in AD hippocampus [132]. Cholesterol is increased in patient astrocyte mitochondria [133]. Sensitive imaging shows significantly higher (34%) cholesterol in cortical layers 3 and 4 [134]. AD pyramidal neurons in the hippocampus show no nucleus translocation (activation) of SREBP2, indicating sterol excess. 40–50% of NFT neurons express nonnuclear SREBP2 [135]. Total cholesterol is increased in a CHO cell line with the FAD-causing presenilin1 mutation [136]. CSF levels of cholesterol correlate with p-tau [137] and secreted APP (both α and β) [138] in patients but not controls. PCSK9, which downregulates LDLR and thus ApoE uptake, was reported to be increased in AD, indicating excess. However, one study reported no changes [139].

Fibroblasts from sporadic AD and FAD patients show markedly higher levels of free cholesterol and cholesterol esters [140]. MAMs, which contain LRs, show a higher number of contacts and upregulated activity (cholesterol esterification and phospholipid synthesis) in sporadic AD and FAD fibroblasts and in mouse models [73]. Patient skin fibroblasts show increased levels of cholesterol esterification enzyme and decreased levels of SREBP2 and ABCA1 mRNA [141]. In addition to showing cholesterol excess, these results are important because they show that the problem can be present in cells other than glia and neurons, shedding light on the core cause and allowing practical biomarkers to be identified.

In many cases, the core of the problem may be lipid trafficking rather than uptake. ApoE4 (and, to a lesser degree, ApoE3) tends to aggregate in and damage endosomes [142], which are crucial for cholesterol homeostasis. Indeed, endosomes are dysregulated in AD, and endosome-related genes such as Bin1, TREM2, PICALM, and SORLA have been highlighted in genome-wide association studies (GWAS) [142].

11.4.3 Polyunsaturated fatty acids

Docosahexanoic acid, the main omega-3 PUFA, is reduced in AD serum and postmortem brain [143]. PUFAs are the main target of lipid peroxidation by reactive oxygen species produced during oxidative stress, and AD brains show higher levels of PUFA oxidation products and oxidative stress (which can stem from chronicity, e.g., chronically high levels of calcium) [143]. Although PUFAs are mainly located outside LRs, some are located inside LRs, and PUFA levels are reduced in LRs in frontal cortex and ETRC in AD [115].

11.4.4 Plasticity agents

Virtually all important plasticity agents are dysregulated in AD, including Ca^{2+} [2], ERK, p38, JNK, Akt, PKA, PKC, GSK3β, PP2B, PP1, PTEN, Cdk5 [144], BDNF, TrkA (the NGF receptor), tPA, MMP9 [145], and PAI-1 (a tPA inhibitor) [18]. Of the listed agents, tau phosphorylation agents (ERK, p38, JNK, GSK3, PP2B, and Cdk5 but not PKA) are chronically increased [144], while PP2A, the main tau dephosphorylation agent, is reduced in AD [86].

Notably, PKC [144] and GluA2 [146], the hallmarks of winner enhancement and stabilized winners, are reduced in AD. In the hippocampus, the greatest decrease in GluA2 occurs in the most vulnerable areas (subiculum, CA1) [146]. Note that PKC is activated by moderate levels of calcium, so chronically high calcium levels (e.g., those induced by membrane Aβ cation channels) should activate it, which would explain the reduction in GluA2 (PKC promotes its endocytosis; see Section 11.2.4). The fact that PKC is reduced and not increased indicates a fundamental non-Aβ problem with winner enhancement processes.

11.4.5 Synapses

Synaptic damage is a well-known early event in AD [7]. This shows that synapses are not formed correctly or are degraded early. Both cases support T*AD.

11.4.6 Brain areas

The earliest areas that show tau pathology in AD are the ETRC, hippocampus, and locus coeruleus (LC) [5]. Among hippocampus fields, the subiculum and CA1 are much more vulnerable than the dentate gyrus (DG) and CA3 [147]. Among thalamic nuclei, the nucleus reuniens, connecting the ETRC, subiculum, CA1, and the medial prefrontal cortex, is one of the most heavily affected nuclei [148]. ETRC and hippocampus represent scenes and events, which due to their richness, present continuous novelty that requires plasticity. The LC, the main norepinephrine center in the brain, is also active in all novel situations. The fact that the areas that show the largest plasticity requirements are those most vulnerable in AD supports T*PL. Moreover, CA1 and subiculum support familiar scenes, while DG and CA3 support the encoding of new ones [149].

Most of our life experiences involve familiar scenes with some element of novelty, explaining why CA1 and subiculum are relatively more vulnerable. ETRC supports both familiar and novel scenes, explaining its central role in early AD.

Early auditory [150], olfactory [151], and retinal [152] sensory cells contain LRs, explaining the early loss of hearing and smell and retinal abnormalities in AD [4]. Of note, statin use is associated with sudden hearing loss in an all-Taiwan insurance database [153], statins are among the drugs that can impair olfaction [154], and cholesterol depletion causes hearing loss in cats and severe cochlear hair cell loss in mice [155].

11.4.7 Genetics

Cholesterol and lipid pathway genes are repeatedly identified as leading clusters in AD GWAS [156]. So are endosome-related genes, as mentioned in Section 11.4.2.

11.4.8 Other diseases

Niemann-Pick disease type C (NPC), which involves dementia and neurodegeneration, is caused by mutations in the NPC1 or NPC2 genes, which support transport of cholesterol from late endosomes and lysosomes [157]. NPC brains show tau-rich NFTs with paired helical filaments identical to those found in AD [157].

Down syndrome patients usually carry three copies of the APP gene and manifest AD-like pathology [158].

11.5 Risk and protective factors

Here, I discuss various factors affecting AD. Many of these factors are associated with aging, increasing the aging-related risk.

11.5.1 Viral infections

Increased human herpesvirus 6A and 7 infections were reported in AD [159], and herpesvirus infection was found to induce a threefold increase in dementia risk [160]. Moreover, in a highly controlled all-Wales setting, herpes zoster vaccination was shown to decrease risk of dementia (all cause except vascular) by 20% [161].

In T*AD, viral infection is a direct AD risk factor because many viruses (including herpesvirus and COVID-19) highjack lipid metabolism to persistently weaken lipid homeostasis, especially LRs [162]. Incidentally, this may explain the long-lasting cognitive symptoms of COVID-19.

11.5.2 Traumatic brain injury

Traumatic brain injury (TBI) can induce a physical disconnect of the ECM, which triggers LR endocytosis [16]. Moreover, it involves strong release and prolonged presence of Cgen agents in the brain [163], which can induce chronic loser removal due to DEP. Indeed, TBI is an AD risk factor and is associated with synaptic dysfunction [163].

11.5.3 Diabetes and obesity

Type 2 diabetes and obesity are AD risk factors [1], and the notion that AD is a third type of diabetes is gaining support [164]. In my view, this notion is not justified. T*AD explains this risk factor via the fact that the synthesis of lipids, including cholesterol and PUFAs, needs PI3K–Akt signaling, which is impaired by IR. Thus, IR can impair LRs and promote chronic cholesterol.

Although IR can exacerbate the situation of people who are at risk of AD, brain IR is just one of many risk factors that can yield LR damage, which is the core mechanism in AD. Note that cholesterol homeostasis is more fundamental in AD than IR, since if IR were the core cause, it should affect ApoE2 homozygotes, who are virtually protected. I conclude that IR is definitely a serious AD risk factor, and it may even suffice for causing dementia, but the dementia classified as AD requires additional factors.

It should be noted that the association between AD and obesity is not that simple, since low body-mass index (BMI) is also associated with increased risk [165]. This supports T*AD, since a low BMI may indicate a tissue-wide problem in lipid synthesis and/or uptake, which can impair LRs.

11.5.4 Vascular impairment

Vascular dementia is the second most common dementia after AD, accounting for 5–10% of cases, and cerebrovascular disease is commonly shown in AD [1]. Cardiovascular disease is also associated with increased AD risk [1]. Vascular impairment can increase AD risk via a reduction in the raw materials needed for lipid synthesis. However, it can also be a consequence of the AD core mechanism, since impaired cholesterol homeostasis yields vascular damage.

Statins suppress cholesterol synthesis and are regularly taken by people at perceived risk of cardiovascular disease. They do not cross the blood–brain barrier, so they should not directly affect AD, but they might reduce risk via the other risk factors. They can also be detrimental in AD in the event of barrier damage.

11.5.5 Immunity

Neuroinflammation is common in AD and is associated with activation of microglia [1,2] and their TREM2 receptors [166]. TREM2 is activated by lipids, and different mutations have been identified that increase AD risk or decrease TREM2–ApoE binding [166]. Microglia might be activated by cholesterol excess and have an initial protective role in AD. However, chronic neuroinflammation promotes neurodegeneration.

11.5.6 Stress

Early-life and lifetime stress are associated with earlier AD onset and faster disease progression [167]. This is consistent with the fact that chronic stress is associated with neurodegeneration in memory-related areas [9]. The mechanisms of damage due to chronic stress may be related to LRs (e.g., cortisol induces endocannabinoid synthesis from PUFAs, which can impair LRs) or be independent of LRs (e.g., calcium excitotoxicity). As a neurosteroid, cortisol requires cholesterol for its synthesis, so chronic cortisol synthesis may promote brain cholesterol depletion.

Oxidative stress and its lipid peroxidation effect are higher in AD (see Section 11.4.3).

11.5.7 Smoking

Smoke exposure and smoking are associated with increased AD risk AZ2023. This can occur via several mechanisms. For example, nicotinic agonists increase p-tau [168].

11.5.8 Education and bilingualism

Formal education is a clear protective factor against AD [1], and so is (less clearly) bilingualism [169]. T*AD explains these data as follows. Both involve memory-related learning, which creates synapses. A denser synaptic space might reduce the number of candidates, which is a function of novelty. It should facilitate the formation of new synapses, because synapse candidates are closer to each other and are thus easier to connect. Therefore, the growth needs of the educated brain are smaller, so smaller amounts of cholesterol are needed for plasticity. Indeed, bilinguals have a larger gray matter volume [170] and increased connectivity [171].

11.5.9 Exercise

Most (not all) data indicate that exercise weakly reduces AD risk [172]. Exercise has positive effects on many of the risk factors discussed here, including brain vasculature, blood flow, brain clearance from chronic agents, obesity, sleep, and cardiovascular disease.

11.6 Discussion

This article presents the first theory of AD that is complete, in the sense that it mechanistically explains all of the major AD phenomena, including etiology, symptoms, pathology, and risk factors. To do this, the article presents a new theory of brain plasticity (T*PL) that explains memory formation and the roles in health and disease of sAPPα, Aβ, tau, growth factors, kinases, phosphatases, cholesterol, and other agents. T*PL enables the development of a coherent theory of AD.

11.6.1 Related theories

Cholesterol has been repeatedly recognized as an important factor in AD [121,173]. However, this was based on its promoting effects of Aβ, its link with cardiovascular disease, and evidence of lipid dysregulation in AD. The point in the present chapter is that cholesterol and its major effects on lipid rafts is the main culprit in the disease. Impaired cholesterol distribution (cytosol vs. plasma membrane) and trafficking have been described as a major event [173], but these were in light of Aβ as a culprit. I found only one paper that points to cholesterol as the central agent in AD [158], but it focuses only on chronically high cholesterol as the driving force behind neurodegeneration, without addressing anterograde memory symptoms and plasticity agents and processes. All of this work presents a negative view of cholesterol (opposite to T*PL) and does not explain the disease mechanisms and pathological process.

Likewise, tau has long been known to be the main pathological factor correlated with symptoms, but no coherent story for why it is phosphorylated in health and disease has been presented. T*PL, which proposes that Cgen requires destabilization and Cres removes losing candidates, naturally explains p-tau and its chronicity-induced accumulation. Many hypotheses have been raised in AD research, including the cholinergic, Aβ, tau propagation, mitochondria, calcium, neurovascular, inflammation, microbe, metal ion, and lymphatic hypotheses [2], and the type 3 diabetes hypothesis [164]. As discussed in Section 11.5, these are factors that affect AD risk but are not fundamental to the disease.

11.6.2 The theory of adaptive response plasticity

Brain plasticity is one of the most heavily researched areas of neuroscience. Competition between spines and the elimination of losing ones is an established idea in plasticity research, with strong evidence supporting it [9]. T*PL is the first theory of plasticity that presents a coherent mechanistic story explaining how initial potentiation switches to consolidation and the first that seamlessly integrates structural plasticity with neurotransmission plasticity and explains the roles of cholesterol, APP, tau, and other agents.

Strong high-level support for T*PL comes from its structural similarity to other biological theories. Notably, candidate generation followed by competition is the cornerstone of the theory of evolution. In immunity, clonal selection of B and T cells can be viewed as candidate generation, while memory T cells result from consolidation. The principle of DEP has some superficial resemblance to the notion of hormesis in toxicology [174]. While the opposite effects of CaMKII versus PP2B and of TrkB and TrkA versus p75 are clearly known, as far as I know, this article is the first in which DEP is phrased as a general biological principle. Note that DEP applies to neuromodulators as well (see the examples involving dopamine and serotonin in section 11.2.1). It also applies to the immune system, with mechanisms that are not described in this article.

This article focuses on the main notions relevant to plasticity and AD, to show the forest rather than a huge number of trees. Additional topics are left for future texts, including the difference between LDLR and LRP1, other LRPs, gangliosides and SPM, Src and Fyn kinases, prion protein, reelin, amyloid precursor protein intracellular cytoplasmic domain, smoking, myelin, metabotropic glutamate receptors, Cdc42, Arc/Arg3.1, adenosine, p38, cofilin and other non-tau cytoskeleton proteins, specific adhesion molecules, α-synuclein, TGF-β, NFkB, homeostatic plasticity, the difference between different Aβ species, etc.

A topic that is of particular importance is the timeline of winner enhancement. For example, CaMKII is autophosphorylated to keep it active without calcium. Does PKC (which is calcium dependent) switch to PKMzeta (which shows constitutive activity) at the same time? It seems that it should, otherwise it would continue to promote sAPPα and inhibit GluA2. In addition, is GluN2A eventually removed from winners, like GluA1? More research is needed on these topics.

Additional research is also needed with respect to LR homeostasis. How precisely does cholesterol get incorporated in PM LRs? One possibility is that it is transported by caveolin1, but the precise mechanisms are still not clear.

11.6.3 Sleep

AD is associated with impaired sleep. Sleep is crucial for memory and plasticity, and the most upregulated genes in sleep support lipid synthesis and transport and LRs [106]. There is some controversy around the synaptic homeostasis hypothesis, in which the goal of sleep (or at least of slow-wave sleep) is to globally downscale synapses. In T*PL, sleep supports the late part of Cres, which indeed involves massive loser removal and reduced calcium entry in winning synapses. However, sleep also strengthens winning synapses.

11.6.4 Neurogenesis

Adult neurogenesis is crucial for memory [175] and occurs in the hippocampus DG, which receives inputs from ETRC reelin neurons; these neurons show specific vulnerability in AD. In T*PL, new neuron candidates are generated during Cgen. New cells require substantial resources to mature, so we expect adult neurogenesis to be impaired in AD, which is indeed the case [176]. Unlike synaptogenesis, which is a ubiquitous process, neurogenesis-related evidence is small. However, its impairment may well be important in AD.

11.6.5 Dementia

This article focuses on AD, but T*PL and T*AD also provide a reasonable explanation for other types of dementia, in particular vascular dementia. In addition, zinc, iron, and copper are fundamental in cellular processes and are dysregulated in AD [2]. Metals interact with ApoE, and the link to LRs and to other types of dementia should be further investigated.

Frontotemporal dementia (FTD) has a major variant that shows tau pathology. Nonetheless, in my view, both the core cause and the disease mechanisms of FTD are different from those of AD. A detailed theory of FTD will be presented elsewhere.

11.6.6 Theory predictions

T*PL and T*AD are supported by very strong evidence, including evidence from patient data and a large number of animal models developed for AD and brain plasticity. This evidence pertains to the details underlying the theories. The main prediction resulting from these theories is that the cause of the human disease diagnosed as AD is reduced cholesterol in neural PM LRs during plasticity. This has not been directly shown yet. One way of showing it would be via clinical trials with the participation of people diagnosed with AD or known to be at a high risk, which is obviously a very long and risky process.

The theory presented here points to several promising directions for treating AD, for example, enhancing the ApoE receptor LDLR by inhibiting PCSK9. I hope that some of these will be taken to help patients, families, and caregivers.

References

[1] Alzheimer's Association, Alzheimer's disease facts and figures, Alzheimer's & Dementia 19 (4) (2023) 1598–1695.

[2] P.P. Liu, Y. Xie, X.Y. Meng, J.S. Kang, History and progress of hypotheses and clinical trials for Alzheimer's disease, Signal Transduction and Targeted Therapy 4 (1) (2019) 29.

[3] G.P. Morris, I.A. Clark, B. Vissel, Questions concerning the role of amyloid-β in the definition, aetiology and diagnosis of Alzheimer's disease, Acta Neuropathologica 136 (5) (2018) 663–689.

[4] C. Murphy, Olfactory and other sensory impairments in Alzheimer disease, Nature Reviews Neurology 15 (1) (2019) 11–24.

[5] S.K. Kaufman, K. Del Tredici, T.L. Thomas, H. Braak, M.I. Diamond, Tau seeding activity begins in the transentorhinal/entorhinal regions and anticipates phospho-tau pathology in Alzheimer's disease and PART, Acta Neuropathologica 136 (1) (2018) 57–67.

[6] E. Area-Gomez, E.A. Schon, Alzheimer disease, Organelle Contact Sites: From Molecular Mechanism to Disease (2017) 149–156.

[7] L. Crews, E. Masliah, Molecular mechanisms of neurodegeneration in Alzheimer's disease, Human Molecular Genetics 19 (R1) (2010) R12–R20.

[8] W.C. Abraham, O.D. Jones, D.L. Glanzman, Is plasticity of synapses the mechanism of long-term memory storage?, NPJ Science of Learning 4 (1) (2019) 1–10.

[9] I.S. Stein, K. Zito, Dendritic spine elimination: molecular mechanisms and implications, The Neuroscientist 25 (1) (2019) 27–47.

[10] J.M. Beaulieu, S. Espinoza, R.R. Gainetdinov, Dopamine receptors–IUPHAR review 13, British Journal of Pharmacology 172 (1) (2015) 1–23.

[11] N.M. Barnes, T. Sharp, A review of central 5-HT receptors and their function, Neuropharmacology 38 (8) (1999) 1083–1152.

[12] E. Bednarek, P. Caroni, β-Adducin is required for stable assembly of new synapses and improved memory upon environmental enrichment, Neuron 69 (6) (2011) 1132–1146.

[13] T. Biederer, P.S. Kaeser, T.A. Blanpied, Transcellular nanoalignment of synaptic function, Neuron 96 (3) (2017) 680–696.
[14] H.J. Chung, J. Xia, R.H. Scannevin, X. Zhang, R.L. Huganir, Phosphorylation of the AMPA receptor subunit GluR2 differentially regulates its interaction with PDZ domain-containing proteins, The Journal of Neuroscience 20 (19) (2000) 7258–7267.
[15] J.W. Fawcett, T. Oohashi, T. Pizzorusso, The roles of perineuronal nets and the perinodal extracellular matrix in neuronal function, Nature Reviews. Neuroscience 20 (8) (2019) 451–465.
[16] O. Muriel, M. Sánchez-Álvarez, R. Strippoli, M.A. Del Pozo, Role of the endocytosis of caveolae in intracellular signaling and metabolism, Endocytosis and Signaling (2018) 203–234.
[17] J. Leschik, R. Eckenstaler, T. Endres, T. Munsch, E. Edelmann, K. Richter, et al., Prominent postsynaptic and dendritic exocytosis of endogenous BDNF vesicles in BDNF-GFP knock-in mice, Molecular Neurobiology 56 (2019) 6833–6855.
[18] M. Hébert, F. Lesept, D. Vivien, R. Macrez, The story of an exceptional serine protease, tissue-type plasminogen activator (tPA), Revue Neurologique 172 (3) (2016) 186–197.
[19] E. Knapska, Kaczmarek L. Matrix, Metalloproteinase 9 (MMP-9) in learning and memory, in: Novel Mechanisms of Memory, Springer, 2016, pp. 161–181.
[20] C. Tapia-Rojas, F. Cabezas-Opazo, C.A. Deaton, E.H. Vergara, G.V. Johnson, R.A. Quintanilla, It's all about tau, Progress in Neurobiology 175 (2019) 54–76.
[21] I. Cervellini, J. Galino, N. Zhu, S. Allen, C. Birchmeier, D.L. Bennett, Sustained MAPK/ERK activation in adult Schwann cells impairs nerve repair, The Journal of Neuroscience 38 (3) (2018) 679–690.
[22] F.K. Ludka, M.P. Cunha, T. Dal-Cim, L.B. Binder, L.C. Constantino, C.M. Massari, et al., Atorvastatin protects from Aβ 1–40-induced cell damage and depressive-like behavior via ProBDNF cleavage, Molecular Neurobiology 54 (2017) 6163–6173.
[23] Q.W. Fan, W. Yu, T. Senda, K. Yanagisawa, M. Michikawa, Cholesterol-dependent modulation of tau phosphorylation in cultured neurons, Journal of Neurochemistry 76 (2) (2001) 391–400.
[24] F.Q. Zhou, J. Zhou, S. Dedhar, Y.H. Wu, W.D. Snider, NGF-induced axon growth is mediated by localized inactivation of GSK-3β and functions of the microtubule plus end binding protein APC, Neuron 42 (6) (2004) 897–912.
[25] C. Itami, F. Kimura, T. Kohno, M. Matsuoka, M. Ichikawa, T. Tsumoto, et al., Brain-derived neurotrophic factor-dependent unmasking of "silent" synapses in the developing mouse barrel cortex, Proceedings of the National Academy of Sciences 100 (22) (2003) 13069–13074.
[26] H. Park, Poo Mm, Neurotrophin regulation of neural circuit development and function, Nature Reviews. Neuroscience 14 (1) (2013) 7–23.
[27] R.A. Nicoll, H. Schulman, Synaptic memory and CaMKII: a review, Physiological Reviews 103 (4) (2023) 2877–2925.
[28] L. Armijo-Weingart, G. Gallo, It takes a village to raise a branch: cellular mechanisms of the initiation of axon collateral branches, Molecular and Cellular Neuroscience 84 (2017) 36–47.
[29] J.M. Henley, K.A. Wilkinson, AMPA receptor trafficking and the mechanisms underlying synaptic plasticity and cognitive aging, Dialogues in Clinical Neuroscience 15 (1) (2013) 11–27.
[30] J.J. Zhu, Y. Qin, M. Zhao, L. Van Aelst, R. Malinow, Ras and rap control AMPA receptor trafficking during synaptic plasticity, Cell 110 (4) (2002) 443–455.
[31] D. Bissen, F. Foss, A. Acker-Palmer, AMPA receptors and their minions: auxiliary proteins in AMPA receptor trafficking, Cellular and Molecular Life Sciences 76 (2019) 2133–2169.
[32] J. Boehm, M.G. Kang, R.C. Johnson, J. Esteban, R.L. Huganir, R. Malinow, Synaptic incorporation of AMPA receptors during LTP is controlled by a PKC phosphorylation site on GluR1, Neuron 51 (2) (2006) 213–225.
[33] Y. Pilpel, M. Segal, Activation of PKC induces rapid morphological plasticity in dendrites of hippocampal neurons via Rac and Rho-dependent mechanisms, European Journal of Neuroscience 19 (12) (2004) 3151–3164.

[34] N. Yamawaki, X. Li, L. Lambot, L.Y. Ren, J. Radulovic, G.M. Shepherd, Long-range inhibitory intersection of a retrosplenial thalamocortical circuit by apical tuft-targeting CA1 neurons, Nature Neuroscience 22 (4) (2019) 618–626.
[35] V. Balmaceda, I. Cuchillo-Ibáñez, L. Pujadas, M.S. García-Ayllón, C.A. Saura, J. Nimpf, et al., ApoER2 processing by presenilin-1 modulates reelin expression, The FASEB Journal 28 (4) (2014) 1543–1554.
[36] A.M. Stranahan, J.R. Erion, M. Wosiski-Kuhn, Reelin signaling in development, maintenance, and plasticity of neural networks, Ageing Research Reviews 12 (3) (2013) 815–822.
[37] R. Van Der Kant, L.S. Goldstein, Cellular functions of the amyloid precursor protein from development to dementia, Developmental Cell 32 (4) (2015) 502–515.
[38] Y.W. Ge, D. Lahiri, Regulation of promoter activity of the APP gene by cytokines and growth factors: implications in Alzheimer's disease, Annals of the New York Academy of Sciences 973 (1) (2002) 463–467.
[39] Y.W.A. Huang, B. Zhou, M. Wernig, T.C. Südhof, ApoE2, ApoE3, and ApoE4 differentially stimulate APP transcription and Aβ secretion, Cell 168 (3) (2017) 427–441.
[40] S.M. Nigam, S. Xu, J.S. Kritikou, K. Marosi, L. Brodin, M.P. Mattson, Exercise and BDNF reduce Aβ production by enhancing α-secretase processing of APP, Journal of Neurochemistry 142 (2) (2017) 286–296.
[41] C. Yang, Y. Liu, X. Ni, N. Li, B. Zhang, X. Fang, Enhancement of the nonamyloidogenic pathway by exogenous NGF in an Alzheimer transgenic mouse model, Neuropeptides 48 (4) (2014) 233–238.
[42] M.D. Ledesma, J.S. Da Silva, K. Crassaerts, A. Delacourte, B. De Strooper, C.G. Dotti, Brain plasmin enhances APP α-cleavage and Aβ degradation and is reduced in Alzheimer's disease brains, EMBO Reports 1 (6) (2000) 530–535.
[43] A. Fragkouli, A.K. Tzinia, I. Charalampopoulos, A. Gravanis, E.C. Tsilibary, Matrix metalloproteinase-9 participates in NGF-induced α-secretase cleavage of amyloid-β protein precursor in PC12 cells, Journal of Alzheimer's Disease 24 (4) (2011) 705–719.
[44] J.D. Buxbaum, S.E. Gandy, P. Cicchetti, M.E. Ehrlich, A.J. Czernik, R.P. Fracasso, et al., Processing of Alzheimer beta/A4 amyloid precursor protein: modulation by agents that regulate protein phosphorylation, Proceedings of the National Academy of Sciences of the United States of America 87 (15) (1990) 6003–6006.
[45] E. Kojro, G. Gimpl, S. Lammich, W. März, F. Fahrenholz, Low cholesterol stimulates the nonamyloidogenic pathway by its effect on the α-secretase ADAM 10, Proceedings of the National Academy of Sciences of the United States of America 98 (10) (2001) 5815–5820.
[46] R. Ehehalt, P. Keller, C. Haass, C. Thiele, K. Simons, Amyloidogenic processing of the Alzheimer β-amyloid precursor protein depends on lipid rafts, The Journal of Cell Biology 160 (1) (2003) 113–123.
[47] W. Wang, A.L. Mutka, U.P. Zmrzljak, D. Rozman, H. Tanila, H. Gylling, et al., Amyloid precursor protein α- and β-cleaved ectodomains exert opposing control of cholesterol homeostasis via SREBP2, The FASEB Journal 28 (2) (2014) 849–860.
[48] S. Jimenez, M. Torres, M. Vizuete, R. Sanchez-Varo, E. Sanchez-Mejias, L. Trujillo-Estrada, et al., Age-dependent accumulation of soluble amyloid β (Aβ) oligomers reverses the neuroprotective effect of soluble amyloid precursor protein-α (sAPPα) by modulating phosphatidylinositol 3-kinase (PI3K)/Akt-GSK-3β pathway in Alzheimer mouse model, Journal of Biological Chemistry 286 (21) (2011) 18414–18425.
[49] X. Wang, S. Yu, S.J. Gao, J.P. Hu, Y. Wang, H.X. Liu, Insulin inhibits Abeta production through modulation of APP processing in a cellular model of Alzheimer's disease, Neuroendocrinology Letters 35 (2014) 224–229.
[50] R.W. Livingstone, M.K. Elder, A. Singh, C.M. Westlake, W.P. Tate, W.C. Abraham, et al., Secreted amyloid precursor protein-alpha enhances LTP through the synthesis and trafficking of Ca2+-permeable AMPA receptors, Frontiers in Molecular Neuroscience 14 (2021) 660208.

[51] M. Hick, U. Herrmann, S.W. Weyer, J.P. Mallm, J.A. Tschäpe, M. Borgers, et al., Acute function of secreted amyloid precursor protein fragment APPsα in synaptic plasticity, Acta Neuropathologica 129 (1) (2015) 21–37.
[52] L.J. Sosa, A. Cáceres, S. Dupraz, M. Oksdath, S. Quiroga, A. Lorenzo, The physiological role of the amyloid precursor protein as an adhesion molecule in the developing nervous system, Journal of Neurochemistry 143 (1) (2017) 11–29.
[53] D. Obregon, H. Hou, J. Deng, B. Giunta, J. Tian, D. Darlington, et al., Soluble amyloid precursor protein-α modulates β-secretase activity and amyloid-β generation, Nature Communications 3 (1) (2012) 1–9.
[54] M. Rohe, M. Synowitz, R. Glass, S.M. Paul, A. Nykjaer, T.E. Willnow, Brain-derived neurotrophic factor reduces amyloidogenic processing through control of SORLA gene expression, Journal of Neuroscience 29 (49) (2009) 15472–15478.
[55] R. Gugustea, Z. Jia, Genetic manipulations of AMPA glutamate receptors in hippocampal synaptic plasticity, Neuropharmacology 194 (2021) 108630.
[56] M. Martin, C.G. Dotti, M.D. Ledesma, Brain cholesterol in normal and pathological aging, Biochimica et Biophysica Acta (BBA)-Molecular and Cell Biology of Lipids 1801 (8) (2010) 934–944.
[57] M.S. Spagnuolo, A. Donizetti, L. Iannotta, V. Aliperti, C. Cupidi, A.C. Bruni, et al., Brain-derived neurotrophic factor modulates cholesterol homeostasis and Apolipoprotein E synthesis in human cell models of astrocytes and neurons, Journal of Cellular Physiology 233 (9) (2018) 6925–6943.
[58] M.R. Strachan-Whaley, K. Reilly, J. Dobson, B.E. Kalisch, Map kinase and PKC signaling pathways modulate NGF-mediated apoE transcription, Neuroscience Letters 595 (2015) 54–59.
[59] J.M. Wang, R.W. Irwin, R.D. Brinton, Activation of estrogen receptor α increases and estrogen receptor β decreases apolipoprotein E expression in hippocampus in vitro and in vivo, Proceedings of the National Academy of Sciences of the United States of America 103 (45) (2006) 16983–16988.
[60] R.W. Mahley, Y. Huang, Apolipoprotein E sets the stage: response to injury triggers neuropathology, Neuron 76 (5) (2012) 871–885.
[61] H. Shimano, R. Sato, SREBP-regulated lipid metabolism: convergent physiology–divergent pathophysiology, Nature Reviews Endocrinology 13 (12) (2017) 710.
[62] Y. Yamazaki, N. Zhao, T.R. Caulfield, C.C. Liu, G. Bu, Apolipoprotein E and Alzheimer disease: pathobiology and targeting strategies, Nature Reviews Neurology 15 (9) (2019) 501–518.
[63] C.R. Mondadori, D.J.F. de Quervain, A. Buchmann, H. Mustovic, M.A. Wollmer, C.F. Schmidt, et al., Better memory and neural efficiency in young apolipoprotein E $\varepsilon 4$ carriers, Cerebral Cortex 17 (8) (2007) 1934–1947.
[64] E. Sezgin, I. Levental, S. Mayor, C. Eggeling, The mystery of membrane organization: composition regulation and roles of lipid rafts, Nature Reviews. Molecular Cell Biology 18 (6) (2017) 361–374.
[65] B.P. Head, H.H. Patel, P.A. Insel, Interaction of membrane/lipid rafts with the cytoskeleton: impact on signaling and function: membrane/lipid rafts, mediators of cytoskeletal arrangement and cell signaling, Biochimica Et Biophysica Acta. Biomembranes 1838 (2) (2014) 532–545.
[66] S.N. Whitehead, S. Gangaraju, A. Aylsworth, S.T. Hou, Membrane raft disruption results in neuritic retraction prior to neuronal death in cortical neurons, BioScience Trends 6 (4) (2012) 183–191.
[67] J.P. Albanesi, B. Barylko, G.N. DeMartino, D.M. Jameson, Palmitoylated proteins in dendritic spine remodeling, Frontiers in Synaptic Neuroscience (2020) 12.
[68] L.J. Pike, Growth factor receptors, lipid rafts and caveolae: an evolving story, Biochimica Et Biophysica Acta. Molecular Cell Research 1746 (3) (2005) 260–273.

[69] J.E. Baenziger, J.A. Domville, J.D. Therien, The Role of Cholesterol in the Activation of Nicotinic Acetylcholine Receptors, Current Topics in Membranes, vol. 80, Elsevier, 2017, pp. 95–137.
[70] D.H. Mauch, K. Nägler, S. Schumacher, C. Göritz, E.C. Müller, A. Otto, et al., CNS synaptogenesis promoted by glia-derived cholesterol, Science 294 (5545) (2001) 1354–1357.
[71] H. Hering, C.C. Lin, M. Sheng, Lipid rafts in the maintenance of synapses, dendritic spines, and surface AMPA receptor stability, Journal of Neuroscience 23 (8) (2003) 3262–3271.
[72] C. Frank, S. Rufini, V. Tancredi, R. Forcina, D. Grossi, G. D'arcangelo, Cholesterol depletion inhibits synaptic transmission and synaptic plasticity in rat hippocampus, Experimental Neurology 212 (2) (2008) 407–414.
[73] E. Area-Gomez, M. del Carmen Lara Castillo, M.D. Tambini, C. Guardia-Laguarta, A.J. De Groof, M. Madra, et al., Upregulated function of mitochondria-associated ER membranes in Alzheimer disease, EMBO Journal 31 (21) (2012) 4106–4123.
[74] M.G. Waugh, Raft-like membranes from the trans-Golgi network and endosomal compartments, Nature Protocols 8 (12) (2013) 2429–2439.
[75] D. Chowdhury, J.W. Hell, Ca2+/calmodulin binding to PSD-95 downregulates its palmitoylation and ampars in long-term depression, Frontiers in Synaptic Neuroscience 11 (2019) 6.
[76] A. Sanz-Clemente, R.A. Nicoll, K.W. Roche, Diversity in NMDA receptor composition: many regulators, many consequences, The Neuroscientist 19 (1) (2013) 62–75.
[77] K. Plant, K.A. Pelkey, Z.A. Bortolotto, D. Morita, A. Terashima, C.J. McBain, et al., Transient incorporation of native GluR2-lacking AMPA receptors during hippocampal long-term potentiation, Nature Neuroscience 9 (5) (2006) 602–604.
[78] E.C. Miller, P.J. Teravskis, B.W. Dummer, X. Zhao, R.L. Huganir, D. Liao, Tau phosphorylation and tau mislocalization mediate soluble Aβ oligomer-induced AMPA glutamate receptor signaling deficits, European Journal of Neuroscience 39 (7) (2014) 1214–1224.
[79] P.W. Liu, T. Hosokawa, Y. Hayashi, Regulation of synaptic nanodomain by liquid–liquid phase separation: a novel mechanism of synaptic plasticity, Current Opinion in Neurobiology 69 (2021) 84–92.
[80] H.Z. Shouval, S.S.H. Wang, G.M. Wittenberg, Spike timing dependent plasticity: a consequence of more fundamental learning rules, Frontiers in Computational Neuroscience 4 (2010) 19.
[81] T. Saneyoshi, H. Matsuno, A. Suzuki, H. Murakoshi, N.G. Hedrick, E. Agnello, et al., Reciprocal activation within a kinase-effector complex underlying persistence of structural LTP, Neuron 102 (6) (2019) 1199–1210.
[82] T.C. Sacktor, A.A. Fenton, What does LTP tell us about the roles of CaMKII and PKMζ in memory?, Molecular Brain 11 (2018) 1–9.
[83] J. Egawa, M.L. Pearn, B.P. Lemkuil, P.M. Patel, B.P. Head, Membrane lipid rafts and neurobiology: age-related changes in membrane lipids and loss of neuronal function, Journal of Physiology 594 (16) (2016) 4565–4579.
[84] L. Bakota, R. Brandt, Why kiss-and-hop explains that tau does not stabilize microtubules and does not interfere with axonal transport (at physiological conditions), Cytoskeleton 81 (1) (2024) 47–52.
[85] Y. Cabrales Fontela, H. Kadavath, J. Biernat, D. Riedel, E. Mandelkow, M. Zweckstetter, Multivalent cross-linking of actin filaments and microtubules through the microtubule-associated protein Tau, Nature Communications 8 (1) (2017) 1981.
[86] C.X. Gong, K. Iqbal, Hyperphosphorylation of microtubule-associated protein tau: a promising therapeutic target for Alzheimer disease, Current Medicinal Chemistry 15 (23) (2008) 2321–2328.
[87] J.M. Sontag, V. Nunbhakdi-Craig, E. Sontag, Leucine carboxyl methyltransferase 1 (LCMT1)-dependent methylation regulates the association of protein phosphatase 2A and Tau protein with plasma membrane microdomains in neuroblastoma cells, Journal of Biological Chemistry 288 (38) (2013) 27396–27405.

[88] L.L. Shen, W.W. Li, Y.L. Xu, S.H. Gao, M.Y. Xu, X.L. Bu, et al., Neurotrophin receptor p75 mediates amyloid β-induced tau pathology, Neurobiology of Disease 132 (2019) 104567.
[89] X. Bai, J. Wu, M. Zhang, Y. Xu, L. Duan, K. Yao, et al., DHCR24 knock-down induced tau hyperphosphorylation at Thr181, Ser199, Thr231, Ser262, Ser396 epitopes and inhibition of autophagy by overactivation of GSK3β/mTOR signaling, Frontiers in Aging Neuroscience 13 (2021) 513605.
[90] M. Merezhko, R.L. Uronen, H.J. Huttunen, The cell biology of tau secretion, Frontiers in Molecular Neuroscience 13 (2020) 569818.
[91] M. Simons, P. Keller, B. De Strooper, K. Beyreuther, C.G. Dotti, K. Simons, Cholesterol depletion inhibits the generation of β-amyloid in hippocampal neurons, Proceedings of the National Academy of Sciences of the United States of America 95 (11) (1998) 6460–6464.
[92] M.O. Grimm, H.S. Grimm, I. Tomic, K. Beyreuther, T. Hartmann, C. Bergmann, Independent inhibition of Alzheimer disease β- and γ-secretase cleavage by lowered cholesterol levels, Journal of Biological Chemistry 283 (17) (2008) 11302–11311.
[93] M.O. Grimm, H.S. Grimm, A.J. Pätzold, E.G. Zinser, R. Halonen, M. Duering, et al., Regulation of cholesterol and sphingomyelin metabolism by amyloid-β and presenilin, Nature Cell Biology 7 (11) (2005) 1118–1123.
[94] Y.Y. Cho, O.H. Kwon, S. Chung, Preferred endocytosis of amyloid precursor protein from cholesterol-enriched lipid raft microdomains, Molecules 25 (23) (2020) 5490.
[95] C. Costantini, R. Weindruch, G. Della Valle, L. Puglielli, A TrkA-to-p75NTR molecular switch activates amyloid β-peptide generation during aging, Biochemical Journal 391 (1) (2005) 59–67.
[96] M. Guglielmotto, D. Monteleone, L. Giliberto, M. Fornaro, R. Borghi, E. Tamagno, et al., Amyloid-β 42 activates the expression of BACE1 through the JNK pathway, Journal of Alzheimer's Disease 27 (4) (2011) 871–883.
[97] H. Hsieh, J. Boehm, C. Sato, T. Iwatsubo, T. Tomita, S. Sisodia, et al., AMPAR removal underlies Aβ-induced synaptic depression and dendritic spine loss, Neuron 52 (5) (2006) 831–843.
[98] M.A. Bruno, W.C. Leon, G. Fragoso, W.E. Mushynski, G. Almazan, A.C. Cuello, Amyloid β-induced nerve growth factor dysmetabolism in Alzheimer disease, Journal of Neuropathology and Experimental Neurology 68 (8) (2009) 857–869.
[99] S. Knafo, J.A. Esteban, PTEN: local and global modulation of neuronal function in health and disease, Trends in Neurosciences 40 (2) (2017) 83–91.
[100] S. Petratos, Q.X. Li, A.J. George, X. Hou, M.L. Kerr, S.E. Unabia, et al., The β-amyloid protein of Alzheimer's disease increases neuronal CRMP-2 phosphorylation by a Rho-GTP mechanism, Brain 131 (1) (2008) 90–108.
[101] J.J. Dougherty, J. Wu, R.A. Nichols, β-Amyloid regulation of presynaptic nicotinic receptors in rat hippocampus and neocortex, Journal of Neuroscience 23 (17) (2003) 6740–6747.
[102] G.L. Zhang, X. Zhang, X.M. Wang, J.P. Li, Towards understanding the roles of heparan sulfate proteoglycans in Alzheimer's disease, BioMed Research International (2014).
[103] C. Di Scala, H. Chahinian, N. Yahi, N. Garmy, J. Fantini, Interaction of Alzheimer's β-amyloid peptides with cholesterol: mechanistic insights into amyloid pore formation, Biochemistry 53 (28) (2014) 4489–4502.
[104] D. Puzzo, L. Privitera, E. Leznik, M. Fa, A. Staniszewski, A. Palmeri, et al., Picomolar amyloid-β positively modulates synaptic plasticity and memory in hippocampus, The Journal of Neuroscience 28 (53) (2008) 14537–14545.
[105] P.S. Finnie, K. Nader, Amyloid beta secreted during consolidation prevents memory malleability, Current Biology 30 (10) (2020) 1934–1940.
[106] B. Rasch, J. Born, About sleep's role in memory, Physiological Reviews 93 (2) (2013) 681–766.
[107] A.N. Lazar, L. Hanbouch, L. Boussicaut, B. Fourmaux, P. Daira, M.J. Millan, et al., Lipid dys-homeostasis contributes to APOE4-associated AD pathology, Cells 11 (22) (2022) 3616.

[108] H.A. Ferris, R.J. Perry, G.V. Moreira, G.I. Shulman, J.D. Horton, C.R. Kahn, Loss of astrocyte cholesterol synthesis disrupts neuronal function and alters whole-body metabolism, Proceedings of the National Academy of Sciences of the United States of America 114 (5) (2017) 1189–1194.
[109] K.L. Stewart, S.E. Radford, Amyloid plaques beyond Aβ: a survey of the diverse modulators of amyloid aggregation, Biophysical Review 9 (4) (2017) 405–419.
[110] E.R. Georgieva, S. Xiao, P.P. Borbat, J.H. Freed, D. Eliezer, Tau binds to lipid membrane surfaces via short amphipathic helices located in its microtubule-binding repeats, Biophysical Journal 107 (6) (2014) 1441–1452.
[111] C.R. Jack Jr, H.J. Wiste, C.G. Schwarz, V.J. Lowe, M.L. Senjem, P. Vemuri, et al., Longitudinal tau PET in ageing and Alzheimer's disease, Brain 141 (5) (2018) 1517–1528.
[112] M.T. Ferretti, M.F. Iulita, E. Cavedo, P.A. Chiesa, A.S. Dimech, A.S. Chadha, et al., Sex differences in Alzheimer disease – the gateway to precision medicine, Nature Reviews Neurology 14 (8) (2018) 457–469.
[113] R.J. Bateman, P.S. Aisen, B. De Strooper, N.C. Fox, C.A. Lemere, J.M. Ringman, et al., Autosomal-dominant Alzheimer's disease: a review and proposal for the prevention of Alzheimer's disease, Alzheimer's Research & Therapy 3 (1) (2011) 1–13.
[114] M.D. Ledesma, J. Abad-Rodriguez, C. Galvan, E. Biondi, P. Navarro, A. Delacourte, et al., Raft disorganization leads to reduced plasmin activity in Alzheimer's disease brains, EMBO Reports 4 (12) (2003) 1190–1196.
[115] N. Fabelo, V. Martín, R. Marín, D. Moreno, I. Ferrer, M. Díaz, Altered lipid composition in cortical lipid rafts occurs at early stages of sporadic Alzheimer's disease and facilitates APP/BACE1 interactions, Neurobiology of Aging 35 (8) (2014) 1801–1812.
[116] M. Molander-Melin, K. Blennow, N. Bogdanovic, B. Dellheden, J.E. Månsson, P. Fredman, Structural membrane alterations in Alzheimer brains found to be associated with regional disease development, increased density of gangliosides GM1 and GM2 and loss of cholesterol in detergent-resistant membrane domains, Journal of Neurochemistry 92 (1) (2005) 171–182.
[117] M. Abdullah, N. Kimura, H. Akatsu, Y. Hashizume, T. Ferdous, T. Tachita, et al., Flotillin is a novel diagnostic blood marker of Alzheimer's disease, Journal of Alzheimer's Disease 72 (4) (2019) 1165–1176.
[118] F. Mesa-Herrera, R. Marín, E. Torrealba, G. Santos, M. Díaz, Neuronal ER-signalosome proteins as early biomarkers in prodromal Alzheimer's disease independent of amyloid-β production and tau phosphorylation, Frontiers in Molecular Neuroscience 15 (2022) 879146.
[119] W.H. Chan, L.F. Yau, X.Y. Meng, K.M. Chan, Z.H. Jiang, J.R. Wang, Robust quantitation of gangliosides and sulfatides in human brain using UHPLC-MRM-MS: method development and application in Alzheimer's disease, Talanta 256 (2023) 124264.
[120] N. Girardot, B. Allinquant, D. Langui, A. Laquerriere, B. Dubois, J.J. Hauw, et al., Accumulation of flotillin-1 in tangle-bearing neurones of Alzheimer's disease, Neuropathology and Applied Neurobiology 29 (5) (2003) 451–461.
[121] P. Foley, Lipids in Alzheimer's disease: a century-old story, Biochimica et Biophysica Acta (BBA)-Molecular and Cell Biology of Lipids 1801 (8) (2010) 750–753.
[122] R.P. Mason, W.J. Shoemaker, L. Shajenko, T.E. Chambers, L.G. Herbette, Evidence for changes in the Alzheimer's disease brain cortical membrane structure mediated by cholesterol, Neurobiology of Aging 13 (3) (1992) 413–419.
[123] H.N. Yassine, Q. Feng, J. Chiang, L.M. Petrosspour, A.N. Fonteh, H.C. Chui, et al., ABCA1-mediated cholesterol efflux capacity to cerebrospinal fluid is reduced in patients with mild cognitive impairment and Alzheimer's disease, Journal of the American Heart Association 5 (2) (2016) e002886.
[124] H. Kölsch, R. Heun, F. Jessen, J. Popp, F. Hentschel, W. Maier, et al., Alterations of cholesterol precursor levels in Alzheimer's disease, Biochimica et Biophysica Acta (BBA)-Molecular and Cell Biology of Lipids 1801 (8) (2010) 945–950.
[125] C.F. Phelix, R.G. LeBaron, D.J. Roberson, R.E. Villanueva, G. Villareal, O.B. Rahimi, et al., In vivo and in silico evidence: hippocampal cholesterol metabolism decreases with aging and

increases with Alzheimer's disease–modeling brain aging and disease, in: 2011 IEEE 11th International Conference on Data Mining Workshops, IEEE, 2011, pp. 1064–1070.
[126] X. Bai, M. Mai, K. Yao, M. Zhang, Y. Huang, W. Zhang, et al., The role of DHCR24 in the pathogenesis of AD: re-cognition of the relationship between cholesterol and AD pathogenesis, Acta Neuropathologica Communications 10 (1) (2022) 35.
[127] V.R. Varma, H. Büşra Lüleci, A.M. Oommen, S. Varma, C.T. Blackshear, M.E. Griswold, et al., Abnormal brain cholesterol homeostasis in Alzheimer's disease–a targeted metabolomic and transcriptomic study, npj Aging and Mechanisms of Disease 7 (1) (2021) 11.
[128] R. Distl, V. Meske, T.G. Ohm, Tangle-bearing neurons contain more free cholesterol than adjacent tangle-free neurons, Acta Neuropathologica 101 (2001) 547–554.
[129] R.G. Cutler, J. Kelly, K. Storie, W.A. Pedersen, A. Tammara, K. Hatanpaa, et al., Involvement of oxidative stress-induced abnormalities in ceramide and cholesterol metabolism in brain aging and Alzheimer's disease, Proceedings of the National Academy of Sciences of the United States of America 101 (7) (2004) 2070–2075.
[130] R.B. Chan, T.G. Oliveira, E.P. Cortes, L.S. Honig, K.E. Duff, S.A. Small, et al., Comparative lipidomic analysis of mouse and human brain with Alzheimer disease, Journal of Biological Chemistry 287 (4) (2012) 2678–2688.
[131] H. Xiong, D. Callaghan, A. Jones, D.G. Walker, L.F. Lue, T.G. Beach, et al., Cholesterol retention in Alzheimer's brain is responsible for high β- and γ-secretase activities and Aβ production, Neurobiology of Disease 29 (3) (2008) 422–437.
[132] A. Akram, J. Schmeidler, P. Katsel, P.R. Hof, V. Haroutunian, Increased expression of cholesterol transporter ABCA1 is highly correlated with severity of dementia in AD hippocampus, Brain Research 1318 (2010) 167–177.
[133] F. Arenas, F. Castro, S. Nuñez, G. Gay, C. Garcia-Ruiz, J.C. Fernandez-Checa, STARD1 and NPC1 expression as pathological markers associated with astrogliosis in post-mortem brains from patients with Alzheimer's disease and Down syndrome, Aging (Albany NY) 12 (1) (2020) 571.
[134] A.N. Lazar, C. Bich, M. Panchal, N. Desbenoit, V.W. Petit, D. Touboul, et al., Time-of-flight secondary ion mass spectrometry (TOF-SIMS) imaging reveals cholesterol overload in the cerebral cortex of Alzheimer disease patients, Acta Neuropathologica 125 (1) (2013) 133–144.
[135] C. Wang, F. Zhao, K. Shen, W. Wang, S.L. Siedlak, H.g. Lee, et al., The sterol regulatory element-binding protein 2 is dysregulated by tau alterations in Alzheimer disease, Brain Pathology 29 (4) (2019) 530–543.
[136] Y.Y. Cho, O.H. Kwon, M.K. Park, T.W. Kim, S. Chung, Elevated cellular cholesterol in Familial Alzheimer's presenilin 1 mutation is associated with lipid raft localization of β-amyloid precursor protein, PLoS ONE 14 (1) (2019) e0210535.
[137] J. Popp, S. Meichsner, H. Kölsch, P. Lewczuk, W. Maier, J. Kornhuber, et al., Cerebral and extracerebral cholesterol metabolism and CSF markers of Alzheimer's disease, Biochemical Pharmacology 86 (1) (2013) 37–42.
[138] J. Popp, P. Lewczuk, H. Kölsch, S. Meichsner, W. Maier, J. Kornhuber, et al., Cholesterol metabolism is associated with soluble amyloid precursor protein production in Alzheimer's disease, Journal of Neurochemistry 123 (2) (2012) 310–316.
[139] M.P. Adorni, M. Ruscica, N. Ferri, F. Bernini, F. Zimetti, Proprotein convertase subtilisin/kexin type 9, brain cholesterol homeostasis and potential implication for Alzheimer's disease, Frontiers in Aging Neuroscience 11 (2019) 120.
[140] J. Montesinos, M. Pera, D. Larrea, C. Guardia-Laguarta, R.R. Agrawal, K.R. Velasco, et al., The Alzheimer's disease-associated C99 fragment of APP regulates cellular cholesterol trafficking, EMBO Journal 39 (20) (2020) e103791.
[141] A. Pani, S. Dessì, G. Diaz, P. La Colla, C. Abete, C. Mulas, et al., Altered cholesterol ester cycle in skin fibroblasts from patients with Alzheimer's disease, Journal of Alzheimer's disease. 18 (4) (2009) 829–841.

[142] Z.P. Van Acker, M. Bretou, W. Annaert, Endo-lysosomal dysregulations and late-onset Alzheimer's disease: impact of genetic risk factors, Molecular Neurodegeneration 14 (1) (2019) 20.
[143] M.O. Grimm, J. Mett, H.S. Grimm, T. Hartmann, APP function and lipids: a bidirectional link, Frontiers in Molecular Neuroscience 10 (2017) 63.
[144] S.H. Chung, Aberrant phosphorylation in the pathogenesis of Alzheimer's disease, BMB Reports 42 (8) (2009) 467–474.
[145] M. Florencia Iulita, A. Claudio Cuello, The NGF metabolic pathway in the CNS and its dysregulation in Down syndrome and Alzheimer's disease, Current Alzheimer Research 13 (1) (2016) 53–67.
[146] T.L. Carter, R.A. Rissman, A.J. Mishizen-Eberz, B.B. Wolfe, R.L. Hamilton, S. Gandy, et al., Differential preservation of AMPA receptor subunits in the hippocampi of Alzheimer's disease patients according to Braak stage, Experimental Neurology 187 (2) (2004) 299–309.
[147] S.A. Small, S.A. Schobel, R.B. Buxton, M.P. Witter, C.A. Barnes, A pathophysiological framework of hippocampal dysfunction in ageing and disease, Nature Reviews. Neuroscience 12 (10) (2011) 585–601.
[148] H. Braak, E. Braak, Alzheimer's disease affects limbic nuclei of the thalamus, Acta Neuropathologica 81 (3) (1991) 261–268.
[149] A. Maass, H. Schütze, O. Speck, A. Yonelinas, C. Tempelmann, H.J. Heinze, et al., Laminar activity in the hippocampus and entorhinal cortex related to novelty and episodic encoding, Nature Communications 5 (1) (2014) 5547.
[150] P.V. Thomas, A.L. Cheng, C.C. Colby, L. Liu, C.K. Patel, L. Josephs, et al., Localization and proteomic characterization of cholesterol-rich membrane microdomains in the inner ear, Journal of Proteomics 103 (2014) 178–193.
[151] J.D. Brady, T.C. Rich, X. Le, K. Stafford, C.J. Fowler, L. Lynch, et al., Functional role of lipid raft microdomains in cyclic nucleotide-gated channel activation, Molecular Pharmacology 65 (3) (2004) 503–511.
[152] C. Munderloh, G.P. Solis, V. Bodrikov, F.A. Jaeger, M. Wiechers, E. Málaga-Trillo, et al., Reggies/flotillins regulate retinal axon regeneration in the zebrafish optic nerve and differentiation of hippocampal and N2a neurons, The Journal of Neuroscience 29 (20) (2009) 6607–6615.
[153] S.D. Chung, C.H. Chen, S.H. Hung, H.C. Lin, L.H. Wang, A population-based study on the association between statin use and sudden sensorineural hearing loss, JAMA Otolaryngology – Head & Neck Surgery 152 (2) (2015) 319–325.
[154] J. Lötsch, C. Knothe, C. Lippmann, A. Ultsch, T. Hummel, C. Walter, Olfactory drug effects approached from human-derived data, Drug Discovery Today 20 (11) (2015) 1398–1406.
[155] M.A. Crumling, L. Liu, P.V. Thomas, J. Benson, A. Kanicki, L. Kabara, et al., Hearing loss and hair cell death in mice given the cholesterol-chelating agent hydroxypropyl-β-cyclodextrin, PLoS ONE 7 (12) (2012) e53280.
[156] H.K. Dong, J.A. Gim, S.H. Yeo, H.S. Kim, Integrated late onset Alzheimer's disease (LOAD) susceptibility genes: cholesterol metabolism and trafficking perspectives, Gene 597 (2017) 10–16.
[157] S. Love, L.R. Bridges, C.P. Case, Neurofibrillary tangles in Niemann-Pick disease type C, Brain 118 (1) (1995) 119–129.
[158] M.A. Castello, S. Soriano, Rational heterodoxy: cholesterol reformation of the amyloid doctrine, Ageing Research Reviews 12 (1) (2013) 282–288.
[159] B. Readhead, J.V. Haure-Mirande, C.C. Funk, M.A. Richards, P. Shannon, V. Haroutunian, et al., Multiscale analysis of independent Alzheimer's cohorts finds disruption of molecular, genetic, and clinical networks by human herpesvirus, Neuron 99 (1) (2018) 64–82.
[160] N.S. Tzeng, C.H. Chung, F.H. Lin, C.P. Chiang, C.B. Yeh, S.Y. Huang, et al., Anti-herpetic medications and reduced risk of dementia in patients with herpes simplex virus infections–a nationwide, population-based cohort study in Taiwan, Neurotherapeutics 15 (2) (2018) 417–429.

[161] M. Eyting, M. Xie, S. Hess, P. Geldsetzer, Causal evidence that herpes zoster vaccination prevents a proportion of dementia cases, medRxiv (2023) 2023-05.
[162] R.F. Itzhaki, M.A. Wozniak, Herpes simplex virus type 1, apolipoprotein E, and cholesterol: a dangerous liaison in Alzheimer's disease and other disorders, Progress in Lipid Research 45 (1) (2006) 73–90.
[163] L. Li, J. Liang, H. Fu, An update on the association between traumatic brain injury and Alzheimer's disease: focus on tau pathology and synaptic dysfunction, Neuroscience and Biobehavioral Reviews (2020).
[164] M. de la Monte SM Tong, J.R. Wands, The 20-year voyage aboard the journal of Alzheimer's disease: docking at 'Type 3 Diabetes', environmental/exposure factors, pathogenic mechanisms, and potential treatments, Journal of Alzheimer's Disease 62 (3) (2018) 1381–1390.
[165] N. Qizilbash, J. Gregson, M.E. Johnson, N. Pearce, I. Douglas, K. Wing, et al., BMI and risk of dementia in two million people over two decades: a retrospective cohort study, The Lancet Diabetes & Endocrinology 3 (6) (2015) 431–436.
[166] J.D. Ulrich, T.K. Ulland, M. Colonna, D.M. Holtzman, Elucidating the role of TREM2 in Alzheimer's disease, Neuron 94 (2) (2017) 237–248.
[167] L. Hoeijmakers, S.L. Lesuis, H. Krugers, P.J. Lucassen, A. Korosi, A preclinical perspective on the enhanced vulnerability to Alzheimer's disease after early-life stress, Neurobiol Stress 8 (2018) 172–185.
[168] E. Hellström-Lindahl, H. Moore, A. Nordberg, Increased levels of tau protein in SH-SY5Y cells after treatment with cholinesterase inhibitors and nicotinic agonists, Journal of Neurochemistry 74 (2) (2000) 777–784.
[169] A.M. Paulavicius, C.C. Mizzaci, D.R. Tavares, A.P. Rocha, V.T. Civile, R.R. Schultz, et al., Bilingualism for delaying the onset of Alzheimer's disease: a systematic review and meta-analysis, European Geriatric Medicine (2020) 1–8.
[170] S. Heim, J. Stumme, N. Bittner, C. Jockwitz, K. Amunts, S. Caspers, Bilingualism and "brain reserve": a matter of age, Neurobiology of Aging 81 (2019) 157–165.
[171] D. Perani, M. Farsad, T. Ballarini, F. Lubian, M. Malpetti, A. Fracchetti, et al., The impact of bilingualism on brain reserve and metabolic connectivity in Alzheimer's dementia, Proceedings of the National Academy of Sciences of the United States of America 114 (7) (2017) 1690–1695.
[172] Q. Meng, M.S. Lin, I. Tzeng, et al., Relationship between exercise and Alzheimer's disease: a narrative literature review, Frontiers in Neuroscience 14 (2020) 131.
[173] L. Puglielli, R.E. Tanzi, D.M. Kovacs, Alzheimer's disease: the cholesterol connection, Nature Neuroscience 6 (4) (2003) 345–351.
[174] M.P. Mattson, Hormesis defined, Ageing Research Reviews 7 (1) (2008) 1–7.
[175] J.T. Gonçalves, S.T. Schafer, F.H. Gage, Adult neurogenesis in the hippocampus: from stem cells to behavior, Cell 167 (4) (2016) 897–914.
[176] E.P. Moreno-Jiménez, M. Flor-García, J. Terreros-Roncal, A. Rábano, F. Cafini, N. Pallas-Bazarra, et al., Adult hippocampal neurogenesis is abundant in neurologically healthy subjects and drops sharply in patients with Alzheimer's disease, Naturalna Medycyna 25 (4) (2019) 554–560.

Chapter 12

The brain's adaptive response process: function and anatomy

12.1 Explaining the brain

How the brain works is one of the most important open problems in science. The role of the brain is to manage the organism's interaction with the external environment, producing external responses to sensory inputs conveying survival threats and opportunities. It also controls internal organs to provide resources for external responses (e.g., increasing heart rate to increase available energy). Hence, the main task in explaining brain function is to explain how it selects and releases responses. The second task is to explain the roles of the various brain anatomical components (cortex, subcortical nuclei, etc.) and how they assist in the main task. Finally, a theory of brain function should show how the brain achieves its main adaptive temporal characteristic, the capacity of learning from experience.

Here I present a simple biological theory that fully addresses these tasks. The brain utilizes a single process for selecting and releasing responses, a process that I call the **adaptive response process (ARP)**. The ARP has two major subprocesses, one for selecting responses and one for releasing them. Each stage in the selection process utilizes different cortical layers and neural types, and is supported by different agents released by specialized nuclei. The release process relies on an architecture that I call "Allow, Restrain, Amplify, Respond (ARAR)" that includes the important subcortical nuclei such as the basal ganglia, habenula, and amygdala. Consequently, the ARP not only explains the brain's main task in abstract terms, but also ties each subfunction to specific anatomical structures, allowing a connection with empirical data and providing strong support for the theory. The anatomical components of each subprocess directly support learning from experience. Another attractive feature of the selection process is that it provides a unified view of the major notions of goals, predictions, and hierarchical sequences, showing how the latter emerge without explicit planning and representations.

12.2 The adaptive response process (ARP)

12.2.1 Response selection

In the present paper, my discussion of response selection will focus on cortex. The same principles apply to responses generated in the spinal cord and other areas.

The Science of the Brain. https://doi.org/10.1016/B978-0-44-345008-2.00018-7

Selection stages. The selection part of the ARP has 4 stages: **sensory inputs**, generation of **competing response candidates (Cgen), competition resolution (Cres)**, and **execution of winning responses**, which are released via a set of Allow-Restrain-Amplify-Respond (ARAR) circuits.

The various ARP stages map into different neuronal networks distinguished by cortical layer, neuron type, and subcortical nucleus. Cortex is arranged in horizontal layers, L1 to L6. ARP selection stages map into these layers and define their functions. **L4 supports sensory inputs** (L2/3 supports inputs in areas with a negligible L4). **L2/3 supports Cgen (candidates)**, while **L5 supports responses**. These layers are referred to as the input network, the Cgen network, and the response network, respectively. L1 and L6 provide auxiliary functions.

Excitatory neurons (ENs) support inputs, Cgen, and response execution. **Inhibitory interneurons (IINs) support Cres and post-Cres execution**. Moreover, IIN subnetworks support different aspects of Cres and execution (i.e., different subnetworks for enhancing winners, suppressing losers, and supporting sustained responses). Projection (non-local) inhibitory neurons (INs) are mainly present in ARAR architecture nuceli and have a different role, see below.

The local minicolumn circuit. Most cortex is arranged in **minicolumns (MCLs)** [1] (for simplicity, I will not distinguish between MCLs, macrocolumns, and columns). These are tight neural sets spanning all cortical layers that are separated from each other by some distance. Each MCL represents a single focused entity (external and internal sensory objects, movements, etc). The role of the ARP is to select the MCLs that represent the desired response to the current input, and execute that response.

Within a single MCL, there is a general well-defined connectivity pattern ("the canonical microcircuit") [2,3]. Sensory inputs (mainly from the thalamus) arrive at L4 (or L2/3 when L4 is thin, and/or L5 when responses are largely automated/learned, see below). L5 is divided into two sublayers, L5a and L5b, the latter being the one driving midbrain and spinal responses. (L5a and L5b support novel/learned responses, see below.) L4 neurons excite L2/3 neurons (and L5b neurons in automaticity). L2/3 excites L5a, which excites L5b. Naturally, things are not that clean, and there are many other connections. Nonetheless, this is the main pattern. MCLs are strongly connected to each other across cortex, via L2/3/5 neurons.

There are other content representation areas besides cortex. For example, the basolateral nucleus of the amygdala (BLA) represents input and action valence, and the hippocampus represents events in space and time (see Table 12.1). As mentioned above, this paper focuses on cortex for clarity.

Bottom-up vs. top-down flow. The basic selection process goes as follows. Sensory inputs yield **bottom-up (feedforward)** flow across cortex. Since the input network excites the candidates network, this activates candidates (apart from state of complete automaticity). The current motivational state (needs, goals) of the organism is generally encoded in frontal areas, which generate **top-down (feedback)** flow to sculpt Cres and execution. The circuits participating in the response are modified by **plasticity** mechanisms, see automaticity/learning below.

12.2.2 Response release: ARAR circuits

Subcortex is arranged in a set of circuits whose goal is to provide specific input types and to release the response selected by the previous ARP stages. These circuits have a uniform architecture comprised of 4 components: **Allow, Restrain, Amplify, and Respond (ARAR), at this order**. The ARAR architecture is detailed in Chapter 13. Each component is implemented by a neural nucleus (usually not by layers as in cortex). The first nucleus ('Allow') is the one receiving most inputs from the responses selected by the first ARP stage. It is comprised of projection INs that, when activated by the selected response, suppress the Restrain nucleus. The 'Restrain' nucleus contains INs that tonically suppress an 'Amplify' nucleus. The Amplify nucleus (mainly containing ENs) targets circuits that actually execute the response by driving muscles and conveying inputs to other circuits, and is capable of strong sustained firing to make sure that the selected and released 'Response' is continuously executed. Thus, activation of the Allow nucleus eventually disinhibits the Amplify nucleus to drive the response.

There are several ARAR circuits, all operating under the same principle. Virtually all of the important nuclei of the brain (besides nuclei whose role is to release specific agents such as dopamine and serotonin) participate in ARAR circuits (Table 12.1). ARAR circuits interact with the selection circuits. They receive response selection inputs, provide inputs to selection circuits, and interact with each other, e.g., by inhibiting other ARAR circuits to promote their own type of response.

As an example, probably the most familiar ARAR circuit is the D1 ('direct') path of the basal ganglia (BG) [4]. It receives cortical, thalamic, amygdalar, hippocampal, and other inputs representing the selected response. Its Allow function is mediated by D1-expressing striatal medium spiny neurons (MSNs), which are projection INs. When activated, these suppress the Restrain nuclei, the internal globus pallidus (GPi) and substantia nigra (SNi). These tonically inhibit the thalamus, which is disinhibited when the selected response is released. The thalamus is a powerful Amplifier that sustains responses via repeated firing and widespread connections [5]. It targets both subcortical (via its CM/Pf nuclei [6]) and cortical circuits to drive the response.

12.2.3 Novel vs. Automated (learned) responses

Learning from past experience is important for the organism's survival. Following response selection and release, the circuits participating in response execution undergo plasticity processes, mainly generation of new synapses and modification of existing ones to make them more stable and make their usage more efficient in terms of time and energy [13].

Technically, the difference between novel and familiar inputs is that learned states involve preceding partial excitation of neurons predicted to participate in the response. Such predictions are a natural consequence of the enhancement of

TABLE 12.1 Summary of the main ARAR circuits. Note that many of the circuits are standalone in the sense that they have dedicated content representations in addition to the ARAR circuits. Many details (e.g., the role of the zona incerta in vigorous movements) are not shown, and some of the listing (e.g., the assigned functions of the Supm and nucleus incertus in the space circuit) should be refined. Other less central circuits having the same structure (e.g., the auditory dorsal cochlear nucleus) are not shown. BG: basal ganglia. STR: striatum. D1s, D2s: D1, D2 dopamine receptor-expressing medium spiny neurons. GPi/GPe: internal/external glubus pallidus. STN: subthalamic nucleus. BLA/CeM: basolateral/centromedial nuclei of the amygdala. BNST: bed nucleus of the stria terminalis. LHthalA: lateral hypothalamic area. PAG: periaqueductal gray. crb: cerebellar. DG: dentate gyrus. CA1: cornu ammonis 1. Lsep/Msep: lateral/medial septum. Supm: supramammillary nucleus. LHb/MHb: lateral/medial habenula. IPN: interpeduncular nucleus. VTA: ventral tegmental area (via the rostromedial tegmental nucleus, RMTg). SCi: intermediate layers of the superior colliculus.

Name	Function	Content	Allow	Restrain	Amplify	Respond
D1 BG path [4]	novel responses	all	STR D1s	GPi, SNr	thalamus	all
D2 BG path [4]	learned responses	all	STR D2s	GPe	STN	all
Extended amygdala [7]	valence, survival responses	BLA, thalamus	CeM	BNST	LHthalA	PAG, other
Cerebellum (CRB) [8]	quick or precise movements	granules	golgis	Purkinjes	deep crb nuclei	crb targets
Hippocampus [9,10]	space time events	CA1-CA3 DG, subiculum	Lsep	Msep	Supm	nucleus incertus
Habenula [11]	switch to defend	many	STR	(some) ventral pallidum	MHb LHb	IPN, VTA
Superior colliculus [12]	saccades	all	STR	SNr	SCi	eye motor nuclei

synapses that have already been used under similar conditions. When neurons that are not partially excited receive novel firing-inducing inputs, they fire strong action potential bursts [14], such that the effect of a surprise is much larger than the effect of a predicted response.

In the ARP, novel inputs induce a stronger bottom-up flow and a larger number of candidates. Conversely, fully automated responses yield a direct activation of the response network by the input network. L2/3 excites L5a but not L5b, L5a is the one sustaining novel responses. The excitation pattern L2/3 →L5a →L5b may be needed because the alternative pattern, L2/3 →L5b, would have caused immediate L5b firing for novel responses. The presence of L5a provides more time for top-down flow to guide inter-candidate competition (Cres).

Acute inputs generate flow in many MCLs (because no MCL is predicted, and they are strongly interconnected), exciting their L2/3 neurons. These MCLs are the response candidates. This stage is called candidate generation (Cgen).

The candidate set includes all MCLs that might be somehow relevant to the selected response, by being the ones that receive the current sensory input or being connected to them.

This means that the next time that similar inputs arrive, there would be fewer candidates activated (because IINs would suppress them faster, see the next section), ENs would be more synchronized, new synapses going directly from the thalamus to L5b might be generated, etc. Automated responses are more energy-efficient than acute ones, are quicker (due to skipping most Cres), and are more stable due to higher synchronization.

12.2.4 Agents

The brain utilizes a large number of agents to calibrate its processes. In the present context, it is imperative to mention 3 of them, which directly support the different ARP stages. **Norepinephrine** is released during sensory inputs to recruit energy and cognitive resources needed to deal with the new input [15]. **Dopamine** is released during novel responses, including 'charge' (sex, predation, 'reward') actions but also strong defensive fight (aversive situations) [16]. **Acetylcholine** [17] works with IINs to support both Cres and post-Cres execution.

Thus, the tight correspondence between the brain's function and anatomy also extends to agent-releasing nuclei, in addition to content and ARAR circuits. We do not have the space to deal with other important agents (e.g., orexin and oxytocin) here. I have detailed general theories of opioids, endocannabinoids and CRH in my papers presenting theories of depression (and bipolar disorder), schizophrenia, and autism, respectively [18–20]. I have also detailed a large number of plasticity-related agents in the context of Alzheimer's Disease [13]. Readers are welcome to consult these papers.

A fourth agent, **serotonin (5-HT)** is usually mentioned along with the other 3 agents. In the theory presented here, the basic role of serotonin is to deal with situations of excess (food, warmth, hyperoxia), e.g., by promoting gut food absorption (about 90% of body serotonin is located in the gut) and glucose uptake by adipose and other tissue [21]. Since dealing with excess is in many ways opposite to the roles of the other 3 agents, which deal with deficiency-induced stress, serotonin can oppose them [22], a capacity that the brain has adapted for additional purposes. For example, in the habenular ARAR circuit, serotonin, via opposition to dopamine, can put a strong brake on vigorous charging actions, effectively switching from charge to strong passive defence.

12.3 IINs: competition resolution (cres) & execution

If the situation is not that urgent to handle, MCLs **compete** until a response emerges [23,24]. Competition is implemented by IINs [24–26]. It is crucial to understand that although IINs are technically "inhibitory" (even this is not always the case, since they are initially excitatory in many areas), their overall role is NOT to inhibit responses. Their role is to synchronize the firing of their EN targets, which includes suppression of losing candidates but also enhancement of winning ones. When an IIN fires onto two ENs that have just fired, it does not inhibit their firing but ensures that they would start charging at the same time, and if they receive comparable inputs, this increases their synchronized firing. IINs inhibit ENs when they fire onto them when they are partially excited, preparing to fire. Thus, **IINs suppress most ENs, but enhance the coordinated firing of the ENs that are most temporally synchronized with the input**. Assuming that IINs are always inhibitory is a big mistake. A good theory-independent term for their role is **coordination**.

To allow their Cres function, IINs receive sensory inputs from the thalamus, from local MCL ENs, and from other IINs. Since IINs are small neurons, they are quick to fire, allowing quick Cres in automated situations. IINs keep their activity to support post-Cres execution, because they need to maintain the winning circuits.

In the MCLs that have won the competition, sustained input, sustained top-down flow from long-range connections, and/or sustained L4 firing (which may be the role of L4), sustain the firing of L2/3 neurons, which in turn excite L5a neurons, which excite L5b neurons to generate the response.

IINs can be classified into many subsets, based on location, connectivity, and agent expression [27]. For our purposes here, it is beneficial to highlight 3 such subsets. First, so-called Martinotti IINs are located in superficial layers and target apical dendrites. They are thus natural candidates to mediate the suppressing aspect of Cres. Second, VIP-expressing IINs located in L1 and L2/3 locally target the Martinotti IINs, thus supporting the winner-promotion aspect of Cres. Finally, parvalbumin-expressing IINs, located in most layers but mostly in the response layers, support post-Cres execution.

12.4 Goals and predictions

Suppose that an MCL has won the competition, and its L5b neurons drive the current response. As a general rule, responses involve external movement. How does the brain know that the movement has attained its purpose so that the muscle contraction that drives it should be stopped? This is a crucial question for understanding motor control, and yet it is surprisingly not asked that often.

Our answer to this question is as follows. When L5b drive responses, L5a or L5b neurons in the same MCL also excite L5a or L5b neurons in other MCLs (L5a and L5b are used in novel and learned responses, respectively). **When a response is executed by an MCL, its L5 neurons excite the L5 neurons of the MCLs that represent the desired sensory consequences of the executed response (the goals)**. For example, if the executed response is to extend your arm in order to reach an apple, then the goal MCLs represent the state in which your fingers touch the apple (or get close to it). These kinds of physical configurations (a limb getting in contact with an external object) are generally represented in the parietal cortex [28].

Why is this technique useful? When the response goal has been met (reaching the apple), sensory inputs encoding this state excite the MCLs that represent it. They also excite other MCLs. However, the L2/3/5 neurons of the "correct" MCLs are already partially excited (by the response MCLs), which gives them a head advantage in winning the competition.

When the sensory inputs denoting the event arrive, the L5b neurons of the goal MCL are activated. This is a type of response. Unlike motor responses, which generate movement, this response indicates that a particular event has occurred in the real world. In other words, it indicates the fulfillment of a **prediction**. When this happens, the activated L5b neurons induce a response that suppresses the movement of the effector (arm) that participates in this MCL's representation.

Note that what the activation of motor MCLs represents are **target sensory configurations**, not just direct muscle contractions [29], plus the sum of external forces needed to sustain the desired configuration [30].

Note also that **the notions of goals and predictions are identical**. Instead of saying that the MCL's L5 neurons represent the goal of the movement, we can say that they represent a prediction for some sensory event (and vice versa).

12.5 The basal ganglia and the cerebellum

BG D2 path. Above, I gave the BG D1 (direct) circuit as a well-known example of an ARAR circuit. Here I devote some space to the circuit known as the D2 (indirect) path of the BG, because its description in virtually all of the scientific literature is simply **wrong** [31]. Its standard description is that D2-expressing MSNs of the striatum suppress the external globus pallidus (GPe), which suppresses the subthalamic nucleus (STN), which excites the BG output nuclei GPi and SNi. The net result is thought to suppress the direct path and movement.

This is not an ARAR circuit, because STN projection neurons are ENs, and they supposedly project to Restrain nuclei, not to a Respond nucleus. **In the present theory, the correct arrangement of this circuit is an Allow nucleus (D2 MSNs) that targets a Restrain nucleus (GPe), which releases an Amplify nucleus (STN) that drives responses**. This conforms with the obvious anatomical data, with the STN taking the Amplify role of the thalamus in the D1 path, while GPe takes that of GPi. **Unlike the BG's D1 path, which supports vigorous "charging" movements (e.g., towards rewards, or for active defence), the role of the D2 circuit is to support learned movement**.

Indeed, the STN projects to brainstem locomotion circuits to produce movement [32], most STN neurons show locomotion-dependent activity increase, and brief optogenetic inhibition slows, dysregulates, and terminates locomotion [33]. Moreover, it is well known that the D2 path is the main learner of habits [34], and that it cooperates with the CRB in the execution of precise, learned movements [35]. Thus, my account here is completely opposite to the standard one, where the D2 path's role is 'stop'. As part of its role, this circuit indeed suppresses the direct BG circuit, but this is in order to prevent vigorous movements from competing with learned ones. Its main role is automated/learned movements. I will not expand upon this point any further in the present paper, deferring it to a detailed discussion of ARAR circuits.

Note that there is **redundancy** in the BG ARAR circuit (and possibly in all ARAR circuits). The number of inputs is larger than the number of neurons in the Allow nucleus, which could be larger than the number of neurons in the Restrain nucleus. This means that the Allowed muscles are not fully determined by the inputs. In my opinion, the ARAR circuit determines a superset of muscles that possibly participate in the response, but the actual muscles participating is selected by sensosry inputs. This is what lets the brain adapt so rapidly to external changes but still maintain its goals.

The BG is the ARAR circuit that controls the release of cortical goal-directed responses, novel and learned. The CRB provides both precision, enabled by its huge set of input content space (granules), and speed (vs. the BG). It is not specialized for kinematics and dynamics (when compared to the BG). The BG can do both, but less accurately and more slowly.

12.6 Hierarchical sequences (HSEQs)

A major issue in motor control is how the brain represents action sequences, including hierarchical ones. The predominant notion is that of optimal control with explicit planning of hierarchical sequences [36]. However, the number of possible meaningful sequences is so large that it is not clear whether the brain has enough space to represent all of them explicitly. Moreover, the brain extremely rapidly recuperates from minor and major obstacles and changes during execution, and it is not clear how this can be done with explicit top-down representations.

Here I present an almost trivial account of HSEQs. There are four keys to this account. First, the fact that motor responses are phrased at the level of goal configurations, not as direct muscle contractions. Second, the fact that the ARP starts with and is guided by external and proprioceptive sensory inputs. Third, the fact that frontal areas continuously receive interoceptive inputs denoting the internal needs of the organism. Finally, the relatively small number of ethologically meaningful high-level sequences, which are learned during early development.

Suppose that the organism needs to eat, and that there is an apple reachable by arm. The visual inputs denoting the apple trigger an ARP, whose winners include frontal nodes activated by the current hunger (because they are partially excited by it so they have an advantage in winning response selection). These frontal nodes receive valence input (based on previous experience) indicating that the apple can satisfy hunger. Thus, the winners include motivational frontal nodes, motor nodes whose responses drive the arm to reach the apple, and sensory nodes representing the fingers touching the apple (or just getting close to it). (Clearly, there should be additional nodes involved, whose identity is a good open question.) Now suppose that someone has moved the apple to the right, or has introduced an obstacle preventing the arm from reaching it. This yields new sensory inputs. Our point is that **there is no need for a renewed top-down plan to reach the apple**. The new inputs simply trigger a new ARP with the same motivation. This ARP yields Cgen, Cres, and probably a new goal winner (because the goal configuration of the arm could be different). This new ARP is resolved just like the previous one, so the brain fixes the problem on-the-fly without any difficulty.

The next response in the sequence is to grab the apple with the fingers, followed by taking it into the mouth. Why are these actions executed? A large part of development time is devoted to acquiring action plans that satisfy needs. In abstract terms, there aren't that many of them, and 'reach, grab, put in mouth' is a basic one. Given the hunger, the nodes that represent grabbing the apple, and those that represent taking it into the mouth (and chewing it), are partially excited by these schemes learned via previous experience, so they win the competition again (unless something more urgent comes up).

In summary, every new sensory input can trigger a new response. Selection of the response is guided by needs and opportunities. The actual movements done in order to execute the response are mainly a function of the existing network structure, which has been learned from past experience. Motor control is definitely not 'optimal', because past experience may have been non-optimal (e.g., early training may have been done with tied arms). It is only optimal from the point of view of the brain, in the sense that if a response has won, it had to win.

12.7 Additional evidence

The evidence supporting the ARP is vast. Here I briefly mention some lines of evidence with some salient references.

Efference copy. A notion that is very close to goals and predictions is the old notion of efference copy (of action commands) [37]. It has been known for a long time that when an action executes, it sends links to sensory nodes. This has been thought to be for suppressing the effects of self-generated movements in order that they do not interfere with required responses to sensory inputs. In the present theory, **a main role of efference copy is to declare the sensory consequences of actions as the goals of the action and prepare the brain for their occurrence**. The effect of this 'copy of an action command' is to partially excite the target, which causes its activation when the event occurs to be smaller than when it is not predicted (as in automaticity). Thus, the efference copy seems to suppress the action's consequences, while in fact it prepares the brain for their efficient activation. It has been shown that it is more likely that the efference copy specifies the sensory goal rather than a copy motor command [38].

It is also possible that some efference copies actually suppress competitors, supporting the full range of goals and predictions during the ARP [39].

Goals and posterior parietal cortex. Supporting our view that goal nodes suppress the current response when its goal has been attained, posterior parietal cortex (PPC) stimulation can generate finger and wrist movement (presumably of the antagonist muscles) [40]. Moreover, PPC firing rates rise before contact, peak at contact, and decline when grasp is secure [41]. It has also been shown that PPC encodes visual goals related to future movements [42].

Place cells. Place cells are neurons that fire in specific spatial locations that the rodent (usually) reaches [43]. They start firing a few cycles earlier, and exhibit interesting properties such as theta phase precession. Place cells provide strong evidence for activation of action goals during execution. The other famous spatial cell type, grid cells, might be goals expressed in internal-limb space.

Goal configurations. An extremely strong line of evidence supporting goals is given by the fact that motor cortex represents goal configurations rather than direct muscle contractions [29].

Event-related potentials (ERPs). The first sensory-induced ERPs are negative, and they then turn positive [44]. Negative ERPs indicate Cgen (activation of the superficial L2/3), while positive ERPs indicate Cres and responses.

BOLD. The central technique of showing brain activity via fMRI BOLD reflects the Cgen stage (BOLD is most salient in the superficial networks).

Sensory flow. There are different feedforward and feedback bidirectional streams, occurring in the superficial (Cgen) and deep (response) networks, respectively. The former flow is stronger and is more point focused [45].

Sensory input drives motor control. There is a wide line of evidence for sensory inputs being essential for all stages of response selection, execution, and learning, showing that top-down planning does not suffice (or does not exist). Sensory feedback is crucial for trained finger sequences [46]. Spinal stretch reflexes support efficient corrective responses, and these depend on goals, not just on muscle stretch [47]. Most S1 neurons induce movements that combine distinct body parts [48]. Rodent barrell cortex controls motor responses directly, like M1 [49]. S1 activity correlates with locomotion. Stimulating S1 increases speed, inhibition slows speed and terminates [50]. Supporting the ARP, new input is immediately reflected in movement strategies [51].

Proprioception (sensory input reporting limb and muscle state) is essential for locomotion [52]. Movement is still possible with lesions impairing proprioception, but only with a lot of training in visually-defined goals [53].

MCL competition. Inter-MCL lateral inhibition has been demonstrated [23]. In addition, the well-known rich line of research of **surround suppression** supports inter-MCL competition [24]. Strong simultaneous stimulation of 4 pyramidal neurons suppressed all pyramides at a MCL distance [26].

Competition between selected and non-selected actions has been demonstrated to be constrained by competitor similarity, showing competition between relatively close alternatives [54]. More excitable neurons win the competition to be included in the response [55].

IIN competition. IINs clearly mediate competition. Martinotti IINs have been shown to mediate inhibitory competition [25]. High frequency (>70 Hz) stimulation of a single pyramidal neuron suppresses others via Martinotti IINs, with suppression of neighboring MCLs [26]. VIP IINs 'poke holes' in the blanket of IIN inhibition, at roughly the radius between MCLs, to promote winners [56]. Supporting our view that they continue to support the winning response, a GABAA receptor antagonist in medial prefrontal cortex impaired effortful execution [57].

Mirror neurons (MNs). MNs are neurons that fire both when the animal performs a certain action and when it sees others perform it, and are claimed to identify an action's intention [58]. They are quite widespread. MNs support the ARP, which interprets them as candidates activated by sensory inputs resulting from the action. Due to the sensory similarity between the two states, activation of overlapping candidates is to be expected. Note that MNs respond to acting on geometric shapes without any high level intentions involved [59].

The attentional blink (AB). In the AB, during rapid presentation of sequences of sensory targets, subjects usually do not report seeing the second of a successive pair of pre-specified targets [60]. The sensory representations of pre-specified targets are activated in goal mode. According to the ARP, during the identification of the first target (i.e., goal attainment), the MCLs representing the goal are suppressed. If the second target arrives quickly, higher level task nodes may fail to reactivate the goal, in which case it would be completely missed when it occurs.

Repetition blindness is a related paradigm in which people cannot keep track of how many times a target appears in a rapid sequence.

12.8 Discussion

This chapter presented a relatively simple mechanistic biological theory that explains how the brain fulfills its main function, response selection and execution. As such, it provides a large step forward towards a full understanding of the brain.

12.8.1 The explanatory power and biological logic of the theory

Given the mystery associated with the brain in all of the scientific, philosophical, and popular literature, it might be difficult to accept that it can be simply explained. However, the ARP as described in this chapter provides a complete account of the major aspects of how the brain works.

The brain is simply another body tissue, its role being to select and release responses that interact with the external environment. It does so via a biological process that organisms use elsewhere as well. For example, the adaptive immune system also receives inputs (presented antigens), generates candidates (clonal expansion), its candidates compete for exit from lymph nodes [61], and the winners execute the response and establish long-term plasticity (memory B and T cells). Even more obviously, Cgen followed by Cres is the main principle of the theory of evolution.

12.8.2 Function and anatomy

Perhaps the main feature of the ARP that makes it a convincing biological theory is the elegant connection that it exposes between the brain's anatomy and its function. At a coarse level, all subcortical ARAR nuclei are arranged in the same architecture that has the same behavior. Each of them supports a different type of response or specific content, but their operating principles are identical. Similarly, the different stages of the response selection part of the ARP all use different cortical layers and different IIN networks, and are supported by different agents released by agent-releasing nuclei. Thus, the present theory provides a simple unified account of both the brain's function and of its anatomy. Naturally, this function-anatomy link enables the design and interpretation of empirical experiments to refine the theory.

12.8.3 Other theories; contribution

There is a very rich literature on brain theories. All of the notions we discussed have been previously discussed, including action-perception integration [62], sophisticated models for motor control [30], action goals, efference copy, cortical networks, subcortical nuclei, etc (see references above). Nonetheless, I am not aware of any theory that has both the explanatory power of the present one, and its clean description of the link between the brain's function and anatomy.

In the recently popular notion of 'predictive coding', the brain adapts to minimize the surprise conveyed by inputs by generating predictions [3]. This agrees with some aspects of this paper, but the present theory is much wider and complete in that it describes a mechanistic process, ties it to anatomy, and explains better the role of predictions and goals.

The initial idea of an ARAR-like architecture has been raised by Swanson, who focused on the extended amygdala [7]. Almost all of my analysis is different from his, sometimes contradictory (e.g., the BG D2 path). "CRB-like structures" such as the dorsal cochlear nucleus have been discussed [63], mainly in fish and mammals.

In summary, the contribution of the ARP over existing notions is as follows. First, the explicit phrasing of ARP stages (Cgen, Cres) unifies many important notions (feedforward vs. feedback, superficial vs. deep layers) using a very simple description. Second, the identification of the correspondence between anatomy and function provides a completely mechanistic account of brain function that is grounded by empirical data that can only be gathered (at least today) via anatomy-related means. 'Anatomy' refers here not just to the role of cortical areas, but to the function of cortical layers (e.g., the difference between L5a and L5b) and subnetworks of inhibitory interneurons. Third, an account of motor control that unifies the notions of goals, predictions and efference copy, and shows how hierarchical sequences are achieved without explicit representations. Finally, the identification of a detailed ARAR architecture, which unifies the anatomy and function of almost all subcortical nuclei.

12.8.4 Action execution, observation, imagery

The focus of this paper is on action execution. Action observation is a simple special case in which the animal does not generate movements, only watches what happens. During watching, motivation and sensory inputs keep arriving, which means that there is an on-going ARP. As explained above, goals and predictions are one and the same, and during observation these are better interpreted as predictions. Thus, it is not surprising that observation has large activity overlap with execution, and that most overlap occurs in relatively high-level areas [64] (see also mirror neurons above).

Imagery (which can be equated with 'thinking') is less immediate to explain. When we imagine a triangle, it has an abstract quality that is definitely devoid of the features of sensory inputs. We should first note that humans are not the only species capable of imagery, as rats simulate spatial paths before executing them [65]. Thus, imagery seems to be a universal feature of brains (at least in some species).

The explanation for imagery is strongly tied to the issue of representation. Cortex has a vast space for representing objects, with strong evidence for visual objects such as faces and letters [66] representation in ventral temporal cortex, and integrated object representations at the anterior temporal lobe (ATL) [67] (my view is that the ATL represents knowledge involving language). These representations provide an abstraction over specific objects conveyed by sensory inputs. Assume for simplicity that 'triangle' is represented by a single MCL (an open issue). To explain imagery, we can make the leap to assume that frontal circuits can activate these object representations without supporting sensory input. This does not contradict the ARP, because these object nodes still receive other inputs. If this account is correct, then external sensory inputs may occur if and only if there are external responses, while thinking/imagery use an ARP without external sensory inputs. It would definitely use interoceptive sensory inputs, because these are the ones that provide the motivation for the whole process.

Humans most likely have a larger imagery capacity than other animals. Although the differences between the human and non-human primate brain are a matter of debate [68], humans clearly have a larger temporal lobe with faster bundles of axons leading to it from frontal circuits [69–71], and they have more connections in the frontal candidate network (L2/3), which can generate powerful flow throughout the brain [72].

A very interesting question related to imagery is how we humans know that we are imagining, as opposed to perceiving reality. We do not have the space to discuss this here.

12.8.5 Language

Language is yet another topic widely considered as mysterious. I think that language is very easy to explain. The role of the brain is to manage the organism's interaction with the external environment. This can be done using your own muscles, or via others' muscles. Language (and communication in general, using hands, eyes, etc) is a way of generating responses that use others' muscles. Since our brains are not connected to theirs, a way of overcoming the neural gap has emerged, and this is language.

What allows human language is 'hardware' for producing and perceiving sounds (with humans at least, sound is the quickest medium), and the evolution of a cortical content space to store linguistic representations (object-like representations for words in Wernicke's area in the temporal lobe, the lateral inferior frontal cortex, with higher level action representations for word sequences, and lateral motor areas for control over speech organs). Everything else about language is managed by the ARP as described here. The often cited capacity for an 'infinite number of sentences' simply parallels the capacity for an infinite number of movement sequences. Obviously, the existence of language dramatically enhances the human capacity for internal movement-less thoughts and enables the rich human culture, so there are endless levels of richness built upon language. However, the biological basis of language is covered by the ARP.

12.8.6 Fully explaining the brain

There are several topics that have not been touched upon here and that are required for a full account of the brain. These include memory recall vs. imagining things that never happened (people normally distinguish between the two, and the mechanism for this needs to be explained), familiarity vs. precise recollection, the precise nature of representations (e.g., is 'me' simply yet another notion that we learn through language and represent as other language-acquired notions, or it is represented by animals as a single notion even without language?), the nature of the representations in the various cortical areas (e.g., the claustrum), the precise representation of time (assuming that space is quite well-understood by now, although there are clearly a host of less understood details), the function of many agents (i.e., neurotensin, CCK), volition, the detailed structure of medullar, pontine and spinal circuits (these operate according to the ARP, but are not layered), the nature of the communication between the two hemispheres, striatum matrix vs. striosomes, oscillations, music, working memory, layer 6, visual stability, etc.

No body tissue is fully understood. In my opinion, the present theory provides the important basis of how the brain works, which puts its on par with other tissue and allows decades of more detailed work.

12.8.7 Consciousness and emotions

Consciousness is yet another mysterious and attractive topic that has generated some highly creative accounts [73]. In my view, consciousness is not difficult to explain. What we call consciousness is an internal report that we make of some sensory state (an idea that has already been raised [73].) Being conscious of being alive is most likely simply a report that heart beat inputs continue reaching the insula, as attested by reports of people with lesions in this area (e.g., with Cotard's syndrome) that they feel dead. Awareness of external objects is a report that a response to perceiving that object has been made. In addition to the mechanisms already described above, I hypothesize that such awareness may involve a switch from the sympathetic nervous system (which conveys alerts to new inputs) to the parasympathetic nervous system (and/or the serotonergic system).

As to the report mechanisms, we humans have language, and language areas receive continuous inputs from all areas of the brain, allowing them to actively generate reports. Whether other animals have a 'language' that allows them reports that yield consciousness that is similar in some sense to ours is an open question. However, note that the fact that animals can produce responses that look like ours is not an indication. We, and dogs, can make very similar faces in response to similar external situations, but these are the responses themselves, not reports. What generates our internal feeling of consciousness are reports, not responses.

In the same vein, emotions are reports that we make to ourselves about our basic survival state. For example, in my theory of depression, feeling dejected and sad occurs when we report that the survival response 'disengage, withdraw' has been executed in the face of stress that we do not know how to resolve [18].

Author's comment

Most of the ideas in this chapter have been described in previous papers I wrote [74,75] (long and short versions respectively). However, these papers were not so accessible. I wrote the present chapter completely from scratch, and it should be viewed as the currently definitive version of my brain theory.

References

[1] V.B. Mountcastle, The columnar organization of the neocortex, Brain 120 (4) (1997) 701–722.
[2] M. Morishima, Y. Kawaguchi, Recurrent connection patterns of corticostriatal pyramidal cells in frontal cortex, The Journal of Neuroscience 26 (16) (2006) 4394–4405.
[3] A.M. Bastos, W.M. Usrey, R.A. Adams, G.R. Mangun, P. Fries, K.J. Friston, Canonical microcircuits for predictive coding, Neuron 76 (4) (2012) 695–711.
[4] A. Graybiel, J. Mink, The basal ganglia and cognition, in: M. Gazzaniga (Ed.), The Cognitive Neurosciences IV, MIT Press, Cambridge, MA, 2009, pp. 565–585.
[5] S.J. Cruikshank, O.J. Ahmed, T.R. Stevens, S.L. Patrick, A.N. Gonzalez, M. Elmaleh, et al., Thalamic control of layer 1 circuits in prefrontal cortex, Journal of Neuroscience 32 (49) (2012) 17813–17823.

[6] Y. Smith, A. Galvan, T.J. Ellender, N. Doig, R.M. Villalba, I. Huerta-Ocampo, et al., The thalamostriatal system in normal and diseased states, Frontiers in Systems Neuroscience (2014) 8.
[7] L.W. Swanson, Cerebral hemisphere regulation of motivated behavior, Brain Research 886 (1–2) (2000) 113–164.
[8] J.M. Prati, A. Pontes-Silva, A.C.L. Gianlorenço, The cerebellum and its connections to other brain structures involved in motor and non-motor functions: a comprehensive review, Behavioural Brain Research (2024) 114933.
[9] M. Tsanov, Differential and complementary roles of medial and lateral septum in the orchestration of limbic oscillations and signal integration, European Journal of Neuroscience 48 (8) (2018) 2783–2794.
[10] S. Martínez-Bellver, A. Cervera-Ferri, J. Martínez-Ricós, A. Ruiz-Torner, A. Luque-García, A. Blasco-Serra, et al., Regular theta-firing neurons in the nucleus incertus during sustained hippocampal activation, European Journal of Neuroscience 41 (8) (2015) 1049–1067.
[11] E.E. Benarroch, Habenula recently recognized functions and potential clinical relevance, Neurology 85 (11) (2015) 992–1000.
[12] B.J. White, D.P. Munoz, The superior colliculus, The Oxford Handbook of Eye Movements 5 (4) (2011) 195.
[13] A. Rappoport, A lipid-raft theory of Alzheimer's disease, Annual Review of Biochemistry (2025) 94.
[14] E. Cheong, Shin HS. T-type, Ca2+ channels in normal and abnormal brain functions, Physiological Reviews 93 (3) (2013) 961–992.
[15] E. Szabadi, Functional neuroanatomy of the central noradrenergic system, Journal of Psychopharmacology 27 (8) (2013) 659–693.
[16] M.O. Klein, D.S. Battagello, A.R. Cardoso, D.N. Hauser, J.C. Bittencourt, R.G. Correa, Dopamine: functions, signaling, and association with neurological diseases, Cellular and Molecular Neurobiology 39 (1) (2019) 31–59.
[17] W. Muñoz, B. Rudy, Spatiotemporal specificity in cholinergic control of neocortical function, Current Opinion in Neurobiology 26 (2014) 149–160.
[18] A. Rappoport, A dynorphin theory of depression and bipolar disorder, arXiv preprint, arXiv: 2408.06763, 2024.
[19] A. Rappoport, A polyunsaturated fatty acid (PUFA) theory of schizophrenia, arXiv preprint, arXiv:2408.06794, 2024.
[20] A. Rappoport, A CRH theory of autism spectrum disorder, arXiv preprint, arXiv:2408.06750, 2024.
[21] J.M. Yabut, J.D. Crane, A.E. Green, D.J. Keating, W.I. Khan, G.R. Steinberg, Emerging roles for serotonin in regulating metabolism: new implications for an ancient molecule, Endocrine Reviews 40 (4) (2019) 1092–1107.
[22] K.B. Fink, M. Göthert, 5-HT receptor regulation of neurotransmitter release, Pharmacological Reviews 59 (4) (2007) 360–417.
[23] Y. Hirata, T. Sawaguchi, Functional columns in the primate prefrontal cortex revealed by optical imaging in vitro, Neuroscience Research 61 (1) (2008) 1–10.
[24] A. Angelucci, M. Bijanzadeh, L. Nurminen, F. Federer, S. Merlin, P.C. Bressloff, Circuits and mechanisms for surround modulation in visual cortex, Annual Review of Neuroscience 40 (1) (2017) 425–451.
[25] G. Silberberg, H. Markram, Disynaptic inhibition between neocortical pyramidal cells mediated by Martinotti cells, Neuron 53 (5) (2007) 735–746.
[26] T.K. Berger, R. Perin, G. Silberberg, H. Markram, Frequency-dependent disynaptic inhibition in the pyramidal network: a ubiquitous pathway in the developing rat neocortex, The Journal of Physiology 587 (22) (2009) 5411–5425.
[27] R. Tremblay, S. Lee, B. Rudy, GABAergic interneurons in the neocortex: from cellular properties to circuits, Neuron 91 (2) (2016) 260–292.

[28] E. Borra, M. Gerbella, S. Rozzi, G. Luppino, The macaque lateral grasping network: a neural substrate for generating purposeful hand actions, Neuroscience and Biobehavioral Reviews 75 (2017) 65–90.
[29] M.S. Graziano, Ethological action maps: a paradigm shift for the motor cortex, Trends in Cognitive Sciences 20 (2) (2016) 121–132.
[30] A.G. Feldman, et al., Referent Control of Action and Perception, Springer, 2015.
[31] A. Rappoport, Basal Ganglia paths support acute vs. automated execution, not movement vs. stopping, https://doi.org/10.20944/preprints201808.0157. preprtingsorg, 2019.
[32] T.K. Roseberry, A.M. Lee, A.L. Lalive, L. Wilbrecht, A. Bonci, A.C. Kreitzer, Cell-type-specific control of brainstem locomotor circuits by basal ganglia, Cell 164 (3) (2016) 526–537.
[33] J.W. Callahan, J.C. Morales, J.F. Atherton, D. Wang, S. Kostic, M.D. Bevan, Movement-related increases in subthalamic activity optimize locomotion, Cell Reports 43 (8) (2024).
[34] Q. Shan, M.J. Christie, B.W. Balleine, Plasticity in striatopallidal projection neurons mediates the acquisition of habitual actions, European Journal of Neuroscience 42 (4) (2015) 2097–2104.
[35] A.C. Bostan, R.P. Dum, P.L. Strick, Cerebellar networks with the cerebral cortex and basal ganglia, Trends in Cognitive Sciences 17 (5) (2013) 241–254.
[36] A.L. Wong, A.M. Haith, J.W. Krakauer, Motor planning, The Neuroscientist 21 (4) (2015) 385–398.
[37] H. Straka, J. Simmers, B.P. Chagnaud, A new perspective on predictive motor signaling, Current Biology 28 (5) (2018) R232–R243.
[38] C.A. Niziolek, S.S. Nagarajan, J.F. Houde, What does motor efference copy represent? Evidence from speech production, Journal of Neuroscience 33 (41) (2013) 16110–16116.
[39] J.D. Greenlee, A.W. Jackson, F. Chen, C.R. Larson, H. Oya, H. Kawasaki, et al., Human auditory cortical activation during self-vocalization, PLoS ONE 6 (3) (2011) e14744.
[40] J.A. Rathelot, R.P. Dum, P.L. Strick, Posterior parietal cortex contains a command apparatus for hand movements, Proceedings of the National Academy of Sciences of the United States of America 114 (16) (2017) 4255–4260.
[41] E.P. Gardner, K.S. Babu, S.D. Reitzen, S. Ghosh, A.S. Brown, J. Chen, et al., Neurophysiology of prehension. I. Posterior parietal cortex and object-oriented hand behaviors, Journal of Neurophysiology 97 (1) (2007) 387–406.
[42] S. Kuang, P. Morel, A. Gail, Planning movements in visual and physical space in monkey posterior parietal cortex, Cerebral Cortex 26 (2) (2016) 731–747.
[43] M. Sosa, A. Gillespie, L. Frank, Neural activity patterns underlying spatial coding in the hippocampus, Current Topics in Behavioral Neurosciences 37 (2018) 43–100.
[44] S.J. Luck, E.S. Kappenman, The Oxford Handbook of Event-Related Potential Components, Oxford University Press, 2012.
[45] N.T. Markov, J. Vezoli, P. Chameau, A. Falchier, R. Quilodran, C. Huissoud, et al., Anatomy of hierarchy: feedforward and feedback pathways in macaque visual cortex, Journal of Comparative Neurology 522 (1) (2014) 225–259.
[46] N.J. Popp, C.R. Hernandez-Castillo, P.L. Gribble, J. Diedrichsen, The role of feedback in the production of skilled finger sequences, Journal of Neurophysiology 127 (4) (2022) 829–839.
[47] J. Weiler, P.L. Gribble, J.A. Pruszynski, Spinal stretch reflexes support efficient control of reaching, Journal of Neurophysiology (2021).
[48] A.C. Halley, M.K. Baldwin, D.F. Cooke, M. Englund, L. Krubitzer, Distributed motor control of limb movements in rat motor and somatosensory cortex: the sensorimotor amalgam revisited, Cerebral Cortex 30 (12) (2020) 6296–6312.
[49] F. Matyas, V. Sreenivasan, F. Marbach, C. Wacongne, B. Barsy, C. Mateo, et al., Motor control by sensory cortex, Science 330 (6008) (2010) 1240–1243.
[50] S.K. Karadimas, K. Satkunendrarajah, A.M. Laliberte, D. Ringuette, I. Weisspapir, L. Li, et al., Sensory cortical control of movement, Nature Neuroscience 23 (1) (2020) 75–84.
[51] C.E. Vargas-Irwin, L. Franquemont, M.J. Black, J.P. Donoghue, Linking objects to actions: encoding of target object and grasping strategy in primate ventral premotor cortex, The Journal of Neuroscience 35 (30) (2015) 10888–10897.

[52] E. Formento, K. Minassian, F. Wagner, J.B. Mignardot, C.G. Le Goff-Mignardot, A. Rowald, et al., Electrical spinal cord stimulation must preserve proprioception to enable locomotion in humans with spinal cord injury, Nature Neuroscience 21 (12) (2018) 1728.
[53] J. Cole, J. Paillard, Living without touch and peripheral information about body position and movement: studies with deafferented subjects, The Body and the Self (1995) 245–266.
[54] L. Labruna, F. Lebon, J. Duque, P.A. Klein, C. Cazares, R.B. Ivry, Generic inhibition of the selected movement and constrained inhibition of nonselected movements during response preparation, Journal of Cognitive Neuroscience 26 (2) (2014) 269–278.
[55] S.A. Josselyn, P.W. Frankland, Memory allocation: mechanisms and function, Annual Review of Neuroscience 41 (2018) 389–413.
[56] M.M. Karnani, J. Jackson, I. Ayzenshtat, A.H. Sichani, K. Manoocheri, S. Kim, et al., Opening holes in the blanket of inhibition: localized lateral disinhibition by VIP interneurons, Journal of Neuroscience 36 (12) (2016) 3471–3480.
[57] P.T. Piantadosi, S. Khayambashi, M.G. Schluter, A. Kutarna, S.B. Floresco, Perturbations in reward-related decision-making induced by reduced prefrontal cortical GABA transmission: relevance for psychiatric disorders, Neuropharmacology. 101 (2016) 279–290.
[58] G. Rizzolatti, C. Sinigaglia, Mirrors in the Brain: How Our Minds Share Actions and Emotions, Oxford University Press, USA, 2008.
[59] C. Press, C. Catmur, R. Cook, H. Widmann, C. Heyes, G. Bird, fMRI evidence of 'mirror' responses to geometric shapes, PLoS ONE 7 (12) (2012) e51934.
[60] J.I. Kawahara, T. Kumada, V. Di Lollo, The attentional blink is governed by a temporary loss of control, Psychonomic Bulletin & Review 13 (5) (2006) 886–890.
[61] G.D. Victora, T.A. Schwickert, D.R. Fooksman, A.O. Kamphorst, M. Meyer-Hermann, M.L. Dustin, et al., Germinal center dynamics revealed by multiphoton microscopy with a photoactivatable fluorescent reporter, Cell 143 (4) (2010) 592–605.
[62] K.R. Ridderinkhof, Neurocognitive mechanisms of perception–action coordination: a review and theoretical integration, Neuroscience and Biobehavioral Reviews 46 (2014) 3–29.
[63] C.C. Bell, V. Han, N.B. Sawtell, Cerebellum-like structures and their implications for cerebellar function, Annual Review of Neuroscience 31 (1) (2008) 1–24.
[64] S.A. Rueschemeyer, M. Ekman, M. van Ackeren, J. Kilner, Observing, performing, and understanding actions: revisiting the role of cortical motor areas in processing of action words, Journal of Cognitive Neuroscience 26 (8) (2014) 1644–1653.
[65] B.E. Pfeiffer, D.J. Foster, Hippocampal place-cell sequences depict future paths to remembered goals, Nature 497 (7447) (2013) 74–79.
[66] K. Grill-Spector, K.S. Weiner, The functional architecture of the ventral temporal cortex and its role in categorization, Nature Reviews. Neuroscience 15 (8) (2014) 536–548.
[67] Y. Wang, J.A. Collins, J. Koski, T. Nugiel, A. Metoki, I.R. Olson, Dynamic neural architecture for social knowledge retrieval, Proceedings of the National Academy of Sciences of the United States of America 114 (16) (2017) E3305–E3314.
[68] A.M. Sousa, K.A. Meyer, G. Santpere, F.O. Gulden, N. Sestan, Evolution of the human nervous system function, structure, and development, Cell 170 (2) (2017) 226–247.
[69] J.K. Rilling, M.F. Glasser, T.M. Preuss, X. Ma, T. Zhao, X. Hu, et al., The evolution of the arcuate fasciculus revealed with comparative DTI, Nature Neuroscience 11 (4) (2008) 426.
[70] S.A. Chance, E.K. Sawyer, L.M. Clover, B. Wicinski, P.R. Hof, T.J. Crow, Hemispheric asymmetry in the fusiform gyrus distinguishes Homo sapiens from chimpanzees, Brain Structure and Function 218 (2013) 1391–1405.
[71] G.H. Patel, D. Yang, E.C. Jamerson, L.H. Snyder, M. Corbetta, V.P. Ferrera, Functional evolution of new and expanded attention networks in humans, Proceedings of the National Academy of Sciences 112 (30) (2015) 9454–9459.
[72] G.N. Elston, R. Benavides-Piccione, A. Elston, B. Zietsch, J. Defelipe, P. Manger, et al., Specializations of the granular prefrontal cortex of primates: implications for cognitive processing, The Anatomical Record 288 (1) (2006) 26–35.

[73] S. Dehaene, Consciousness and the Brain: Deciphering How the Brain Codes Our Thoughts, Penguin, 2014.
[74] A. Rappoport, The brain, explained: a comprehensive theory of brain function, Neuroscience and Neurology (2018), https://doi.org/10.20944/preprints201805.0137.v1.
[75] A. Rappoport, Short version of 'the brain, explained': a response process theory of brain function, Biology and Life Sciences Neuroscience and Neurology (2018), https://doi.org/10.20944/preprints201806.0092.

Chapter 13

The brain's 'Allow, Restrain, Amplify, Respond' (ARAR) architecture

13.1 Introduction

The brain responds to sensory inputs by a two-stage adaptive response process (ARP) that starts with selecting a response, followed by allowing it to execute. In this paper I show that the allowing circuits all have a similar architecture, comprised of four nuclei. First, Content representations (the selected response) innervate a GABAergic 'Allow' nucleus, which, then activated, suppresses a GABAergic 'Restrain' nucleus. The neurons in the restrain nucleus are tonically active, suppressing, an 'Amplify' nucleus. When the response is to be allowed, the Allow nucleus suppression of the Restrain one disinhibits the Amplify nucleu. This nucleus makes sure that the response executes strongly. I call this architecture the Allow-Restrain-Amplify-Respond (ARAR) architecture. Most subcortical nuclei participate in this architecture.

Response selection. The ARP response selection stage selects the muscles that are candidates to be activated as part of the response. The precise identity of those that are activated depends on sensory inputs (see below).

ARAR nuclei. In ARAR, the first nucleus ('Allow') is the one receiving most inputs from the response contents selected by the first ARP stage. It is comprised of projection interneurons (INs) that, when activated by the selected response, suppress the Restrain nucleus. INs are generally GABAergic. Thus, there is a difference between GABAergic INs and between local GABAergic interneurons that serve for competition between competing responses during response selection. In some cases, the selected content representations directly innervate other ARAR nuclei, by-passing the Allow nucleus, to ensure a rapid response.

ARAR circuits. There are several ARAR circuits, all operating under the same principle (Table 13.1). Virtually all of the important nuclei of the brain (besides nuclei whose role is to release specific agents such as dopamine and serotonin) participate in ARAR circuits. ARAR circuits also interact with each other, e.g., by inhibiting other ARAR circuits to promote their own type of response.

In this chapter I expand upon the two basal ganglia circuits, D1 and D2, and provide shorter summaries for the other circuits. These enjoy a rich literature and merit their own dedicated descriptions.

The Science of the Brain. https://doi.org/10.1016/B978-0-44-345008-2.00019-9

TABLE 13.1 Summary of the main ARAR circuits. Note that many of the circuits are standalone in the sense that they have dedicated content representations in addition to the ARAR circuits. Many details (e.g., the role of the zona incerta in vigorous movements) are not shown, and some of what is shown (e.g., the assigned functions of the septum, Supm and nucleus incertus in the space circuit) should be refined. Other less central circuits having the same structure (e.g., the auditory dorsal cochlear nucleus) are not shown. BG: basal ganglia. STR: striatum. D1s, D2s: D1, D2 dopamine receptor-expressing medium spiny neurons. GPi/GPe: internal/external glubus pallidus. STN: subthalamic nucleus. BLA/CeM: basolateral/centromedial nuclei of the amygdala. BNST: bed nucleus of the stria terminalis. LHthalA: lateral hypothalamic area. PAG: periaqueductal gray. crb: cerebellar. Lsep/Msep: lateral/medial septum. Supm: supramammillary nucleus. LHb/MHb: lateral/medial habenula. IPN: interpeduncular nucleus. VTA: ventral tegmental area (via the rostromedial tegmental nucleus, RMTg). SCi: intermediate layers of the superior colliculus.

Name	Function	Content	Allow	Restrain	Amplify	Respond
D1 BG path [1]	novel responses	all	STR D1s	GPi, SNr	thalamus	all
D2 BG path [1]	learned responses	all	STR D2s	GPe	STN	all
Extended amygdala [2]	valence, survival responses	BLA, thalamus	CeM	BNST	LHthalA	PAG, other
Cerebellum (CRB) [3]	quick or precise movements	granules	golgis	Purkinjes	deep crb nuclei	crb targets
Hippocampus [4,5]	space time events	CA1-CA3 subiculum	Lsep	Msep	Supm	nucleus incertus
Habenula [6]	switch to defend	many	STR	(some) ventral pallidum	MHb LHb	IPN, VTA
Superior colliculus [7]	saccades	all	STR	SNr	SCi	eye motor nuclei

13.2 The D1 ARAR circuit

The best-known ARAR circuit is the D1 ('direct') path of the basal ganglia (BG) [1] (Fig. 13.1, left, left). It receives cortical, thalamic, amygdalar, hippocampal, and other inputs representing the selected response. Its Allow function is mediated by D1-expressing striatal medium spiny neurons (MSNs), which are projection INs. When activated, these suppress the Restrain nuclei, the internal globus pallidus (GPi) and the internal substantia nigra (SNi). These tonically inhibit the thalamus, which is disinhibited when the selected response is released. The thalamus is a powerful Amplifier that sustains responses via repeated firing and widespread connections [8]. It targets both subcortical (via its CM/Pf nuclei [9]) and cortical circuits to drive the response.

The role of the D1 circuit is to support DA-based responses when DA acts via the D1 (or D5) receptor. DA is released when an unexpected stimulus appears, and D1 provides vigor to charge the stimulus (for food, sex, or defence) [10].

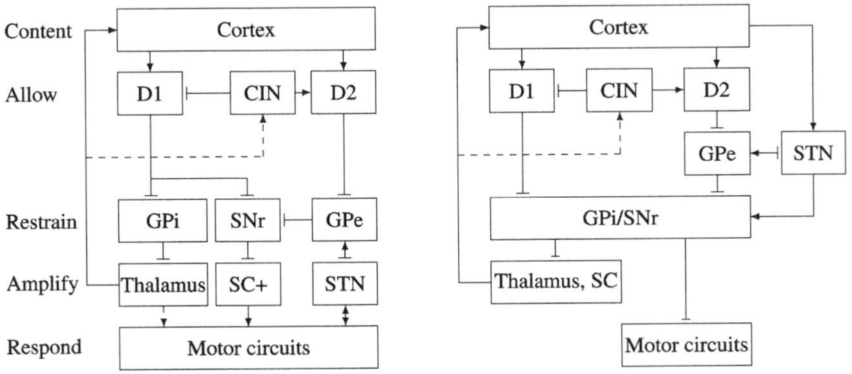

FIGURE 13.1 Basal ganglia (BG) architectures. **Right**: The classical view. The GPi and SNr are the BG output nuclei. The D1 ('direct') path supports movement, the D2 ('indirect') path suppresses it. **Left**: The view proposed here. The GPe is an output Restrain nucleus of the BG. The STN is an Amplify nucleus sustaining Response sequences mediated by motor circuits. CINs are part of the D2 path. The roles of the D1 and D2 paths are to support novel and learned (automated) responses, respectively. The SNr is a Restrain nucleus for many subcortical motor Responses. Its Amplify function for saccades is mediated by the intermediate SC layers. D1/D2: dopamine receptor 1/2-expressing striatal medium spiny neurons. CIN: striatal cholinergic interneurons. GPi/GPe: internal/external glubus pallidus. SNr: substantia nigra pars reticulata. STN: subthalamic nucleus. SC+: superior colliculus and other innate motor nuclei. Dashed lines: targets of the thalamic intralaminar nuclei (CM/Pf). For clarity, some links are not shown (e.g., STN to GPi).

This is why D1 is commonly associated with 'reward', although in its defence role it deals with 'aversion'.

13.3 The D2 circuit: automated (learned) responses

One of the most important functions of the brain is to learn from past experience. Following response selection and release, the circuits participating in response execution undergo plasticity processes, mainly involving the generation of new synapses and the modification of existing ones to make them more stable and make their usage more efficient in terms of time and energy [11].

Unlike novel inputs, familiar (learned) inputs involve preceding partial excitation of neurons predicted to participate in the response. Such predictions are a natural consequence of the enhancement of synapses that have already been used under similar conditions. When neurons that are not partially excited receive novel firing-inducing inputs, they fire strong action potential bursts [12], such that the effect of a surprise is much larger than the effect of a predicted response.

13.3.1 The circuit

In light of the important of learned responses, there are ARAR circuits that specialize in them. The D2-expressing MSNs of the striatum (the indirect path) constitute an Allow nucleus for automated responses.

Here I devote some space to this circuit, because its description in virtually all of the scientific literature is simply wrong [13]. Its standard description is that D2-expressing MSNs of the striatum suppress the external globus pallidus (GPe), which suppresses the subthalamic nucleus (STN), which excites the BG output nuclei GPi and SNi. The net result is thought to suppress the direct path and movement.

I arrange the nuclei of the D2 path of the basal ganglia differently, as follows. The D2 MSNs are an Allow nucleus. They suppress the external globus pallidus (GPe), paralleling the suppressive action of the D1s over the internal globus pallidus (GPi). The GPe restrains the subthalamic nucleus, which is an Amplify nucleus for responses executed in the pons and spinal cord.

Note that my proposed architecture (Fig. 13.1, left side) is very different from the accepted view of the indirect path (Fig. 13.1, right side). Likewise, the role of the D2 path is universally assumed to be the suppression of movement, while in my ARAR theory its role is to support automated responses.

13.3.2 Problems with the standard D2 account

The standard account for the role of the D2 path in movement suppression is widely accepted. However, accumulating evidence of different types contradicts it, there are theoretical arguments against it, and some arguments supporting it are conceptually flawed.

Evidence of path cooperation during execution. If the indirect path terminates movements, it should be active only at the end of a movement. Conversely, if it suppresses competitors, it should be active only at the beginning of movement. However, several labs have shown that both paths are active throughout movement [14–17]. Moreover, clusters of direct and indirect neurons seem to encode specific movement types and are of similar size [16], while the competitor suppression variant predicts a larger participation of indirect MSNs [18].

In addition, the two paths cooperate during reward-related execution [19], which involves phasic DA that activates the direct/D1R path.

A possible answer here is that the movements terminated and/or selected by the indirect path are low-level ones that are replaced at a high pace. However, this explanation does not conform to the experimental arguments cited in support of the standard account. In addition, there is large flow convergence along the cortex-STR-SNr/GPi axis [20], reducing the likelihood that low-level actions are supported by different BG neurons.

BG outputs can recruit the thalamus. Focused GPi excitation in low DA states (i.e., the states in which the direct path is inactive and the indirect path can be active) can induce excitatory thalamic motor signals [21]. This result undermines the logic behind the anatomical and DA arguments for the standard account.

The STN. In the standard account, the STN induces stopping by exciting the indirect path. Indeed, it excites the GPi, which should enhance its firing and suppress movement. However, the STN also excites the GPe, which inhibits the GPi and should allow movement. A possible answer is that GPe suppresses the STN, but this does not explain why the STN excites the GPe. A more elaborate account posits that the STN (the hyperdirect path) participates in the first of three stages of response suppression, and is suppressed by the indirect path in the third stage [22]. However, this still does not explain why the STN and GPe should oppose each other.

The DA argument. In a variant of the standard account, indirect MSNs suppress competing action plans. Since the DA surge inhibits indirect MSNs, this suppression needs to occur before the DA surge. However, the DA surge is extremely rapid, and it is not reasonable to expect that competition is always resolved before it occurs. In fact, there are two DA surges, a short latency one due to surprise [23] and a longer latency one due to valence (reward) [24]. This means that DA affects the BG for a relatively long time, starting almost immediately after the event starts, which does not allow time for resolving competitions.

Substance P (SP). SP is an excitatory peptide via the neurokinin-1 receptor, which binds to Gq. It is released in situations requiring sustained, effortful need-driven action, such as pain inputs and sexual approach [25]. SP is expressed by direct path MSNs, but excites the indirect path. It excites the so-called prototypical GPe neurons that project to the STN [26], and enhances STR cholinergic interneurons (CINs) [27]. Prolonged excitation of the indirect path by the direct path is incompatible with the standard account.

Parkinson's disease. Motor PD symptoms appear only after near complete depletion of DA. Since the affinity of D2R is higher than that of D1R, this means that amounts of DA that can activate only the indirect path can support behavior for quite some time without any discernible impairment. Thus, daily activity, not stopping, seems to be supported by the indirect path.

In summary, although the standard account is supported by some evidence, it is contradicted by strong evidence from multiple modalities and its logic is undermined by architectural considerations.

13.3.3 Evidence supporting a learned movement role of the D2 path

The STN projects to brainstem locomotion circuits to produce movement [28], most STN neurons show locomotion-dependent activity increase, and brief optogenetic inhibition slows, dysregulates, and terminates locomotion [29]. Moreover, it is well known that the D2 path is the main learner of habits [30], and that it cooperates with the cerebellum (CRB) in the execution of precise, learned movements [31].

There is clear evidence that the indirect path is associated with learned motor execution. In a behavioral task, the direct path was essential for the initiation of attended actions, but execution of learned sequences mostly used the indirect path [32]. In a motor training paradigm, autoradiography showed strong dorsomedial STR (dmSTR) D1 reduction after the first execution, while the sensorimotor dorsolateral STR (dlSTR) D2 (and DA transporter mRNA) showed progressive reduction after extended training [33]. Using D2R antagonism [34] and direct electrophysiological recording [30], habit learning was shown to preferably induce LTP in the indirect dlSTR path. Sensory and valence cortical areas, which are more involved in action initiation, preferably target the direct path, while motor areas target the indirect path [35,36].

Thus, my account here is completely opposite to the standard one, where the D2 path's role is 'stop'. As part of its role, this circuit indeed suppresses the direct BG circuit, but this is in order to prevent vigorous movements from competing with learned ones. Its main role is automated/learned movements.

Note that there is **redundancy** in the BG ARAR circuit (and possibly in all ARAR circuits). The number of inputs is larger than the number of neurons in the Allow nucleus, which could be larger than the number of neurons in the Restrain nucleus. This means that the Allowed muscles are not fully determined by response selection inputs. In my opinion, the ARAR circuit determines a superset of muscles that possibly participate in the response, but the actual muscles participating are selected by sensosry inputs. This is what lets the brain adapt so rapidly to external changes but still maintain its goals.

Huntington's disease (HD). The role of the indirect path in cognition is strongly supported by evidence from HD, where the earliest pathology is a specific degeneration of the indirect path, and cognitive symptoms related to thinking appear before motor symptoms [37].

Dopamine. DA is released in the STR by neurons located in two nuclei, substantia nigra compacta (SNc) and ventral tegmental area (VTA). These receive wide topographic inputs from all over the brain, including from L5b.

Consider novel acute events, which involve a large number of competing neurons firing at high frequency. This activation induces the phasic DA response and a DA surge in the STR. High arousal also yields high DA, via projections of orexin neurons to the VTA [38]. The DA surge can activate the lower affinity D1Rs in addition to the higher affinity D2Rs. Thus, in acute events, DA suppresses the indirect path and allows the direct path. The paths passing through the BG are topographic, giving rise to cortico-BG-thalamo-cortical loops [1]. Thalamic neurons innervate the apical dendrites of the L5 neurons, providing these large neurons with sufficient energy to fire responses.

Now consider fully automated responses. Here, only a small number of DA-projecting neurons are activated, and at a lower frequency. They still excite DA neurons, which may result in DA release. There are two possibilities. First, the resulting DA may be at a high enough concentration to activate D2Rs. In this case, the neurons implementing automated responses are suppressed after response execution (note that this is different from the first variant of the standard account, in which D2Rs terminate *all* responses). Since the execution pace of automated responses is relatively slow, there may not be any noticeable effect to this activation of D2Rs (in fact, this D2-mediated suppression may be essential for the execution of the next response in the sequence). A second possibility is that the resulting DA is so low that it does not activate any receptor. This accords with the quick sensory driven nature of fully automated responses; they do not need to be suppressed, because they are activated if and only if their sensory triggers actually occur.

In both scenarios, thalamic neurons can synchronize with the indirect path and innervate their cortical targets. The resulting cortico-BG-thalamo-cortical loop stabilizes the executing path and sustains its prolonged synchronous firing. During movement, DA neurons participate in this focused loop. The activation of GABAergic VTA IINs plays a crucial role in DA firing during nicotine-induced activity, probably by enhancing rebound [39], providing strong evidence that GABAergic IINs can synchronize execution and do not always suppress it.

In both acute and automated execution, *the role of D2 receptors is to terminate automated responses*. This is done before action selection in acute responses and after action execution in automated responses.

Experimental 'reward' paradigms usually involve learning (conditioning) to associate a cue with food, which excites DA release via beta-endorphin, directly and indirectly [40]. The surprising appearance of the cue induces phasic DA release, explaining why direct (indirect) MSNs increase (decrease) activity with reward value [41].

Cholinergic interneurons. The STR contains a population of CINs [42]. These are small in number (about 3-5% of STR neurons) but are extensively arbored, receiving inputs from the thalamic centromedian-parafascicular (cmpf) complex, whose source of innervation is incoming sensory flow. The CINs release ACh, suppressing/exciting direct/indirect MSNs via presynaptic M2, M4/M1 muscarinic AChRs, respectively [43].

Following surprise, cmpf bursts strongly activate the CINs, yielding a large excitation of the indirect path, and of IINs throughout the BG via nicotinic AChRs, followed by a pause induced by D2Rs [44] and afterhyperpolarization. The burst interferes with any synchronized ongoing action executing through the BG, and the pause releases direct MSNs from the CIN's suppression to let them support coarse acute responses. After competition resolution, the CINs return to their tonic (automated) activity, which excites the indirect path. This explains the CIN firing pattern. Synchronized CIN activity induces direct axonal DA release in the STR [45,46], to terminate automated actions via D2R.

STN. In our account, *a major role of the STN is to Amplify and sustain the focused execution path used by indirect path neurons during execution,* in addition to stopping movement in case of surprise. Cortico-STN projections are mostly from collaterals of L5b neurons [47], which implement responses and recruit

DA. Thus, the STN is excited exactly when responses are made, supporting its role as providing energy and predictions to the chain implementing the next response in a sequence.

The STN is known for rapidly stopping actions in case of surprise (see above). This occurs because surprises induce high-frequency firing (e.g., in medial prefrontal cortex, a STN major input), which impairs the slow synchronous firing in the indirect path. Notably, the STN can stop actions in learned tasks too [48], supporting a role in learned responses.

STN neurons have a strong autonomous spiking capacity, continuously exciting the BG output neurons. Unlike most other neurons, the main effect of their inputs is not to generate action potentials but to modify their timing [48], further supporting our view of the STN as supporting a narrow synchronized channel.

Suppression of the STN by lesions or pharmacological intervention can lead to dyskinesia and involuntary ballistic movements [49]. This may be caused by the removal of the continuous unsynchronized excitation by the STN of non-executing output neurons, which guarantees the suppression of BG targets (see PD below). Without this restraint, thalamic and other motor neurons can be accidentally recruited by noisy activation of motor cortical neurons, amplifying noisy activity and making it capable of driving motoneurons.

Another major STN role is to communicate with other motor centers, e.g., the CRB [31].

Gene expression. The extracellular signal-regulated kinases (ERK) and mitogen-activated protein kinase (MAPK) pathway is activated by ligand-receptor binding and regulates DNA protein transcription and translation, promoting proliferation and growth. It has been shown that cortico-STR stimulation induces ERK1/2/MAPK only in indirect MSNs, in both the DA-intact and DA-depleted STR [50]. This shows that although both paths undergo plasticity, some learning processes are stronger in the indirect path.

Adenosine (ADN). ADN is a by-product of astrocytic and neuronal energy utilization. It affects the BG via A1 and A2A receptors targeting the direct and indirect paths, respectively. A1 is inhibitory, while A2A is excitatory and reverses the effect of D2 in MSNs [51]. A key role of ADN is to promote sleep, to restore homeostatic health and performance [52]. A2AR promotes the participation of the indirect path in the restoring global oscillations of slow-wave sleep. Indeed, A2ARs are essential for long-term potentiation of indirect cortico-STR synapses [53], and their STR-specific deletion impairs habit learning [54].

As part of their sleep-promoting role, A2ARs counter the action of D2Rs in the indirect path [51], which impairs immediate performance, especially when the indirect path is damaged. Indeed, inactivation of A2ARs reverses working memory deficits in early Huntington's disease models [55].

DYN, ENK. The selective expression of ENK and DYN in the indirect and direct paths (respectively) seems to support the standard account. DYN promotes innate freeze [56], so it suppresses movements by suppressing the direct path. ENK promotes innate cardiorespiratory effort (i.e., running) [57], so it suppresses the indirect path to neutralize movement suppression. However, ENK and DYN support our account as well. ENK does not suppress the indirect path to overcome its suppression of movement, but to overcome its promotion of *automated* movements, which are relaxed and slow. DYN does not suppress the direct path to overcome any movement, but to overcome the strong *engage* (approach) movements promoted by D1. In any case, retrograde transmission can affect inputs to both paths, suppressing adaptive responses to promote innate ones.

In summary, the evidence favors a 'learned responses' role for the D2 path.

13.4 The extended amygdala ARAR circuit

The extended amygdala includes amygdala nuclei and the bed nucleus of the stria terminalis (BNST). The content space of the amygdala (the parallel of cortex) is the basolateral amygdala (BLA). BLA innervates the central amygdala (CeA), which is the Allow nucleus. The BNST is a major Restrain nucleus, with lateral hypothalamus area being an Amplify nucleus. The periaqueductal gray (PAG) is also a Restrain nucleus.

The role of the extended amygdala ARAR circuit is to support survival responses, with an emphasis on countering predators in the PAG [58], and on reproduction in the BNST [59]. Indeed, BNST GABAergic neurons suppress lateral hypothalamus area glutamatergic neurons [60]. BNST activation decreases social motivation, and suppression enhances [61,62]. Optogenetic activation of BNST CRH neurons promotes avoid and aversion [63].

With respect to the PAG, tonic dorsal PAG GABAergic neurons target vglut2 dorsal PAGs that implement escape. Their firing increases during escape, peaking at termination [58]. As a threat gets closer, activity shifts from vmPFC to the PAG. It is highest when more pain is expected, inducing a freeze response in humans [64].

13.5 The habenula ARAR circuit

The habenula (HBN) is an epithalamic nucleus comprised of two parts, lateral (LHb) and medial (MHb) [6]. LHb receives excitatory inputs from the border area of the globus pallidus, the prefrontal cortex, ventral pallidum, lateral preoptic area, lateral hypothalamic area, and lateral septum. It projects to the rostromedial tegmental nucleus (RMTg), which sends inhibitory projections to the DA neurons of the substantia nigra pars compacta (SNc) and ventral tegmental area (VTA). MHb receives inputs from the medial septum and diagonal band of Broca, and projects to the interpeduncular nucleus (IPN). Both IPN and LHb directly target the serotonin (SER) neurons of the dorsal and medial raphe nuclei.

LHb is excited by aversive stimuli during goal-directed responses, and excites RMTg to suppress VTA DA [65]. LHb stops current execution and disengages from DA-based reward seeking behavior [66]. Medial PFC inputs to LHb indicate stressful events [67], and the HBN suppresses social play [68].

The HBN is an Amplify nucleus in this circuit, as indicated by its epithalamus location and the identity of its neurons. It is Restrained by parts of the Ventral Pallidum, which are in turn Allowed by part of the basal ganglia striatum.

In summary, the HBN is activated when DA actively promotes goal-directed actions, which then turn out to be wrong or dangerous. In this case, the HBN suppresses DA via RMTg, and promotes SER. SER opposes DA, mediating a rapid halt over DA charging action, moving to a defensive mode.

For example, in the habenular ARAR circuit, serotonin, via opposition to dopamine, can put a strong brake on vigorous charging actions, effectively switching from charge to strong passive defence.

13.6 The superior colliculus ARAR circuit

This circuit is a special kind of goal-directed movement, controling eye movements. The intermediate layer of the superior colliculus (SCi) is an Amplify nucleus for eye movements [69]. Saccades are induced by striatum-SNr disinhibition of the SC. This circuit's Allow nucleus is the striatum, and its Restrain nucleus is the SNr (like the D1 path) [7].

13.7 The hippocampus ARAR circuit

The organization of the hippocampus as an ARAR circuit is not fully clear [4]. The hippocampus fields (DG, CA3, CA2, CA1, subiculum) provide the content space from which responses are selected, representing space-time events [4,5]. We can tentatively assign the following functions. Lateral septum is an Allow nucleu. Its lesions decrease active coping, promote stress levels [70]. Social play involves increased lateral septum glutamate and GABA [71]. Medial septum is a Restrain nucleus. There is not much functional evidence to support this hypothesis, which is mainly supported by the pallidal location of the medial septum in the basal forebrain (all Restrain nuclei are pallidal). The Amplify nucleus is the supramammillary nucleus of the hypothalamus, which projects to the hippocampus [72]. Its projections to the dentate gyrus/the CA2 field support contextual novelty and social encounters [73]. The Respond nucleus is the pontine nucleus incertus, which is a strong mediator of the theta rhythm [74]. Sustained stimulation of the incertus activates theta neurons that are almost silent in baseline [5]. Incertus neuromedinB activity tightly correlates with locomotor speed, arousal level, hippo theta power [75].

13.8 The cerebellum ARAR circuit

The CRB behaves like an ARAR circuit, but it is not organized in separate nuclei. Rather, the ARAR functions are arranged according to cell type. In the CRB, granule cells represent content used for action selection [3]. Granules innervate Golgi cells, which are an Allow population. Golgis target Purkinje cells, which are a Restrain population. When they are released, they disinhibit the deep cerebellar nuclei [76], which are the circuit's Amplify nuclei, with targets that implement responses.

It is useful to compare the functions of the basal ganglia and the CRB. The BG is the ARAR circuit that controls the release of cortical (non-innate) goal-directed responses, novel and learned. The CRB provides both precision, enabled by its huge set of input content space (granules), and speed (vs. the BG). It is not specialized for kinematics and dynamics (when compared to the BG). The BG can do both, but less accurately and more slowly. Nonetheless, since both circuits deal with learned movements, they are connected and cooperating [31,77].

13.9 Discussion

This chapter presented a mechanistic biological theory that explains how the brain fulfills the second part of its main function, allowing response to execute after they have been selected. This constitutes a large step towards a full understanding of the brain.

The D2 circuit. Possibly the main contribution of this paper is the reconceptualization of the basal ganglia's D2 (indirect) path. In the standard accepted view, its nuclei are arranged as in Fig. 13.1 (right), and its role is to suppress movement. In our view, the nuclei are arrange differently (Fig. 13.1, left), more symmetrically (e.g., GPe is at the same level and role as GPi, and similarly for the subthalamic nucleus and the thalamus), and its role is to support learned (automated) movements. Since there are important disorder centered in the basal gangalia, such as Parkinson's Disease and Huntington's Disease, this new view can lead to breakthroughs in patient treatment. The D1 and D2 circuits are also central sites of dopamine action, with its effect on schizophrenia, bipolar disorder, and depression.

The extended amygdala circuit. While the general architecture of the amygdala and its relationship with the PAG are basically known, the role of the BNST in this architecture is currently not clear. Our account, which assigns BNST the function of a Restrain nucleus, sheds light on its roles in social interaction and clarifies many open issues related to reproduction and social play.

The habenula circuit. The HBN is known to participate in aversive events, via some known mechanisms related to dopamine, but there is currently no uniform theory covering its function. Such a theory is provided in this paper. This is especially relevant for the role of serotonin, which switches from charging movements mediated by dopamine to defensive movements.

The superior colliculus circuit. The similarity between the D1 circuit and the SC one has been already noted [69]. This paper extends it to the D2 circuit and shows the fundamental similarity between these ARAR circuits.

The cerebellum circuit. The CRB has been the subject of many experiments and reviews. The fact that it is an ARAR circuit strengthens its relationship with the rest of the brain, and resolves some pertinent open questions (e.g., it was not fully clear until now that responses by the deep CRB nuclei are disinhibited by Purkinje cells).

The hippocampus circuit. The hippocampus shows several signs of being arranged in an ARAR architecture, but the details are not fully clear, and there might be differences from the other ARAR circuits. In any case, our view strengthens the case for the nucleus incertus being the meditor of the theta rhythm, and for the supramammillary nucleus to be an Amplifier. It also provides important hints as to the roles of the lateral and medial septum (Allow and Restrain respectively). These are fertile areas for further research.

Other theories. There is a very rich literature on brain theories. However, I found only one precedent for the idea promoted here. The initial idea of a pallidum ARAR-like architecture has been raised by Swanson, who focused on the extended amygdala [2]. Almost all of my analysis is different from his, sometimes contradictory (e.g., the BG D2 path).

"CRB-like structures" such as the dorsal cochlear nucleus have been discussed [78], mainly in fish and mammals.

In summary, the contribution of the ARAR concept over existing notions is as follows. First, the explicit phrasing of four response allowance stages unifies many open and semi-open questions using a very simple description. Second, the identification of a detailed ARAR architecture, unifies the anatomy and function of almost all subcortical nuclei. Third, ARAR provides a direction to guide future research on the functions and anatomy of subcortical nuclei such as the subthalamic nucleus, BNST, habenula, and septum.

References

[1] A. Graybiel, J. Mink, The basal ganglia and cognition, in: M. Gazzaniga (Ed.), The Cognitive Neurosciences IV, MIT Press, Cambridge, MA, 2009, pp. 565–585.

[2] L.W. Swanson, Cerebral hemisphere regulation of motivated behavior, Brain Research 886 (1–2) (2000) 113–164.

[3] J.M. Prati, A. Pontes-Silva, A.C.L. Gianlorenço, The cerebellum and its connections to other brain structures involved in motor and non-motor functions: a comprehensive review, Behavioural Brain Research (2024) 114933.

[4] M. Tsanov, Differential and complementary roles of medial and lateral septum in the orchestration of limbic oscillations and signal integration, European Journal of Neuroscience 48 (8) (2018) 2783–2794.

[5] S. Martínez-Bellver, A. Cervera-Ferri, J. Martínez-Ricós, A. Ruiz-Torner, A. Luque-García, A. Blasco-Serra, et al., Regular theta-firing neurons in the nucleus incertus during sustained hippocampal activation, European Journal of Neuroscience 41 (8) (2015) 1049–1067.

[6] E.E. Benarroch, Habenula recently recognized functions and potential clinical relevance, Neurology 85 (11) (2015) 992–1000.

[7] B.J. White, D.P. Munoz, The superior colliculus, The Oxford Handbook of Eye Movements 5 (4) (2011) 195.

[8] S.J. Cruikshank, O.J. Ahmed, T.R. Stevens, S.L. Patrick, A.N. Gonzalez, M. Elmaleh, et al., Thalamic control of layer 1 circuits in prefrontal cortex, Journal of Neuroscience 32 (49) (2012) 17813–17823.

[9] Y. Smith, A. Galvan, T.J. Ellender, N. Doig, R.M. Villalba, I. Huerta-Ocampo, et al., The thalamostriatal system in normal and diseased states, Frontiers in Systems Neuroscience (2014) 8.

[10] M.O. Klein, D.S. Battagello, A.R. Cardoso, D.N. Hauser, J.C. Bittencourt, R.G. Correa, Dopamine: functions, signaling, and association with neurological diseases, Cellular and Molecular Neurobiology 39 (1) (2019) 31–59.

[11] A. Rappoport, A lipid-raft theory of Alzheimer's disease, Annual Review of Biochemistry (2025) 94.

[12] E. Cheong, Shin HS. T-type, Ca2+ channels in normal and abnormal brain functions, Physiological Reviews 93 (3) (2013) 961–992.

[13] A. Rappoport, Basal ganglia paths support acute vs. automated execution, not movement vs. stopping, https://doi.org/10.20944/preprints201808.0157. preprtingsorg, 2019.

[14] G. Cui, S.B. Jun, X. Jin, M.D. Pham, S.S. Vogel, D.M. Lovinger, et al., Concurrent activation of striatal direct and indirect pathways during action initiation, Nature 494 (7436) (2013) 238–242.

[15] G. Barbera, B. Liang, L. Zhang, C.R. Gerfen, E. Culurciello, R. Chen, et al., Spatially compact neural clusters in the dorsal striatum encode locomotion relevant information, Neuron 92 (1) (2016) 202–213.

[16] J.G. Parker, J.D. Marshall, B. Ahanonu, Y.W. Wu, T.H. Kim, B.F. Grewe, et al., Diametric neural ensemble dynamics in parkinsonian and dyskinetic states, Nature 557 (2018) 177–182.

[17] Sheng Mj, D. Lu, Shen Zm, Poo Mm, Emergence of stable striatal D1R and D2R neuronal ensembles with distinct firing sequence during motor learning, Proceedings of the National Academy of Sciences of the United States of America 116 (22) (2019) 11038–11047.

[18] T. Wichmann, Models of Parkinson's disease revisited, Nature 557 (2018) 169–170.

[19] Y. Isomura, T. Takekawa, R. Harukuni, T. Handa, H. Aizawa, M. Takada, et al., Reward-modulated motor information in identified striatum neurons, Journal of Neuroscience 33 (25) (2013) 10209–10220.

[20] I. Bar-Gad, G. Morris, H. Bergman, Information processing, dimensionality reduction and reinforcement learning in the basal ganglia, Progress in Neurobiology 71 (6) (2003) 439–473.

[21] J. Kim, Y. Kim, R. Nakajima, A. Shin, M. Jeong, A.H. Park, et al., Inhibitory basal ganglia inputs induce excitatory motor signals in the thalamus, Neuron 95 (5) (2017) 1181–1196.

[22] A. Nambu, H. Tokuno, M. Takada, Functional significance of the cortico–subthalamo–pallidal 'hyperdirect' pathway, Neuroscience Research 43 (2) (2002) 111–117.

[23] P. Redgrave, K. Gurney, The short-latency dopamine signal: a role in discovering novel actions?, Nature Reviews. Neuroscience 7 (12) (2006) 967–975.

[24] M. Joshua, A. Adler, H. Bergman, The dynamics of dopamine in control of motor behavior, Current Opinion in Neurobiology 19 (6) (2009) 615–620.

[25] K. Asahina, K. Watanabe, B.J. Duistermars, E. Hoopfer, C.R. González, E.A. Eyjólfsdóttir, et al., Tachykinin-expressing neurons control male-specific aggressive arousal in Drosophila, Cell 156 (1) (2014) 221–235.

[26] K. Mizutani, S. Takahashi, S. Okamoto, F. Karube, F. Fujiyama, Substance P effects exclusively on prototypic neurons in mouse globus pallidus, Brain Structure and Function (2017) 1–22.

[27] G. Govindaiah, Y. Wang, C.L. Cox, Substance P selectively modulates GABA A receptor-mediated synaptic transmission in striatal cholinergic interneurons, Neuropharmacology 58 (2) (2010) 413–422.
[28] T.K. Roseberry, A.M. Lee, A.L. Lalive, L. Wilbrecht, A. Bonci, A.C. Kreitzer, Cell-type-specific control of brainstem locomotor circuits by basal ganglia, Cell 164 (3) (2016) 526–537.
[29] J.W. Callahan, J.C. Morales, J.F. Atherton, D. Wang, S. Kostic, M.D. Bevan, Movement-related increases in subthalamic activity optimize locomotion, Cell Reports 43 (8) (2024).
[30] Q. Shan, M.J. Christie, B.W. Balleine, Plasticity in striatopallidal projection neurons mediates the acquisition of habitual actions, European Journal of Neuroscience 42 (4) (2015) 2097–2104.
[31] A.C. Bostan, R.P. Dum, P.L. Strick, Cerebellar networks with the cerebral cortex and basal ganglia, Trends in Cognitive Sciences 17 (5) (2013) 241–254.
[32] L. Agnoli, P. Mainolfi, R.W. Invernizzi, M. Carli, Dopamine D1-like and D2-like receptors in the dorsal striatum control different aspects of attentional performance in the five-choice serial reaction time task under a condition of increased activity of corticostriatal inputs, Neuropsychopharmacology 38 (5) (2013) 701–714.
[33] W.H. Sommer, R.M. Costa, A.C. Hansson, Dopamine systems adaptation during acquisition and consolidation of a skill, Frontiers in Integrative Neuroscience 8 (2014) 87.
[34] H.H. Yin, S.P. Mulcare, M.R. Hilário, E. Clouse, T. Holloway, M.I. Davis, et al., Dynamic reorganization of striatal circuits during the acquisition and consolidation of a skill, Nature Neuroscience 12 (3) (2009) 333–341.
[35] N.R. Wall, M. De La Parra, E.M. Callaway, A.C. Kreitzer, Differential innervation of direct- and indirect-pathway striatal projection neurons, Neuron 79 (2) (2013) 347–360.
[36] A. Reiner, N.M. Hart, W. Lei, Y. Deng, Corticostriatal projection neurons–dichotomous types and dichotomous functions, Frontiers in Neuroanatomy (2010) 4.
[37] P. Dayalu, R.L. Albin, Huntington disease: pathogenesis and treatment, Neurologic Clinics 33 (1) (2015) 101–114.
[38] T. Sakurai, The role of orexin in motivated behaviours, Nature Reviews. Neuroscience 15 (11) (2014) 719–731.
[39] S. Tolu, R. Eddine, F. Marti, V. David, M. Graupner, S. Pons, et al., Co-activation of VTA DA and GABA neurons mediates nicotine reinforcement, Molecular Psychiatry 18 (3) (2013) 382.
[40] H.L. Fields, E.B. Margolis, Understanding opioid reward, Trends in Neurosciences 38 (4) (2015) 217–225.
[41] J.H. Shin, D. Kim, M.W. Jung, Differential coding of reward and movement information in the dorsomedial striatal direct and indirect pathways, Nature Communications 9 (1) (2018) 404.
[42] K.K. Gonzales, Y. Smith, Cholinergic interneurons in the dorsal and ventral striatum: anatomical and functional considerations in normal and diseased conditions, Annals of the New York Academy of Sciences (2015).
[43] J.B. Ding, J.N. Guzman, J.D. Peterson, J.A. Goldberg, D.J. Surmeier, Thalamic gating of corticostriatal signaling by cholinergic interneurons, Neuron 67 (2) (2010) 294–307.
[44] N. Chuhma, S. Mingote, H. Moore, S. Rayport, Dopamine neurons control striatal cholinergic neurons via regionally heterogeneous dopamine and glutamate signaling, Neuron 81 (4) (2014) 901–912.
[45] S. Threlfell, T. Lalic, N.J. Platt, K.A. Jennings, K. Deisseroth, S.J. Cragg, Striatal dopamine release is triggered by synchronized activity in cholinergic interneurons, Neuron 75 (1) (2012) 58–64.
[46] R. Cachope, Y. Mateo, B.N. Mathur, J. Irving, H.L. Wang, M. Morales, et al., Selective activation of cholinergic interneurons enhances accumbal phasic dopamine release: setting the tone for reward processing, Cell Reports 2 (1) (2012) 33–41.
[47] T. Kita, H. Kita, The subthalamic nucleus is one of multiple innervation sites for long-range corticofugal axons: a single-axon tracing study in the rat, The Journal of Neuroscience 32 (17) (2012) 5990–5999.

[48] M.D. Bevan, The subthalamic nucleus, in: H. Steiner, K.Y. Tseng (Eds.), Handbook of the Basal Ganglia Structure and Function, 2nd ed., Elsevier, 2017, pp. 277–292.
[49] C. Hamani, J.A. Saint-Cyr, J. Fraser, M. Kaplitt, A.M. Lozano, The subthalamic nucleus in the context of movement disorders, Brain 127 (1) (2004) 4–20.
[50] C.R. Gerfen, S. Miyachi, R. Paletzki, P. Brown, D1 dopamine receptor supersensitivity in the dopamine-depleted striatum results from a switch in the regulation of ERK1/2/MAP kinase, The Journal of Neuroscience 22 (12) (2002) 5042–5054.
[51] K. Azdad, D. Gall, A.S. Woods, C. Ledent, S. Ferré, S.N. Schiffmann, Dopamine D2 and adenosine A2A receptors regulate NMDA-mediated excitation in accumbens neurons through A2A–D2 receptor heteromerization, Neuropsychopharmacology 34 (4) (2009) 972–986.
[52] T. Porkka-Heiskanen, A.V. Kalinchuk, Adenosine, energy metabolism and sleep homeostasis, Sleep Medicine Reviews 15 (2) (2011) 123–135.
[53] W. Shen, M. Flajolet, P. Greengard, D.J. Surmeier, Dichotomous dopaminergic control of striatal synaptic plasticity, Science 321 (5890) (2008) 848–851.
[54] C. Yu, J. Gupta, J.F. Chen, H.H. Yin, Genetic deletion of A2A adenosine receptors in the striatum selectively impairs habit formation, The Journal of Neuroscience 29 (48) (2009) 15100–15103.
[55] W. Li, H.B. Silva, J. Real, Y.M. Wang, D. Rial, P. Li, et al., Inactivation of adenosine A2A receptors reverses working memory deficits at early stages of Huntington's disease models, Neurobiology of Disease 79 (2015) 70–80.
[56] H.T. Guo, R.H. Zhang, L.Y. Huang, J. Li, Y.L. Liu, H. Bi, et al., Mechanisms involved in the hypotensive effect of a κ-opioid receptor agonist in hypertensive rats, Archives of Medical Research 38 (7) (2007) 723–729.
[57] G.M. Denning, L.W. Ackermann, T.J. Barna, J.G. Armstrong, L.L. Stoll, N.L. Weintraub, et al., Proenkephalin expression and enkephalin release are widely observed in non-neuronal tissues, Peptides 29 (1) (2008) 83–92.
[58] A.V. Stempel, D.A. Evans, O.P. Arocas, F. Claudi, S.C. Lenzi, E. Kutsarova, et al., Tonically active GABAergic neurons in the dorsal periaqueductal gray control the initiation and execution of instinctive escape, bioRxiv (2023) 2023-11.
[59] K. Hashikawa, Y. Hashikawa, A. Falkner, D. Lin, The neural circuits of mating and fighting in male mice, Current Opinion in Neurobiology 38 (2016) 27–37.
[60] J.H. Jennings, G. Rizzi, A.M. Stamatakis, R.L. Ung, G.D. Stuber, The inhibitory circuit architecture of the lateral hypothalamus orchestrates feeding, Science 341 (6153) (2013) 1517–1521.
[61] R. Emmons, T. Sadok, N.G. Rovero, M.A. Belnap, H.J. Henderson, A.J. Quan, et al., Chemogenetic manipulation of the bed nucleus of the stria terminalis counteracts social behavioral deficits induced by early life stress in C57BL/6J mice, Journal of Neuroscience Research 99 (1) (2021) 90–109.
[62] J.T. Jacobs, R.S. Maior, H.F. Waguespack, C. Campos-Rodriguez, P.A. Forcelli, L. Malkova, Pharmacological inactivation of the bed nucleus of the stria terminalis increases affiliative social behavior in rhesus macaques, The Journal of Neuroscience 43 (18) (2023) 3331–3338.
[63] H.M. Baumgartner, J. Schulkin, K.C. Berridge, Activating corticotropin-releasing factor systems in the nucleus accumbens, amygdala, and bed nucleus of stria terminalis: incentive motivation or aversive motivation?, Biological Psychiatry 89 (12) (2021) 1162–1175.
[64] D. Mobbs, P. Petrovic, J.L. Marchant, D. Hassabis, N. Weiskopf, B. Seymour, et al., When fear is near: threat imminence elicits prefrontal-periaqueductal gray shifts in humans, Science 317 (5841) (2007) 1079–1083.
[65] A.M. Stamatakis, G.D. Stuber, Activation of lateral habenula inputs to the ventral midbrain promotes behavioral avoidance, Nature Neuroscience 15 (8) (2012) 1105–1107.
[66] R.J. Post, D.A. Bulkin, R.B. Ebitz, V. Lee, K. Han, M.R. Warden, Tonic activity in lateral habenula neurons acts as a neutral valence brake on reward-seeking behavior, Current Biology 32 (20) (2022) 4325–4336.

[67] V.P. Mathis, M. Williams, C. Fillinger, P.J. Kenny, Networks of habenula-projecting cortical neurons regulate cocaine seeking, Science Advances 7 (45) (2021) eabj2225.
[68] L.J. Vanderschuren, E.M. Achterberg, V. Trezza, The neurobiology of social play and its rewarding value in rats, Neuroscience and Biobehavioral Reviews 70 (2016) 86–105.
[69] O. Hikosaka, GABAergic output of the basal ganglia, Progress in Brain Research 160 (2007) 209–226.
[70] G.M. Singewald, A. Rjabokon, N. Singewald, K. Ebner, The modulatory role of the lateral septum on neuroendocrine and behavioral stress responses, Neuropsychopharmacology 36 (4) (2011) 793–804.
[71] R. Bredewold, J. Schiavo, M. van der Hart, M. Verreij, A. Veenema, Dynamic changes in extracellular release of GABA and glutamate in the lateral septum during social play behavior in juvenile rats: implications for sex-specific regulation of social play behavior, Neuroscience 307 (2015) 117–127.
[72] W.X. Pan, N. McNaughton, The supramammillary area: its organization, functions and relationship to the hippocampus, Progress in Neurobiology 74 (3) (2004) 127–166.
[73] S. Chen, L. He, A.J. Huang, R. Boehringer, V. Robert, M.E. Wintzer, et al., A hypothalamic novelty signal modulates hippocampal memory, Nature 586 (7828) (2020) 270–274.
[74] A. Nunez, A. Cervera-Ferri, F. Olucha-Bordonau, A. Ruiz-Torner, Nucleus incertus contribution to hippocampal theta rhythm generation, European Journal of Neuroscience 23 (10) (2006) 2731–2738.
[75] L. Lu, Y. Ren, T. Yu, Z. Liu, S. Wang, L. Tan, et al., Control of locomotor speed, arousal, and hippocampal theta rhythms by the nucleus incertus, Nature Communications 11 (1) (2020) 262.
[76] T. Ishikawa, S. Tomatsu, Y. Tsunoda, J. Lee, D.S. Hoffman, S. Kakei, Releasing dentate nucleus cells from Purkinje cell inhibition generates output from the cerebrocerebellum, PLoS ONE 9 (10) (2014) e108774.
[77] D. Milardi, A. Arrigo, G. Anastasi, A. Cacciola, S. Marino, E. Mormina, et al., Extensive direct subcortical cerebellum-basal ganglia connections in human brain as revealed by constrained spherical deconvolution tractography, Frontiers in Neuroanatomy 10 (2016) 29.
[78] C.C. Bell, V. Han, N.B. Sawtell, Cerebellum-like structures and their implications for cerebellar function, Annual Review of Neuroscience 31 (1) (2008) 1–24.

Chapter 14

A comprehensive biological theory of sleep

14.1 Introduction

Sleep and dreaming have fascinated humanity for thousands of years, and are the subject of intense scientific study [1]. While advances have been made in understanding many aspects of sleep [2], it is at present still largely a mystery [3,4].

A comprehensive theory of sleep must answer at least the following questions. First, sleep is evidently crucial for survival. It disconnects the animal from its environment in a way that can put it in danger, yet it exists in some form in virtually all animals [5]. What is the important role of sleep that justifies this? Second, sleep has two main stages, rapid eye movement sleep (REMS) and non-REM sleep (NREMS), the latter exhibiting several EEG phenomena, including spindles, slow wave activity, and sharp wave ripples [6]. What are their roles and mechanisms? Third, sleep is known to be important for memory and learning [7]. What is the exact nature of the connection? Fourth, anesthesia can induce a sleep-like state. How do anesthetics work, and in what ways are they similar to and different from sleep? Finally, sleep involves unique consciousness states, both a sense of reality during dreams and a complete lack of consciousness otherwise. How can this be explained? Specifically, what are the roles and mechanisms of dreaming?

Many theories of the role of sleep have been proposed, including memory consolidation, synaptic homeostasis, energy replenishment and saving, and intracellular and extracellular clearance [8,9]. However, none of these theories addresses all or even most of the questions above. Here, I present a comprehensive theory of sleep, having three main contributions. First, it is the first theory that addresses all of these questions, presenting a coherent story of what sleep is, how it relates to brain function, and how it is implemented. Second, it is the first mechanistic theory of dreaming. Third, it presents a novel account of the plasticity changes occurring in sleep, thereby reconciling ongoing debates.

14.2 Theory overview

During wake, the organism generates responses to sensory inputs conveying internal and external needs and threats. The brain mediates the muscle contraction

The Science of the Brain. https://doi.org/10.1016/B978-0-44-345008-2.00020-5

aspect of this process. To support the response process, the brain utilizes **arousal** agents, the main ones being orexin, norepinephrine, histamine, dopamine, serotonin and **acetylcholine (ACh)**, each having a specific response process role. The role of ACh is to support **focused responses**, generated via competition between response candidates after which neuronal winners are enhanced and executed while losers are suppressed. Executed focused responses are **learned** (automated) via long-term **plasticity** processes. The term 'memory' refers to a specific type of learned content.

Body tissues depend on an **optimal homeostatic state** for health and performance. Wake activity induces deviations from the optimal state, and these can damage cells and impair tissue function. Reactive species resulting from metabolism, excessive intracellular calcium ions (**Ca^{2+}**), and extracellular debris can all be toxic, mainly via the apoptosis arm of the **unfolded protein response (UPR).** Tissues and individual cells possess state restoration mechanisms, but these are not fully effective as long as activity continues. *Sleep is a brain-managed state that enforces the cessation of activity and promotes efficient restoration of the optimal state, especially of cytosolic, mitochondria, and endoplasmic reticulum Ca^{2+}*. As such, it enhances all aspects of brain function, including both responses and plasticity, and is essential for tissue health. *The role of NREMS is to efficiently restore large neuronal populations via sustained global firing.* All arousal neurons except ACh neurons are restored via tonic firing during wake. *The role of REMS is to restore ACh neurons via firing.*

NREM sleep is induced by circadian circuits and activity- and immune-induced sleep pressure. First, circadian areas such as the **suprachiasmatic nucleus** can suppress arousal neurons. Second, energy metabolism and the immune system (via prostaglandin D2) induce the accumulation of an agent conveying sleep pressure, **adenosine (ADN)**, in the extracellular space. Via the A1 receptor, ADN activates **potassium channels** to suppress cells, including arousal neurons. Via the A2A receptor and A1R-mediated disinhibition, ADN excites neuronal groups in the **preoptic area** that mutually inhibit arousal neurons. The suppression of arousal neurons and the decrease of sensory inputs due to reduced activity relieve the drive to form focused responses. Together with an increased neural excitability due to degradation of the optimal state, this enables the emergence of fast corticothalamic oscillations (spindles) followed by **slow wave activity (SWA)**, slow oscillations of large neuronal populations mediated by the synchronizing drive capacity of the **thalamus**. Neural firing during SWA restores the intracellular space, and prompts restoration of the extracellular space via **glia cells, blood vessels**, the **cerebrospinal fluid (CSF)** and the **glymphatic system**.

SWA alleviates the block on firing induced by state degradation. At some point, neurons can escape thalamic control to start firing individually. The first to do so are those most strongly affected by prior wake activity, hippocampal and (later) ACh neurons. The former induce a sequential activation shown as EEG **sharp wave ripples (SWRs)** that spreads to cortical areas. The firing of

ACh neurons yields **REM sleep**. REMS terminates SWA, because ACh opposes coordinated activation of large neuronal populations due to its support of focused responses. The plasticity effect of ACh is to enhance focused paths and suppress losing competitors and noise. The enhanced paths are those involved in focused responses during wake, marked by intracellular cation accumulation. This explains why sleep is important for **memory** (learning).

The REMS state is assisted by pontine **sublaterodorsal nucleus (SLD)** neurons, which counter the wake effects of ACh by suppressing movement, and by brainstem and hypothalamic neurons that suppress other arousal neurons.

Neural firing during REMS and NREMS degrades the optimal state, yielding additional **cycles** of the same process until the suppression of arousal neurons cannot be maintained. In the healthy brain, this occurs when brain neurons have been sufficiently restored.

The cortical and hippocampal activity during SWRs and REMS is focused, and comprises neurons that represent real percepts and events during wake. Those are the neurons that represent the content of **dreams**. Hence, dreams involve the general themes present during wake. However, they generally do not recapitulate wake events, since these depend on the coordinated activity of neurons in many brain areas and on precise temporal sequencing, while dreams are driven by deviations from the optimal state. Once started, neural activations during dreams can take a life of their own. For this reason, dreams can include illogical or impossible events.

Our sense of **reality** during wake depends upon the activation of neurons that represent specific perceptual content, and consciousness involves neurons that support the reporting of perceptual content. Both content perception and reporting are focused responses, hence are neutralized during SWA and allowed during REMS and SWR (and possibly spindles). This explains why these sleep stages involve a lack of consciousness and a sense of reality, respectively.

Anesthetics work by preventing focused responses. Many of them utilize the same brain mechanisms used by sleep, and induce a sleep-like state. Some anesthetics utilize different mechanisms, and induce a trance-like state.

14.3 Wake activity

Sleep cannot be understood without a model of wake activity. During wake, the brain receives internal and external sensory inputs, and finds and executes movement responses. Four cell classes are involved in this process. Excitatory neurons represent content, inhibitory interneurons (IINs) support response coordination, agent-releasing neurons manage the different process stages, and glia cells provide energy, protection and plasticity.

Response content. Excitatory (mostly pyramidal) neurons represent perceptual, action, and valence (approach/avoid) content. In general, neural representations are specific, in that every particular neuron is activated in a relatively small number of events. Sensory inputs of different types reach highly specific areas

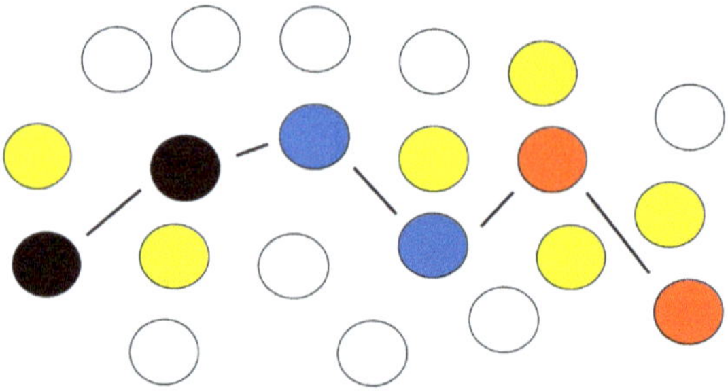

FIGURE 14.1 A top cortical view of a focused response path. Circles: microcolumns. Lines: local connections (long-distance connections are not shown). Red, blue and black: sensory, motor and valence (need) representations. Yellow: candidates that have lost the competition due to IINs. White: representations not taking part in the current response.

of the brain, and muscle contraction responses are also generated by specific neurons. Although response generation may initially involve widespread neural excitation, response execution is eventually done by a relatively small number of neurons. Thus, a major aspect of brain function is to discover and enhance a neural subset that connects inputs to outputs, and to suppress other neurons (Fig. 14.1). We say that the selected neurons form a **focused response** path.[1]

Focused responses are generated via a **response process**. Sensory inputs can trigger innate responses. If this does not happen, they flow into cortex, which is the main area of adaptive representations. In cortex, sensory inputs generate widespread alerting bottom-up flow, mainly in layers 2-4, which is answered by top-down (TD) flow in layers 2/3/5. In novel situations, the TD flow activates a (possibly large) number of response candidates, which respond to features of the current input learned due to the execution of past responses. If an urgent response is required, a coarse response is rapidly executed. Otherwise, the response candidates compete, and the winners constitute a focused response ('center') that is executed by neurons in layers 5/6. Layer 5b contains the cortical neurons projecting to motor centers that actually drive responses. The losing candidates are suppressed. The focused response is sustained by the basal ganglia and thalamus, which can provide strong synchronizing drive throughout cortex.

This description integrates several prominent existing theories that rely on a large body of evidence, including biased competition [10], the action perception cycle [11], predictive coding [12], and the reverse hierarchy theory [13]. To cite just one important piece of evidence, consider EEG event-related potential (ERP) components [14]. The activation of candidates in the superficial layers is what generates negative ERPs such as the N170 associated with face perception and the N400 associated with semantics (especially in language). Surprises yield increased negative ERP amplitude, because they induce the activation of more

[1] The selected neurons are distributed, not linearly connected as may be implied by 'path'. We use this term to emphasize the fact that the selected subset is relatively small and focused.

candidates. Competition and its resolution, which involve neurons in the deep layers, are associated with positive ERP components. For example, the language P600 ERP is larger when the ending of a sentence requires reinterpretation.

Coordination. The selection of the winning subset and the execution of responses by it are assisted by **inhibitory interneurons (IINs)** releasing GABA or glycine. These agents open ion channels that let Cl^- enter the cell and polarize it, suppressing its firing.[2] Although this effect is technically inhibitory, it is misleading to say that the function of IINs is inhibition. When an IIN fires just before its targets are about to fire, it indeed inhibits them. However, when an IIN fires just after its targets have fired, it only resets their charging states. If these targets accumulate charge at approximately the same rate, the effect is to **synchronize** their firing, making it more efficient and powerful. Thus, IINs implement a 'join-or-stop' selection mechanism whereby some neurons (winners) are enhanced while others (losers) are suppressed. Moreover, after the winners are selected, IINs continue synchronizing winner firing to support efficient sustained execution. Thus, a more accurate term for the role of local GABAergic and glycinergic neurons is response **coordination**.

Mechanistically, coordination is done as follows. When flow reaches an area, it activates some excitatory neurons. These excite IINs located around them, which may be viewed as sending **coordination requests**. IINs target the whole local neighborhood indiscriminately, establishing a join-or-stop positive feedback loop. This mechanism is fundamental in creating the well-known phenomenon of surround suppression [15].

There are several IIN classes, each supporting a different aspect of this process [16]. Soma-targeting IINs expressing parvalbumin (PV) are fast spiking due to high expression of calcium-permeable (CP) AMPA receptors [17], inducing a rapid powerful effect over the whole cell. PV binds Ca^{2+} with high affinity, allowing rapid repeated excitation at gamma frequency (30-80 Hz) [18]. Cholecystokinin (CCK)-expressing IINs also target cell somas and express calcium binding proteins (calbindin and PV). Thus, these IINs are suitable for sustaining intense synchronous activity. Non-fast spiking IINs expressing somatostatin (SOM) target apical dendrites of pyramidal neurons, to suppress specific losing synapses during path selection. IINs expressing vasoactive intestinal polypeptide (VIP) suppress the SOMs to disinhibit (enhance) the winning centers [19,20]. Neurogliaform cells (NGFCs) complement VIPs by inducing broad suppression of surrounding neurons [21]. Finally, Chandelier IINs targeting the axon initial segment induce rapid response suppression.

Management agents. The brain's response process is assisted by various agents, each supporting a specific process stage. The main **arousal agents** and their main roles are as follows. Orexin (hypocretin) conveys general needs, e.g., for food, and excites the dopamine system [22]. Vasopressin indicates the need

---

2 In addition, they can induce longer-term inhibition via G protein-coupled receptors.

for water and various social needs [23]. Histamine conveys the need to activate the immune system and to remove pathogens by itch [24]. Norepinephrine (NEP) is triggered by surprises and internal needs to induce global alert and energy recruitment (increased heart rate, vasoconstriction in the skin and gut, vasodilation in muscle and airways, glycogenolysis) [25]. Dopamine (DA) is triggered by strong need cues to support goal-setting [26] and immediate coarse responses [27]. Serotonin (SER) restrains rapid responses to promote slower, more patient, flexible planning [28].

All of these agents promote the formation of responses, so oppose the coordinated activity of large neuronal populations. Hence they need to be suppressed to allow sleep.

ACh. ACh has a unique role in sleep and is hence discussed at greater depth here. Its role in the response process is to support the selection and execution of focused responses. ACh acts via two receptor families, nicotinic (nAChR) and muscarinic (mAChR) receptors. nAChRs are ionotropic and excitatory. They have two common forms, alpha7, which is CP, and alpha4beta2, which is not permeable to calcium. The latter have a higher agonist affinity and desensitize rapidly, supporting efficient automated execution. mAChRs are G protein-coupled receptors with two sub-types, M1/3/5, which bind to Gq and suppress potassium channels to promote sustained activation, and M2/4, which bind to Gi/o to suppress the cell via potassium channels and reduced energy production.

Brain ACh is released by nuclei groups in the basal forebrain (BF, midbrain) and the brainstem [29]. The former send widespread innervation throughout cortex and hippocampus, while the latter innervate subcortical areas, including the thalamus, basal ganglia, agent nuclei and motor areas. The BF group is heavily innervated by cortex, most notably prefrontal cortex (PFC). ACh is released in a precise spatiotemporal manner [30], targeting both excitatory neurons and IINs. It increases glutamate release by excitatory neurons via alpha7 nAChRs [31], affects SOM IINs [32], PV IINs via presynaptic alpha4beta2 nAChRs [33], VIP IINs via nAChRs [34], and NGFC IINs via mAChRs [35]. Thus, **ACh promotes the emergence and sustenance of focused responses** by its strong effect on IINs and through a positive feedback loop with executing content neurons.

The strong relationship between ACh and focused execution is beyond doubt. It is the agent used by the motor unit to induce muscle contraction, and by the parasympathetic autonomic nervous system (ANS) to end the alert mode and support execution. It is known to promote attended execution and its ensuing plasticity [36].

The unfolded protein response (UPR). ACh has a strong effect on plasticity. In fact, its effect should be stronger than that of other agents, because the goal of plasticity is to automate the responses that were executed (this is the overarching principle of Hebbian learning), and ACh is the agent that directly promotes the winning, executing subset.

ACh promotes intracellular calcium, which is the main trigger of plasticity processes. ACh promotes direct Ca^{2+} entry into its target cells via alpha7 nAChRs, recruitment of Ca^{2+} from intracellular stores (endoplasmic reticulum) via M1/3/5 mAChRs, and indirect entry via M1/3 and all nAChRs by activating voltage-gated calcium channels (VGCCs) [30]. PV IINs, which are excited by alpha4beta2 nAChRs, enjoy calcium entry via highly expressed CP-AMPARs. ACh promotes the generation and release of nitric oxide (NO), which produces vasodilation to increase blood flow and also suppresses the Na^+/K^+-ATPase pump in choroid plexus cells, countering pump-dependent calcium extrusion [37]. Indeed, alpha7 nAChR is essential for ontogenic development [38], and neurogenesis, an extreme form of brain plasticity, is enhanced by M1 mAChR [39].

ACh-dependent response execution utilizes ATP. During execution, the endoplasmic reticulum and mitochondria form contact points (mitochondria-associated endoplasmic reticulum membrane) that serve for transfer of Ca^{2+} and lipids into mitochondria. This may deplete the endoplasmic reticulum of calcium, which triggers the UPR. Indeed, sleep deprivation increases interaction between endoplasmic reticulum and mitochondria and leads to ER stress [40]. The UPR can stall translation to make sure that things are managed, or can trigger apoptosis when there is no hope in fixing the situation.

We note that not all focused responses depend on ACh. Acute responses do, but automated (learned) responses utilize accurate contextual predictions, which minimize ACh-dependent competition. Novel responses involve Ca^{2+}, so utilize NMDA glutamate receptors, CP-AMPARs, and alpha7 nAChR, while automated responses utilize CI receptors.

In summary, brain operation consists of focused responses, selected and maintained by IINs with the essential support of ACh in case of novel (non-automated) responses.

14.4 Homeostasis and its restoration

The optimal state. Body tissues have an optimal homeostatic state, defined by extracellular and intracellular (cytoplasmic and intra-organelle) levels of various agents (ions, proteins, molecular debris, reactive oxygen species (ROS), neurotransmitters, neuromodulators etc.). The optimal state is important for both tissue health and performance.

Deviation from the optimal state can damage cells. Metabolism yields by-products that can damage cells via oxidative stress, and cells can accumulate agents (e.g., Ca^{2+}) that are toxic under many conditions [41]. Activity triggers genomic processes that can take hours and are easily impaired by activity-induced agents. Remnants of normal and pathogenic agents can aggregate and impair processing, and activate the immune system to induce inflammation.

Deviation from the optimal state is not only harmful in the long-term, but also impairs short-term performance. Brain function depends on neural responsiveness, which requires specific levels of ion concentration gradients and protein expression.

Ca^{2+} clearance is essential. During activity, Ca^{2+} enters brain cells in large amounts, due to the large concentration gradient across the cell's membrane and the presence of calcium-permeable channels. In addition, calcium is recruited from internal stores into the cytoplasm. Due to the internal gradients induced by proton pumping, Ca^{2+} enters mitochondria, where it signals the need for increased ATP production [42]. Ca^{2+} can rapidly accumulate in mitochondria, because the sodium-calcium exchanger that extrudes Ca^{2+} is slower than its uniporter. Excessive Ca^{2+} enhances the generation of ROS, and triggers Ca^{2+} extrusion via the mitochondria permeability transition pore, which can induce cytochrome c release and apoptosis [43].

Wake activity depends on the availability of ATP from mitochondria. To facilitate this, there is transfer of Ca^{2+} from the endoplasmic reticulum to mitochondria. Mitochondria Ca^{2+} enhances ATP production, but also depletes the endoplasmic reticulum of calcium, which can trigger **the unfolded protein response (UPR)** [44]. The UPR has two arms, one that slows down translation (protein synthesis) in order to allow the cell to recuperate from the intense utilization of resources, and another that involves apoptosis. The restoration done during sleep aims to increase the former and decrease the latter.

In this sense, **possibly the main role of sleep is to handle the second phase of plasticity, translation for protein synthesis** (the first being initial transcription of the needed proteins).

Wake activity induces a rapid rise in brain extracellular K^+ and a decrease in extracellular Ca^{2+} and extracellular volume [45], supporting a wake-induced neural accumulation of Ca^{2+}. Direct evidence for such accumulation has been found [46], where prolonged wake induced a sustained increase in intracellular Ca^{2+} and synaptic plasticity markers in sleep-inducing Drosophila R2 neurons.

Restoration mechanisms. Cells possess intricate mechanisms that restore the optimal state, including antioxidant enzymes, ion pumps, DNA repair processes, the unfolded protein response, degradation and clearance pathways (e.g., autophagy), and anti-inflammatory cytokines. Tissues possess restoration mechanisms beyond those of individual cells. The lymphatic system cleans the interstitial fluid of debris. In the brain, astrocytes maintain the perisynaptic environment, and microglia and astrocytes monitor inflammatory agents. Agents can diffuse into the extrasynaptic space, where they are generally out of the reach of astrocytes and can escape microglia but can affect cells via extrasynaptic receptors. The extrasynaptic space is continuously cleared via blood vessels, the CSF, and the glymphatic system [47].

However, this continuous restoration is insufficient, because as long as activity continues, these mechanisms cannot be fully utilized and are thus not fully effective. This holds for basically all tissue. I and others (see below) propose that the solution that evolution has found to this problem is to enforce a period of minimal activity, sleep. Indeed, sleep deprivation has been shown to be harmful to the cardiovascular, immune and endocrine systems [48,49], to muscle [50], and to the liver, lung, and small intestine [51].

State deviation, the brain, and ACh. The brain may need restoration more than other tissue. Its function depends on large ion concentration gradients, yielding high energy requirements and ROS production, yet its antioxidant mechanisms are relatively small compared to other tissue [52]. This issue pertains most strongly to ACh-supported paths, since these support prolonged focused execution that does not allow parallel effective maintenance. ACh neurons themselves are especially vulnerable. The number of ACh neurons is much smaller than the number of neurons in supported paths, so the load on each ACh neuron is high. Indeed, ACh neurons are impaired in almost all neuron degeneration disorders, as well as in normal aging [53].

State deviation increases excitability. In the optimal state, neurons are kept polarized, with pumps maintaining the large ion concentration gradients across membranes. As the optimal state degrades, neural excitability increases. The wake-induced decrease in brain extracellular Mg^{2+}, Ca^{2+} and H^+ [45] implies an increased permeability of NMDA receptors to Ca^{2+}, increased accumulation of cations in cells, and therefore increased cell depolarization and excitability.

Neuronal firing facilitates restoration. The exit of Ca^{2+} from the ER is triggered by increased cytoplasmic Ca^{2+} levels. Ca^{2+} clearance from mitochondria is primarily done by the sodium-calcium exchange pump (NCX). Since neural firing involves the cytoplasmic entry of Ca^{2+} via VGCCs and of sodium (Na^+) via VGSCs and HCN channels (Ih), firing quickly improves the conditions enabling the clearance of Ca^{2+} from internal stores. Firing also recruits astrocytes to clear the synaptic cleft and to promote neurovascular communication. As long as firing does not involve substantial Ca^{2+} entry, it does not have high energy requirements and its effect is to clear mitochondria from calcium. Under these conditions, firing supports restoration more effectively than pump operation alone.

Note that the increased neural excitability during wake constitutes a restoration mechanism, by promoting spontaneous neural firing from time to time. Some neurons are indeed restored by tonic firing (e.g., DA neurons, see below). Apparently, this mechanism is not sufficient for restoring neurons supporting sustained focused responses or the extracellular space.

Additional evidence. There is substantial evidence that sleep deprivation increases oxidative stress. Sleep deprivation with 36 hour survival training impaired antioxidant enzymes, induces muscle damage, and increased lipid peroxidation [50]. Sleep deprivation increased oxidative stress in PV IINs [54]. A single night of sleep deprivation in humans significantly reduced antioxidants, ATP, and morning cortisol [55]. Short sleep drosophila suffer from increased oxidative stress and shorter survival [56]. Some experiments found no oxidative damage following sleep deprivation [57], but the weight of the evidence points otherwise. A recent review concluded that the molecular correlates of sleep deprivation are related to ER stress, protein misfolding, and oxidative stress [58].

There is also evidence showing a direct benefit of sleep on homeostatic measures. Sleep increases chromosome dynamics, reducing accumulating neuronal DNA damage [59]. A comprehensive study found that the genes upregulated during sleep are mostly related to anabolic processes (cholesterol and protein synthesis, lipid transport, vesicle pools), antioxidation, and energy regulation [60].

14.5 NREM sleep

NREMS mechanisms are a relatively well-understood aspect of sleep [6,61], so here we only summarize the important points. Sleep is induced by suppressing arousal neurons, and involves reduced sensory input. NEP, OX and histamine amplify bottom-up sensory flow conveying needs, so their suppression is essential for sleep. DA and SER support top-down responses to sensory inputs, and can be allowed to continue their tonic firing. Indeed, DA neurons retain their mean firing rate during sleep (and can fire in bursts during REMS) [62], and the effect of SER on sleep is equivocal, generally promoting wake and suppressing REMS but also enhancing sleep in some situations [63].

When bottom-up flow is suppressed, the brain is left without triggers that drive the formation of focused responses. Thalamic neurons possess an inherent oscillation capacity due to ion channels and the interaction between excitatory neurons and inhibitory reticular nucleus (TRN) neurons [64], and can exert a strong excitatory drive over all cortical areas [65].

At the initial stage of sleep (N2), local corticothalamic interactions induce fast (10-15 Hz) EEG oscillations called spindles. An additional EEG phenomenon at this stage is the K-complex, sharp negative EEG deflections commonly having an external sensory (usually auditory) origin. As explained above, IINs tend to synchronize the neurons around them that receive dominant flow while suppressing others. When the flow conveyed by the thalamus is generated by inherent capacity (due to reduced sensory inputs), its cortical targets receive approximately the same flow, and the system gets into a global synchronous mode. This is slow-wave sleep (SWS). SWS is the exact opposite of wake and REMS, in that it involves the synchronous activity of large neuronal populations rather than of small focused paths.

Adenosine (ADN), a by-product of energy production, is the main agent conveying sleep pressure [66]. As more energy is produced, higher amounts of ADN are released into the extracellular space. ADN acts in two ways. First, the A1 receptor (A1R) suppresses ATP production via Gi/o and activates **potassium channels (KCs)**, most notably G protein-coupled inwardly-rectifying KCs (GIRK channels) [67]. KCs are normally activated after neural firing as part of the return to the cell's optimal state, and are important for SWA. The activation of KCs enables burst firing due to T-type VGCCs causing a low-threshold spike, on top of which a series of high frequency action potentials can ride [68]. Indeed, SWA is characterized by cycles comprised of a relatively long down state followed by a bursty up state [6]. SWA spindles are bursts and are probably induced by the TRN [69].

Importantly, ADN has a particularly strong effect in the basal forebrain, where ACh and sleep-inducing preoptic neurons are located. Following 3 hours of sleep deprivation, A1R-induced NFkB nuclear translocation occurs almost only in the ACh neurons of the basal forebrain [70]. A meta-analysis and an experiment showed that ADN accumulation is specifically high in the BF [71]. ACh inhibits the M-current, a potassium current, via M1 mAChRs, so the suppression of ACh release by ADN allows KC activation.

A second effect of ADN is that the A2A receptor (A2AR), which is excitatory, excites sleep-active neurons in selected areas. Important areas include the basal forebrain **ventral lateral preoptic area (VLPO)** and the **median preoptic area (MnPN)** [72], which mutually inhibit ACh, SER, and NEP neurons, and inhibit histamine neurons. VLPO neurons are also disinhibited by the effect of A1R on GABAergic neurons.

The projection neurons of the striatum nucleus of the basal ganglia (BG) oscillate between up and down states during sleep [73]. The BG contain two paths, D1 and D2. The D1 path, which participates in acute DA (D1R)-dependent responses, is suppressed by A1R as part of its arousal suppression role. The D2 path is suppressed by DA via D2Rs. ADN excites this path via A2A, which also reverses the effect of D2R [74], ensuring its restoration during sleep.

Consistent with slow-wave sleep being driven by a factor that gradually diminishes, it is most prominent in the first sleep cycle, decreasing in duration with further cycles.

It may be asked how SWS restores neurons if it involves bursty up-states, since bursts are associated with surprise and acute responses. There are at least three answers. First, extracellular Ca^{2+} and Mg^{2+} increase during sleep, which increases the probability of neurotransmitter release but decreases the opening of NMDARs [45]. This means that action potentials are facilitated but involve relatively little calcium influx, so their net effect is to clean cells. In other words, SWS bursts trigger intracellular restoration mechanisms while accumulation of harmful agents is greatly reduced compared to wake.[3] A second answer is that SWS does not involve sustained high-frequency (e.g., gamma range) firing of any single neuron, since SWS down states are relatively long. Finally, recording in non-human primates showed that SWS involves low firing rates and slow oscillations between cortical down and up states [75], so it is possible that the overall effect of bursts is small.

In addition to restoring neurons, SWA promotes the restoration of the extracellular space by facilitating blood flow via astrocytes, which improves clearing via the glymphatic system [76]. The vascular and glymphatic systems restore the extracellular space during both wake and sleep, but their action may be more efficient during sleep.

3 Accumulation via VGCCs may still occur, which may be another reason why several sleep cycles are required.

Additional evidence. The effect of ADN on sleep pressure is supported by a large amount of evidence [77]. For example, mice lacking the primary metabolizing enzyme of ADN show enhanced sleep drive, and A1 knockout significantly decreases sleep drive [78]. ADN inhibits all ACh neurons [67].

With respect to KCs, mutations in the Shaker KC and its promoters Hyperkinetic and sleepless reduce sleep and increase excitability in drosophila [79,80]. The sleepless gene antagonizes nAChRs, and lynx1, a mammalian homolog, can partially restore normal sleep to mutants [81]. Sleep duration decreased in 14 types of leak KC knockout mice, and a computational model showed that leak KCs can regulate SWA-like EEG along with Ca^{2+} channels [82]. The same group also showed that impaired Ca^{2+}-dependent KCs and VGCCs decrease sleep duration, while impaired plasma membrane Ca^{2+} ATPase increases sleep duration [83]. Finally, KCs are activated by most anesthetics [84].

An elegant demonstration of the role of specific wake activity in inducing sleep is given by the phenomenon of local sleep [85]. When an arm was immobilized during the day, during subsequent sleep, SWA over the corresponding cortical area was markedly reduced. Complementing this result, a learning task involving a specific brain region produced a local increase in sleep SWA.

The important role of slow wave activity in clearing the extracellular space was shown in [86], where a specific disruption of SWA increased CSF amyloid beta.

14.6 REM sleep

A recent review described the adaptive role of REMS as still being a complete mystery [4]. In the present theory, the main role of REMS is to restore ACh neurons. As explained above, ACh neurons are especially sensitive to deviations from the optimal state. However, they cannot be restored by SWA, because their inclusion would introduce a strong drive for competition and focused paths, preventing the global synchronous oscillations of SWA. For the same reason, they cannot be restored by tonic firing during wake. REM sleep follows SWS and restores ACh neurons through firing. Indeed, prolonged REMS deprivation specifically decreases ACh neuron size [87].[4]

Mechanistically, REMS is triggered by SWS-induced restoration of the extracellular space, which clears it from ADN. Since ADN most strongly affects the basal forebrain, its clearance disinhibits BF ACh neurons (and also brainstem ACh neurons). ACh neurons accumulate cations during wake, and are also excited by cortical projections during SWS. As a result, when they are disinhibited, they start firing. This firing drives the activation of focused sequences, which terminates SWS and induces dreaming (see below).

The hallmark of REMS are rapid eye movements. These occur because ACh supports attended execution, which involves saccades to attended spatial locations. The claustrum, which takes part in attending to spatial locations [89], is

[4] It also affects NE and SER neurons, but in an opposite manner [88].

activated during REMS and excites cortex [90], contributing to ACh-induced activations.

ACh-driven focused responses can induce strong muscle contraction. To prevent this, glutamatergic REMS SLD neurons innervate glycinergic neurons in the raphe magnus, the ventral and alpha gigantocellular nuclei, and the lateral paragigantocellular nucleus, which suppress spinal, facial and trigeminal motor neurons [91]. This induces muscle atonia. The circuits activating these SLD neurons during REMS are not fully clear. They are suppressed during wake, possibly via tonic GABAergic inputs arriving from the brainstem ventrolateral periaqueductal grey (vlPAG) and the dorsal (or deep) mesencephalic reticular nucleus (dMeRN).

The suppression of arousal neurons must continue during REMS, otherwise they would induce wake. A population of GABAergic/galaninergic neurons in the extended VLPO suppresses the DRN (SER), LC (NEP) and vlPAG/dMeRN [2]. Neurons in the dorsal paragigantocellular reticular and lateral paragigantocellular nuclei also suppress LC NEP neurons during REMS.

MCH. Lateral hypothalamic (HT) melanin-concentrating hormone (MCH) neurons fire during sleep, and mediate object exploration, eating, maternal behavior, and olfaction [92,93]. They mutually suppress NEP, suppress orexin, histamine, SER and wake-only ACh neurons, and are excited by HT oxytocin neurons [94,95]. Thus, MCH promotes satisfaction and terminates need-induced arousal. The former explains the activity of MCH neurons during sleep, and the latter explains the association between sleep and **satiety**. Since MCH neurons promote object exploration, they participate in focused responses, explaining why they are mostly active during REMS [96].

SWRs. Sharp-wave ripples [97] occur during both wake and sleep. In sleep, they occur mostly during NREM, but they bear a greater resemblance to REMS activity than to SWA. They occur at the final stages of SWS, when the brain has been sufficiently restored to allow some neurons to escape from the synchronous oscillations imposed by the thalamus.

As in REMS, the first neurons to fire individually are those that have accumulated more cations during previous wake activity. Some evidence for this is provided by the fact that the source of SWRs are the principal neurons in the CA3 field of the hippocampus. These neurons are unique in the brain in that during acute responses they are excited not only by Ca^{2+} but also by Zn^{2+} [98]. Zinc is a strong promoter of proliferation and plasticity, so zinc-innervated neurons are expected to be among the first to fire. Their activation ripples through the hippocampus CA1 field and into cortical areas.

SWRs have been shown to be capable of recapitulating wake sequences. However, 'replay' is just one pattern among many exhibited by SWRs [99].[5] Both data points support our account, because firing order during sleep is determined by cation accumulation and does not necessarily recapitulate wake order, although it may do so (see dreaming below).

[5] Wake SWRs (at least some of them) are involved in planning future actions [100].

14.7 Consciousness

Possibly the most perplexing features of sleep are the complete lack of consciousness during SWA, and the sense of reality felt during dreaming. The scientific examination of consciousness is a deep and contentious field of study [101]. Because consciousness is a subjective feeling, it is currently accessible to science only via **reporting** (by words or actions) [102]. Fortunately, to explain the relationship between consciousness and sleep, we only need an aspect of consciousness that we hope would be relatively uncontested, the fact that it involves focused responses.

The key observation is that consciousness involves **specific content**. We can be conscious of the external world, in which case we perceive specific objects and events. We can be conscious of internal brain activations (silent speech, music, static or dynamic imagery) without external sensory inputs, and these are specific as well (silent speech involves a sequence of well-defined words in a particular order, imagery has well-defined visual components, etc.).[6] Finally, it can be argued that consciousness of being alive is the core consciousness feeling and that it is different from thinking. The feeling of being alive depends on attending to interoceptive sensory inputs, possibly cardiorespiratory inputs, which arrive at highly specific cortical locations [103]. This is supported by Cotard's syndrome, in which patients deny being alive and which is associated with right frontal (especially insular) lesions [104]. Note that the right insula receives the strongest heart inputs.

Since the content of consciousness is specific, it involves the activation of a small and focused set of neurons representing this content. With respect to reporting, regardless of whether it is only a scientific way to investigate consciousness or is its crucial defining aspect, it clearly involves focused responses. In other words, *both the content of consciousness and its reporting require focused responses.*

Using this observation, the lack of consciousness during SWA is readily explained by the fact that the synchronous activity of large neuronal populations prevents focused responses. Note that a similar situation occurs during epileptic seizures.

A serious theory of consciousness posits that it requires a global broadcast of information in cortex [102], which may seem to oppose focused paths. However, the broadcast of this theory exactly corresponds to the our activation of candidates competing for inclusion in a focused response. Thus, the two accounts are complementary.[7]

Dreaming. In REMS, the main sleep stage associated with dreaming, focused paths are strongly encouraged by ACh. Focused paths can emerge during NREM

[6] This argument holds regardless of how exactly imagery and thought are implemented in the brain.

[7] Note that we do not equate focused responses with consciousness. For example, highly automated and/or unattended responses are focused but involve very little competition, and it is indeed common not to remember (be aware of) having performed such actions.

without ACh to yield SWRs, since firing excitatory neurons send coordination requests to local IINs. When the synchronizing power of the thalamus diminishes, this can induce competition with focused winners. As during wake and REMS, competition resolution quickly induces forward activations, explaining the association between SWRs at the final NREM stage and dreaming [105].

The sense of consciousness felt during dreaming arises because the neurons activated during dreaming include content neurons that are activated in focused paths during wake.

A fake sense of reality (i.e., one independent of external reality) is not unique to sleep. It can occur during wake, and can be easily induced in healthy people by various hallucinogens [106]. Since a sense of reality requires focused paths, disrupting the signaling of any agent that supports these, including ACh, SER and DA, can induce hallucinations. Conversely, the nAChR agonist nicotine generally sharpens attention (reality).

Thus, the question unique to sleep (the lack or presence of consciousness of reality) is readily answered: sleep suppresses (during SWS) or activates (during REMS) the same neurons inducing the sense of reality during wake. The questions pertaining to both wake and sleep (which neurons are these, what mechanisms are used) are not answered here.[8] In other words, the core issue is not the fact that sleep can obliterate or induce a sense of reality, but the sense of reality itself.

Dreams rarely recapitulate the events experienced during wake [107]. This may seem at odds with our theory, because the drive of neuronal firing during dreams is cations accumulated during wake events. However, real events are represented by a highly distributed network of neurons firing at precise temporal sequences, and the various neurons involved do not accumulate cations at the same rate. Thus, the content of dreams is strongly inspired by the components of wake events, but does not recapitulate their order or logic.

Dream stories are commonly not logical or are plainly impossible (e.g., flying), and develop without a sense of control [105]. This is what we would expect, since the brain can clearly conjure up illogical imagery as long as it can represent its individual components. Dreams are also commonly highly emotional, which can be explained by the strong activity of emotion circuits during wake, reflected by a high activation of the amygdala during REMS [107]. Lucid dreamers are people who are aware that they are dreaming while they do so, and some can exert some control over dream content. Awareness of one's situation involves a report, and the focused responses that allow reports are in principle possible during sleep (similarly to dream content). The capacity of exerting control over dream content points to a higher than normal activation of control areas (e.g., dlPFC) during dreaming, possibly due to increased innervation by ACh or DA. DA is the agent supporting goal-setting, which is a major component of the sense of control. DA neurons continue firing during sleep, and

8 Although the natural conclusion of our discussion is that consciousness can be fully explained as reports of interoceptive representations, implemented in the same way as other reporting actions.

can fire bursts during REMS [62]. Being aware of dreaming may be based on short term memory of getting ready to sleep and the plausibility of the dream scenario.

People usually forget their dreams soon after waking up. This supports our argument that neuronal firing during sleep involves relatively little Ca^{2+} influx (see bursts above), since the latter would initiate long-term plasticity processes. Recalling a dream after waking up relies on short-term cellular excitability, which is restored quickly during wake.

Dreaming is a completely different brain mode from visual imagery during wake. Dreaming involves the activation of the same neurons activated when experiencing reality, while imagery most likely does not. Indeed, images in dreams are described as more vivid than in imagery [105].

Dreams can be useful for finding creative solutions to problems that occupy the dreamer during wake [1]. This occurs because dreams search the solution space in an unrestrained way, while during wake it is searched via focused responses, which are shaped by habitual ways of thinking, preconceptions and specific goals.

In summary, dreams are a side-effect of optimal state restoration. They have no particular role, but can be useful for creativity. Their content reflects the dreamer's wake activities and thoughts, and is experienced as real because the neurons involved in wake perception and dreaming are the same neurons.

Additional evidence. ACh, the agent supporting focused responses, has been described as the 'neurotransmitter correlate of consciousness', based on its effects on attention, disorders, and anesthesia [108]. A recent review concluded that the minimal set of neurons required for a conscious percept includes a temporo-parieto-occipital area associated with perceptual experiences, and a frontal area associated with thought-like (i.e., reporting) experiences [109]. During dreaming, posterior areas generally exhibit reduced low frequency EEG activity, with high frequency activity being associated with specific content [109]. A meta-analysis showed that dreaming involves increased activation in posterior parietal cortex, mPFC, and hippocampus (all of which are heavily innervated by ACh), and reduced activation in dlPFC, inferior frontal gyrus, and OFC (all DA-dominated areas) [110]. In addition, lack of consciousness (albeit via propofol, which blocks NEP) was characterized by disintegration of interareal synchrony, which is a property of focused responses [111].

14.8 Memory and plasticity

Sleep is clearly important for learning [7]. Sleep deprivation impairs, and sleep enhances, learning. Several theories view memory consolidation or plasticity as the main role of sleep [1,8].

In the present theory, improved learning is a natural result of restoration of the optimal homeostatic state, which improves all brain processes. Specifically, restoration of the intracellular space is essential for the genomic processes triggered by wake activity. In addition, the significant ACh flow into cortex during REMS serves as a powerful plasticity catalyst.

The synaptic homeostasis hypothesis (SHY) [112] argues that wake activity strengthens synapses and that this process cannot go on indefinitely due to increased energy requirements, decreased performance (signal to noise), and saturated learning. In SHY, the role of sleep is to normalize plasticity by synapse weakening. Indeed, SHY cites evidence that synapse sizes and numbers decrease only if flies are allowed to sleep, and that sleep/wakefulness yield net spine loss/gain, respectively. Conversely, much evidence counters SHY. For example, sleep involves both synaptic strengthening and weakening [113], most cortical synapses are upregulated during SWS [114], and there is LTP during SWS [115]. Behaviorally, sleep induces both memory consolidation and forgetting [116].

The notion of focused responses, emphasized by the present theory, bridges these two accounts. Recall that focused responses result from competition between a possibly large number of candidates. Thus, the number of losing synapses is much larger than the number of winning ones. Moreover, acute responses induce intracellular Ca^{2+}, which stimulates the formation of new spines, and many of those are associated with losers. Post-execution plasticity weakens or removes the losers and enhances the winners. Our account predicts that synapse weakening should statistically dominate, but that some synapses would be strengthened or retained.

This is exactly what the evidence shows. In [117], sleep induced a GluA1 (an AMPAR subunit) increase in some spines, but a reduction in a larger number of spines. In [118], the axon-dendritic spine contact area decreased by about 20% during sleep, but this held only for the smaller 80% of the spines. In other words, stronger synapses were not downscaled. According with the strengthening of some synapses, NREMS involved the removal of CP-AMPARs, which make synapses more labile [119]. Sleep augmented the connectivity and firing rates of stimulus-selective neurons, and decreased those of less selective (i.e., competition losing) neurons [120]. In [121], REMS pruned new spines created after motor learning, facilitated subsequently generated spines, and strengthened a fraction of new spines. Reactivation of task-specific neurons during NREMS was involved in forming new synapses after learning [122]. Firing rate responses to stimuli are potentiated during sleep, not wake, and are blocked by sleep deprivation [123]. Finally, LTP yields increased spine size, but also an overall decreased spine density, via local competition between stimulated spines [124].

Mechanistically, whether a synapse or spine is weakened or enhanced can be based on Ca^{2+} amplitude, duration, or influx location [125], and on the effect of neurotrophic agents. BDNF enhances synapses via the TrkB receptor, while proBDNF weakens them via the p75 receptor [126].

Another piece of evidence that supports our account is that waking rest also contributes to memory consolidation [127]. Waking rest allows restoration, which has a positive effect on plasticity.

It should be mentioned that glucocorticoids (cortisol in humans) are released during sleep (albeit in small amounts), and so is testosterone in males. Both of these agents support plasticity.

14.9 Anesthesia

Anesthetics are exogenous drugs and discussing each of them at depth is out of the scope of this paper. Nonetheless, their general mechanisms of action, and their effects on consciousness, are readily explained by the present theory. Anesthesia is usually defined via the end-points of unconsciousness, amnesia, analgesia, and immobility. Like sleep, anesthesia is considered to be mysterious [128]. It is perplexing that a relatively large and structurally diverse group of molecules can induce a similar sleep-like state.

The theory here explains anesthesia by noting that each family of anesthetics makes use of a mechanism that is either used by sleep or prevents focused responses by other means. Classical anesthetics activate the sleep-inducing VLPO neurons [129]. Most general anesthetics target potassium channels (KCs) and other ion channels [84,128]. For example, isoflurane and sevoflurane activate KCs, while propofol suppresses VGSCs. Propofol also suppresses NEP, the main arousal agent. These are the same mechanisms that promote sleep.

Most anesthetics potentiate GABAA-induced currents and directly activate GABAA receptors at higher concentrations. While GABA is not a sleep-specific agent, wide activation of GABARs recruits their suppressive action and does not allow focused responses. Note that GABAB receptors activate KCs via Gi/o.

Anesthetics are commonly applied when normal sleep pressure is not strong enough, and when strong sensory input (pain) is generated. Hence, they must be continuously provided in order to sustain anesthesia, but there are cases of intraoperative awareness during anesthesia.

Ketamine, xenon and nitrous oxide are commonly viewed as special cases. They (especially the first two) inhibit NMDARs, possibly by competing with the co-agonist glycine. Ketamine blocks calcium-permeable (CP) glutamate receptors, but promotes calcium-impermeable AMPARs [130]. Thus, it suppresses acute responses, but can increase spontaneous neural firing. This counters normal consciousness and thinking, but the effect is not sleep-like. Indeed, ketamine yields a trance-like state, while other anesthetics induce a sleep-like state. Nitrous oxide and xenon inhibit alpha7nAChR [131], the CP ACh receptor that most strongly promotes focused responses.

14.10 Discussion

This chapter presented the first comprehensive biological theory of sleep. Our main thesis is that sleep serves to restore the optimal homeostatic state, which degrades during wake, with an emphasis on restoring endoplasmic reticulum Ca^{2+} in order to prevents the UPR's apoptosis arms and continue supporting translation. All major aspects of sleep can be explained by understanding the central role of focused responses in wake activity and of the cation accumulation that they induce. ADN and circadian circuits apply sleep pressure by suppressing arousal neurons, and this lets the thalamus and cortex self-organize in an oscillatory SWA pattern that restores the optimal state. In general, REMS restores ACh neurons, while NREMS restores other neurons and the extracellular space. Optimal state restoration facilitates all brain processes, including memory consolidation and overall plasticity. Global oscillations do not allow consciousness during SWS, while the sense of reality associated with dreaming results from the activation of neurons implementing focused responses during both wake and dreams.

Relationship with existing theories. I agree with the benefits of sleep proposed by previous theories cited above. Sleep restores intracellular energy stores, whose usage is triggered by NEP, which is suppressed during sleep. Sleep lets the glymphatic and other systems clear the extracellular space. By restoring the optimal state, it counters wake-induced performance degradation, improves cell health, reduces oxidative stress, and improves plasticity. The specific aspects that are novel in the present theory are the emphasis on and mechanistic description of focused responses and Ca^{2+} accumulation, the role of ACh, the account of consciousness and dreaming, and the realization that these are sufficient to present a complete story.

It has been proposed that sleep promotes creativity and downregulates the emotional aspects of events to support calm planning and reduce anxiety and false alerts [1]. The former indeed holds (see creativity and dreams above). The latter requires clarification. Sleep enhances the responses executed during wake. Normally, these are focused responses that suppress their emotional triggers via the parasympathetic ANS (promoted by ACh). In these cases, sleep would indeed enhance TD control over learned emotional reactions. However, sometimes the nature of alerts is such that they trigger innate responses or coarse adaptive responses. In this case, plasticity processes, and thus sleep as well, would enhance these responses, yielding emotional hyper-sensitivity (as occurs e.g. in PTSD). Recollection of emotional events involves a far smaller activation of the sympathetic ANS than when the event occurs, but this is not due to sleep but to the lack of surprising bursts and emotion-inducing sensory inputs.

Other tissue. In this paper we emphasized brain processes, because the sleep state is managed by the brain. Nonetheless, sleep is important for restoring other body tissues as well. For example, sleep promotes immune memory consolidation and restores immune cells [132] (see above for additional tissues).

Note that the function of the immune system is close to that of sleep. Sleep restores degradation resulting from normal activity, while the immune system generally addresses degradation resulting from abnormal situations (direct threats, damage to blood vessels, etc.). However, the dividing line is diffuse, because the presence of excessive levels of normal agents, even if resulting from normal activity, can activate the immune system. In such cases, sleep and immunity would cooperate towards the same goal.

Animals get sleepy after eating. The gut may use unique mechanisms to trigger sleep after eating, but at least some of the association can be explained via MCH (see above). In addition, OX neurons, which provide a major part of arousal input, are suppressed by glucose. When OX neurons are silent, the excitation of DA and NEP neurons is reduced and that of MCH neurons is increased, inducing further suppression of arousal.

Restoration of DA, NEP, SER, and OX neurons. The arousal neurons releasing OX, DA, NEP and SER widely innervate the brain to support acute responses during wake and are thus in need of restoration. However, NEP and OX neurons are suppressed during all sleep stages, and the data with respect to DA and SER is equivocal, which seems to contradict our main thesis. This issue is resolved by noting that all of these neurons are tonically active during wake, and at least DA neurons are tonically active during sleep as well. We propose that their restoration is assisted by this tonic firing. ACh neurons are different because they are under heavier load, are more important for plasticity, and their tonic firing could promote the erroneous formation of focused responses. Most of these arousal neurons express suppressive autoreceptors (alpha2-NER, D2R, SER1a, M2/4 mAChR), providing another protection mechanism.

Some cortical areas strongly innervated by DA (e.g., dlPFC) are normally not heavily innervated by ACh. These areas undergo plasticity just as the rest of the brain (possibly more, since development of frontal areas is disproportional during adolescence, a critical period in brain plasticity). DA neurons fire bursts during REMS (see above), which may indicate that NREM is not sufficient for plasticity. Indeed, although specific REMS suppression does not always induce a strong behavioral effect [4], several experiments showed that it induces neuronal apoptosis and mitochondrial damage [133]. Thus, REMS may indeed be crucial for memory.

Restoration vs. plasticity. The role assigned to sleep here is state restoration, while plasticity (memory consolidation) was presented as a side-effect. Note that we could have said that the root cause of sleep is that the body is an adaptive (learning) system based on Ca^{2+}. Since Ca^{2+} signaling is metabolically demanding, increases oxidative stress, and can trigger apoptotic processes, it has also promoted the evolution of a special state to undo these undesired side-effects. Thus, memory and restoration are tightly interconnected.

Sleep disorders. Sleep involves many mechanisms, and an impairment in each of them can impair it. For example, impairments in the OX or neurovascular systems can interfere with the normal sleep-wake cycle. Discussing sleep disorders at any reasonable depth is out of the scope of this paper.

Sleep across species. This chapter focused on sleep in humans. REMS and NREMS are unique to mammals and avian species, and are the phenomena that make sleep so fascinating to us. Sleep can be defined across species via EEG and behavior, and the results are highly correlated, showing that both invertebrates and vertebrates exhibit sleep-like states [134]. Although some research was done on a few model species (e.g., roundworms, fruit flies and zebrafish), not much is known for the majority of species. It is a theory prediction that restoration is what drives sleep states in all species, but the mechanisms may be different, just as brain anatomy, limbs and hormones are different across species. For example, dolphins exhibit unihemispheric sleep [5]. Nonetheless, the fact that sleep is strongly affected by potassium channels even in drosophila [79] points to a potentially high degree of shared basic principles between different species.

Future work. Most aspects of the theory here are supported by solid experimental evidence. The existence and nature of focused responses, their promotion by ACh, the degradation of homeostasis induced by sleep, the damages associated with it, and the positive effect of sleep on homeostasis and plasticity are beyond doubt. Many of the circuits and agents involved in transition between sleep stages have been mapped.

Future research should provide more evidence for the following. First, direct evidence that what triggers neuronal firing during SWRs and REMS is cation accumulation is needed. Second, it is important to discover the exact location of the representations giving rise to the sense of reality, during both wake and sleep. In addition to pure science, such a discovery could be of enormous practical use for making informed decisions for and possibly treating patients in comatose situations. Third, the mechanistic circuits promoting NREMS and REMS have not been fully mapped (e.g., it is not clear what activates REMS SLD neurons). In addition, sleep-active neurons exist in many brain areas [135], and have not been fully elucidated yet. Fourth, ADN may not be the only agent conveying sleep pressure; other agents (e.g., ROS) could complement its action. Fifth, zinc is probably important for sleep [136], but its role is not fully clear. Sixth, our understanding of sleep mechanisms in different species is only rudimentary. Finally, a theory of sleep should have implications for the treatment of sleep disorders.

14.11 Conclusion

In summary, I have presented the first comprehensive theory of sleep. By focusing on a small number of key notions, the most important of which being the notion of focused responses, it allows the integration of existing knowledge to provide a concrete biological account of all major aspects of sleep. Sleep is not a mystery but a biological state with a clear biological logic and well-defined mechanisms.

Acknowledgment

I thank Prof. Marcos G. Frank for comments on the first published version of this paper.

References

[1] M. Walker, Why We Sleep: Unlocking the Power of Sleep and Dreams, Simon and Schuster, 2017.

[2] T.E. Scammell, E. Arrigoni, J.O. Lipton, Neural circuitry of wakefulness and sleep, Neuron 93 (4) (2017) 747–765.
[3] W.J. Joiner, Unraveling the evolutionary determinants of sleep, Current Biology 26 (20) (2016) R1073–R1087.
[4] J.M. Siegel, REM sleep: a biological and psychological paradox, Sleep Medicine Reviews 15 (3) (2011) 139.
[5] S. Miyazaki, C.Y. Liu, Y. Hayashi, Sleep in vertebrate and invertebrate animals, and insights into the function and evolution of sleep, Neuroscience Research 118 (2017) 3–12.
[6] R.E. Brown, R. Basheer, J.T. McKenna, R.E. Strecker, R.W. McCarley, Control of sleep and wakefulness, Physiological Reviews 92 (3) (2012) 1087–1187.
[7] B. Rasch, J. Born, About sleep's role in memory, Physiological Reviews 93 (2) (2013) 681–766.
[8] J.M. Krueger, M.G. Frank, J.P. Wisor, S. Roy, Sleep function: toward elucidating an enigma, Sleep Medicine Reviews 28 (2016) 46–54.
[9] V.M. Hill, R.M. O'connor, M. Shirasu-Hiza, Tired and stressed: examining the need for sleep, European Journal of Neuroscience 51 (1) (2020) 494–508, https://doi.org/10.1111/ejn.14197.
[10] R. Desimone, J. Duncan, Neural mechanisms of selective visual attention, Annual Review of Neuroscience 18 (1) (1995) 193–222.
[11] J. Fuster, The Prefrontal Cortex, 5th ed., Academic Press, 2015.
[12] R.A. Adams, S. Shipp, K.J. Friston, Predictions not commands: active inference in the motor system, Brain Structure and Function 218 (3) (2013) 611–643.
[13] M. Ahissar, S. Hochstein, The reverse hierarchy theory of visual perceptual learning, Trends in Cognitive Sciences 8 (10) (2004) 457–464.
[14] B. Kotchoubey, Event-related potentials, cognition, and behavior: a biological approach, Neuroscience and Biobehavioral Reviews 30 (1) (2006) 42–65.
[15] S.N. Chettih, C.D. Harvey, Single-neuron perturbations reveal feature-specific competition in V1, Nature (2019) 334–340.
[16] R. Tremblay, S. Lee, B. Rudy, GABAergic interneurons in the neocortex: from cellular properties to circuits, Neuron 91 (2) (2016) 260–292.
[17] H.X. Wang, W.J. Gao, Development of calcium-permeable AMPA receptors and their correlation with NMDA receptors in fast-spiking interneurons of rat prefrontal cortex, Journal of Physiology 588 (15) (2010) 2823–2838.
[18] Henzl MT. Parvalbumin, in: Encyclopedia of Metalloproteins, Springer, 2013, pp. 1669–1678.
[19] J.J. Letzkus, S.B. Wolff, A. Lüthi, Disinhibition, a circuit mechanism for associative learning and memory, Neuron 88 (2) (2015) 264–276.
[20] M.M. Karnani, J. Jackson, I. Ayzenshtat, A.H. Sichani, K. Manoocheri, S. Kim, et al., Opening holes in the blanket of inhibition: localized lateral disinhibition by VIP interneurons, The Journal of Neuroscience 36 (12) (2016) 3471–3480.
[21] X. Jiang, G. Wang, A.J. Lee, R.L. Stornetta, J.J. Zhu, The organization of two new cortical interneuronal circuits, Nature Neuroscience 16 (2) (2013) 210–218.
[22] Q. Chen, L. de Lecea, Z. Hu, D. Gao, The hypocretin/orexin system: an increasingly important role in neuropsychiatry, Medicinal Research Reviews 35 (1) (2015) 152–197.
[23] R. Stoop, Neuromodulation by oxytocin and vasopressin, Neuron 76 (1) (2012) 142–159.
[24] H.L. Haas, O.A. Sergeeva, O. Selbach, Histamine in the nervous system, Physiological Reviews 88 (3) (2008) 1183–1241.
[25] G. Santulli, The adrenergic system in cardiovascular metabolism and aging, in: A. Lymperopoulos (Ed.), The Cardiovascular Adrenergic System, Springer, 2015, pp. 97–116.
[26] J.D. Salamone, M. Correa, The mysterious motivational functions of mesolimbic dopamine, Neuron 76 (3) (2012) 470–485.
[27] S.A. Sharples, K. Koblinger, J.M. Humphreys, P.J. Whelan, Dopamine: a parallel pathway for the modulation of spinal locomotor networks, Frontiers in Neural Circuits 8 (2014) 55.
[28] J.W. Dalley, J. Roiser, Dopamine, serotonin and impulsivity, Neuroscience 215 (2012) 42–58.

[29] M.M. Mesulam, Cholinergic circuitry of the human nucleus basalis and its fate in Alzheimer's disease, Journal of Comparative Neurology 521 (18) (2013) 4124–4144.
[30] W. Muñoz, B. Rudy, Spatiotemporal specificity in cholinergic control of neocortical function, Current Opinion in Neurobiology 26 (2014) 149–160.
[31] J.L. Yakel, Nicotinic ACh receptors in the hippocampal circuit, functional expression and role in synaptic plasticity, Journal of Physiology 592 (19) (2014) 4147–4153.
[32] E.E. Fanselow, K.A. Richardson, B.W. Connors, Selective, state-dependent activation of somatostatin-expressing inhibitory interneurons in mouse neocortex, Journal of Neurophysiology 100 (5) (2008) 2640–2652.
[33] E.X. Albuquerque, E.F. Pereira, M. Alkondon, S.W. Rogers, Mammalian nicotinic acetylcholine receptors: from structure to function, Physiological Reviews 89 (1) (2009) 73–120.
[34] Y. Fu, J.M. Tucciarone, J.S. Espinosa, N. Sheng, D.P. Darcy, R.A. Nicoll, et al., A cortical circuit for gain control by behavioral state, Cell 156 (6) (2014) 1139–1152.
[35] A. Brombas, L.N. Fletcher, S.R. Williams, Activity-dependent modulation of layer 1 inhibitory neocortical circuits by acetylcholine, The Journal of Neuroscience 34 (5) (2014) 1932–1941.
[36] M. Sarter, C. Lustig, A.S. Berry, H. Gritton, W.M. Howe, V. Parikh, What do phasic cholinergic signals do?, Neurobiology of Learning and Memory 130 (2016) 135–141.
[37] D.Z. Ellis, J.A. Nathanson, K.J. Sweadner, Carbachol inhibits Na+-K+-ATPase activity in choroid plexus via stimulation of the NO/cGMP pathway, American Journal of Physiology. Cell Physiology 279 (6) (2000) C1685–C1693.
[38] C.C. Fernandes, A.F. Lozada, D.K. Berg, Nicotinic signaling in development, in: Nicotinic Receptors, Springer, 2014, pp. 115–135.
[39] J.M. Van Kampen, C.B. Eckman, Agonist-induced restoration of hippocampal neurogenesis and cognitive improvement in a model of cholinergic denervation, Neuropharmacology 58 (6) (2010) 921–929.
[40] A. Aboufares El Alaoui, E. Buhl, S. Galizia, J.J. Hodge, L. de Vivo, M. Bellesi, Increased interaction between endoplasmic reticulum and mitochondria following sleep deprivation, BMC Biology 21 (1) (2023) 1.
[41] N.M. Connolly, J.H. Prehn, The metabolic response to excitotoxicity–lessons from single-cell imaging, Journal of Bioenergetics and Biomembranes 47 (1–2) (2015) 75–88.
[42] M. Gleichmann, M.P. Mattson, Neuronal calcium homeostasis and dysregulation, Antioxidants & Redox Signalling 14 (7) (2011) 1261–1273.
[43] P.S. Brookes, Y. Yoon, J.L. Robotham, M. Anders, S.S. Sheu, Calcium, ATP, and ROS: a mitochondrial love-hate triangle, American Journal of Physiology. Cell Physiology 287 (4) (2004) C817–C833.
[44] N. Naidoo, Sleep loss and the unfolded protein response, in: Sleep and Its Disorders: Translational Medicine, Springer, 2022, pp. 127–147.
[45] F. Ding, J. O'Donnell, Q. Xu, N. Kang, N. Goldman, M. Nedergaard, Changes in the composition of brain interstitial ions control the sleep-wake cycle, Science 352 (6285) (2016) 550–555.
[46] S. Liu, Q. Liu, M. Tabuchi, M.N. Wu, Sleep drive is encoded by neural plastic changes in a dedicated circuit, Cell 165 (6) (2016) 1347–1360.
[47] N.A. Jessen, A.S.F. Munk, I. Lundgaard, M. Nedergaard, The glymphatic system: a beginner's guide, Neurochemical Research 40 (12) (2015) 2583–2599.
[48] H. Liu, A. Chen, Roles of sleep deprivation in cardiovascular dysfunctions, Life Sciences 219 (2019) 231–237.
[49] J. Orzeł-Gryglewska, Consequences of sleep deprivation, International Journal of Occupational Medicine and Environmental Health 23 (1) (2010) 95–114.
[50] E. Jówko, P. Różański, A. Tomczak, Effects of a 36-h survival training with sleep deprivation on oxidative stress and muscle damage biomarkers in young healthy men, International Journal of Environmental Research and Public Health 15 (10) (2018) 2066.

[51] C.A. Everson, C.J. Henchen, A. Szabo, N. Hogg, Cell injury and repair resulting from sleep loss and sleep recovery in laboratory rats, Sleep 37 (12) (2014) 1929–1940.
[52] J.N. Cobley, M.L. Fiorello, D.M. Bailey, 13 reasons why the brain is susceptible to oxidative stress, Redox Biology 15 (2018) 490–503.
[53] R. Schliebs, T. Arendt, The cholinergic system in aging and neuronal degeneration, Behavioural Brain Research 221 (2) (2011) 555–563.
[54] J.H. Harkness, P.N. Bushana, R.P. Todd, W.C. Clegern, B.A. Sorg, J.P. Wisor, Sleep disruption elevates oxidative stress in parvalbumin-positive cells of the rat cerebral cortex, Sleep (2018), 42(1):zsy201<doi>10.1093/sleep/zsy201.</doi>.
[55] M.S. Trivedi, D. Holger, A.T. Bui, T.J. Craddock, J.L. Tartar, Short-term sleep deprivation leads to decreased systemic redox metabolites and altered epigenetic status, PLoS ONE (2017), 12(7):e0181978.
[56] V.M. Hill, R.M. O'Connor, G.B. Sissoko, I.S. Irobunda, S. Leong, J.C. Canman, et al., A bidirectional relationship between sleep and oxidative stress in Drosophila, PLoS Biology 16 (7) (2018) e2005206.
[57] A. Gopalakrishnan, L.L. Ji, C. Cirelli, Sleep deprivation and cellular responses to oxidative stress, Sleep 27 (1) (2004) 27–35.
[58] N. Naidoo, Sleep loss and neuronal stress, in: Sleep, Memory and Synaptic Plasticity, Springer, 2019, pp. 57–76.
[59] D. Zada, I. Bronshtein, T. Lerer-Goldshtein, Y. Garini, L. Appelbaum, Sleep increases chromosome dynamics to enable reduction of accumulating DNA damage in single neurons, Nature Communications 10 (1) (2019) 895.
[60] M. Mackiewicz, K.R. Shockley, M.A. Romer, R.J. Galante, J.E. Zimmerman, N. Naidoo, et al., Macromolecule biosynthesis: a key function of sleep, Physiological Genomics 31 (3) (2007) 441–457.
[61] G.T. Neske, The slow oscillation in cortical and thalamic networks: mechanisms and functions, Frontiers in Neural Circuits 9 (2016) 88.
[62] P. Torterolo, L. Benedetto, J.M. Monti, Functional interactions between MCHergic and dopaminergic neurons: role in the control of wakefulness and sleep, in: Dopamine and Sleep, Springer, 2016, pp. 47–63.
[63] J.M. Monti, Serotonin control of sleep-wake behavior, Sleep Medicine Reviews 15 (4) (2011) 269–281.
[64] J.R. Huguenard, D.A. McCormick, Thalamic synchrony and dynamic regulation of global forebrain oscillations, Trends in Neurosciences 30 (7) (2007) 350–356.
[65] F. Clascá, P. Rubio-Garrido, D. Jabaudon, Unveiling the diversity of thalamocortical neuron subtypes, European Journal of Neuroscience 35 (10) (2012) 1524–1532.
[66] T. Porkka-Heiskanen, A.V. Kalinchuk, Adenosine, energy metabolism and sleep homeostasis, Sleep Medicine Reviews 15 (2) (2011) 123–135.
[67] D.G. Rainnie, H.C. Grunze, R.W. McCarley, R.W. Greene, Adenosine inhibition of mesopontine cholinergic neurons: implications for EEG arousal, Science 263 (5147) (1994) 689–692.
[68] E. Cheong, Shin HS. T-type, Ca^{2+} channels in normal and abnormal brain functions, Physiological Reviews 93 (3) (2013) 961–992.
[69] A. Lüthi, Sleep spindles: where they come from, what they do, The Neuroscientist 20 (3) (2014) 243–256.
[70] V. Ramesh, H.S. Thatte, R.W. McCarley, R. Basheer, Adenosine and sleep deprivation promote NF-κB nuclear translocation in cholinergic basal forebrain, Journal of Neurochemistry 100 (5) (2007) 1351–1363.
[71] C.H. Leenaars, S.A. Savelyev, S. Van der Mierden, R.N. Joosten, M. Dematteis, T. Porkka-Heiskanen, et al., Intracerebral adenosine during sleep deprivation: a meta-analysis and new experimental data, Journal of Circadian Rhythms 16 (2018) 11, https://doi.org/10.5334/jcr.171.
[72] T. Gallopin, P.H. Luppi, B. Cauli, Y. Urade, J. Rossier, O. Hayaishi, et al., The endogenous somnogen adenosine excites a subset of sleep-promoting neurons via A2A receptors in the ventrolateral preoptic nucleus, Neuroscience 134 (4) (2005) 1377–1390.

[73] S. Mahon, N. Vautrelle, L. Pezard, S.J. Slaght, J.M. Deniau, G. Chouvet, et al., Distinct patterns of striatal medium spiny neuron activity during the natural sleep–wake cycle, The Journal of Neuroscience 26 (48) (2006) 12587–12595.
[74] K. Azdad, D. Gall, A.S. Woods, C. Ledent, S. Ferré, S.N. Schiffmann, Dopamine D2 and adenosine A2A receptors regulate NMDA-mediated excitation in accumbens neurons through A2A–D2 receptor heteromerization, Neuropsychopharmacology 34 (4) (2009) 972–986.
[75] W. Xu, F. de Carvalho, A. Jackson, Sequential neural activity in primary motor cortex during sleep, The Journal of Neuroscience 39 (19) (2019) 3698–3712.
[76] H. Mestre, L.M. Hablitz, A.L. Xavier, W. Feng, W. Zou, T. Pu, et al., Aquaporin-4-dependent glymphatic solute transport in the rodent brain, eLife 7 (2018) e40070.
[77] Z.L. Huang, Z. Zhang, W.M. Qu, Roles of Adenosine and Its Receptors in Sleep–Wake Regulation, International Review of Neurobiology, vol. 119, Elsevier, 2014, pp. 349–371.
[78] T.E. Bjorness, N. Dale, G. Mettlach, A. Sonneborn, B. Sahin, A.A. Fienberg, et al., An adenosine-mediated glial-neuronal circuit for homeostatic sleep, The Journal of Neuroscience 36 (13) (2016) 3709–3721.
[79] R. Allada, C. Cirelli, A. Sehgal, Molecular mechanisms of sleep homeostasis in flies and mammals, Cold Spring Harbor Perspectives in Biology (2017), 9(8):a027730.
[80] K. Koh, W.J. Joiner, M.N. Wu, Z. Yue, C.J. Smith, A. Sehgal, Identification of SLEEPLESS, a sleep-promoting factor, Science 321 (5887) (2008) 372–376.
[81] M. Wu, J.E. Robinson, W.J. Joiner, SLEEPLESS is a bifunctional regulator of excitability and cholinergic synaptic transmission, Current Biology 24 (6) (2014) 621–629.
[82] K. Yoshida, S. Shi, M. Ukai-Tadenuma, H. Fujishima, Ri Ohno, H.R. Ueda, Leak potassium channels regulate sleep duration, Proceedings of the National Academy of Sciences of the United States of America 115 (40) (2018) E9459–E9468.
[83] F. Tatsuki, G.A. Sunagawa, S. Shi, E.A. Susaki, H. Yukinaga, D. Perrin, et al., Involvement of Ca2+-dependent hyperpolarization in sleep duration in mammals, Neuron 90 (1) (2016) 70–85.
[84] Y. Li, J. Xu, Y. Xu, X.Y. Zhao, Y. Liu, J. Wang, et al., Regulatory effect of general anesthetics on activity of potassium channels, Neuroscience Bulletin (2018) 1–14.
[85] R. Huber, M.F. Ghilardi, M. Massimini, F. Ferrarelli, B.A. Riedner, M.J. Peterson, et al., Arm immobilization causes cortical plastic changes and locally decreases sleep slow wave activity, Nature Neuroscience 9 (9) (2006) 1169.
[86] Y.E.S. Ju, S.J. Ooms, C. Sutphen, S.L. Macauley, M.A. Zangrilli, G. Jerome, et al., Slow wave sleep disruption increases cerebrospinal fluid amyloid-β levels, Brain 140 (8) (2017) 2104–2111.
[87] S. Majumdar, B. Mallick, Cytomorphometric changes in rat brain neurons after rapid eye movement sleep deprivation, Neuroscience 135 (3) (2005) 679–690.
[88] A. Ranjan, S. Biswas, B.N. Mallick, Cytomorphometric changes in the dorsal raphe neurons after rapid eye movement sleep deprivation are mediated by noradrenalin in rats, Behavioral and Brain Functions 6 (1) (2010) 62.
[89] Y. Goll, G. Atlan, A. Citri, Attention: the claustrum, Trends Neuroscis 38 (8) (2015) 486–495.
[90] P.H. Luppi, F. Billwiller, P. Fort, Selective activation of a few limbic structures during paradoxical (REM) sleep by the claustrum and the supramammillary nucleus: evidence and function, Current Opinion in Neurobiology 44 (2017) 59–64.
[91] P.H. Luppi, C. Peyron, P. Fort, Not a single but multiple populations of GABAergic neurons control sleep, Sleep Medicine Reviews 32 (2017) 85–94.
[92] C. Blanco-Centurion, S. Luo, D.J. Spergel, A. Vidal-Ortiz, S. Oprisen, A.N. Van den Pol, et al., Dynamic network activation of hypothalamic MCH neurons in REM sleep and exploratory behavior, The Journal of Neuroscience 39 (25) (2019) 4986–4998.
[93] L. Alhassen, A. Phan, W. Alhassen, P. Nguyen, A. Lo, H. Shaharuddin, et al., The role of olfaction in MCH-regulated spontaneous maternal responses, Brain Research (2019).

[94] J.M. Monti, S.R. Pandi-Perumal, P. Torterolo, The effects of melanin-concentrating hormone on neurotransmitter systems involved in the generation and maintenance of wakefulness, in: Melanin-Concentrating Hormone and Sleep, Springer, 2018, pp. 109–120.
[95] J.A. González, P. Iordanidou, M. Strom, A. Adamantidis, D. Burdakov, Awake dynamics and brain-wide direct inputs of hypothalamic MCH and orexin networks, Nature Communications (2016) 7:10.1038/ncomms11395.
[96] R. Vetrivelan, D. Kong, L.L. Ferrari, E. Arrigoni, J.C. Madara, S.S. Bandaru, et al., Melanin-concentrating hormone neurons specifically promote rapid eye movement sleep in mice, Neuroscience 336 (2016) 102–113.
[97] G. Buzsáki, Hippocampal sharp wave-ripple: a cognitive biomarker for episodic memory and planning, Hippocampus 25 (10) (2015) 1073–1188.
[98] S.G. Ji, Y.V. Medvedeva, H.L. Wang, H.Z. Yin, J.H. Weiss, Mitochondrial Zn2+ accumulation: a potential trigger of hippocampal ischemic injury, The Neuroscientist 25 (2) (2019) 126–138.
[99] A.S. Gupta, M.A. van der Meer, D.S. Touretzky, A.D. Redish, Hippocampal replay is not a simple function of experience, Neuron 65 (5) (2010) 695–705.
[100] D.K. Roumis, L.M. Frank, Hippocampal sharp-wave ripples in waking and sleeping states, Current Opinion in Neurobiology 35 (2015) 6–12.
[101] C. Koch, The Quest for Consciousness: A Neuroscientific Approach, Roberts & Co, 2004.
[102] S. Dehaene, Consciousness and the Brain: Deciphering How the Brain Codes Our Thoughts, Penguin, 2014.
[103] A. Craig, How do You Feel?: an Interoceptive Moment with Your Neurobiological Self, Princeton University Press, 2014.
[104] A. Sahoo, K.A. Josephs, A neuropsychiatric analysis of the Cotard delusion, The Journal of Neuropsychiatry and Clinical Neurosciences 30 (1) (2017) 58–65.
[105] F. Siclari, G. Tononi, Sleep and dreaming, in: The Neurology of Conciousness, Elsevier, 2016, pp. 107–128.
[106] Nichols DE. Psychedelics, Pharmacological Reviews 68 (2) (2016) 264–355.
[107] M. Schredl, Researching Dreams: The Fundamentals, Springer, 2018.
[108] E. Perry, M. Walker, J. Grace, R. Perry, Acetylcholine in mind: a neurotransmitter correlate of consciousness?, Trends in Neurosciences 22 (6) (1999) 273–280.
[109] C. Koch, M. Massimini, M. Boly, G. Tononi, Neural correlates of consciousness: progress and problems, Nature Reviews. Neuroscience 17 (5) (2016) 307.
[110] K.C. Fox, S. Nijeboer, E. Solomonova, G.W. Domhoff, K. Christoff, Dreaming as mind wandering: evidence from functional neuroimaging and first-person content reports, Frontiers in Human Neuroscience 7 (2013) 412, https://doi.org/10.3389/fnhum.2013.00412.
[111] L.D. Lewis, V.S. Weiner, E.A. Mukamel, J.A. Donoghue, E.N. Eskandar, J.R. Madsen, et al., Rapid fragmentation of neuronal networks at the onset of propofol-induced unconsciousness, Proceedings of the National Academy of Sciences of the United States of America 109 (49) (2012) E3377–E3386.
[112] G. Tononi, C. Cirelli, Sleep and the price of plasticity: from synaptic and cellular homeostasis to memory consolidation and integration, Neuron 81 (1) (2014) 12–34.
[113] M.G. Frank, R. Cantera, Sleep, clocks, and synaptic plasticity, Trends Neuroscis 37 (9) (2014) 491–501.
[114] I. Timofeev, S. Chauvette, Sleep slow oscillation and plasticity, Current Opinion in Neurobiology 44 (2017) 116–126.
[115] S. Chauvette, J. Seigneur, I. Timofeev, Sleep oscillations in the thalamocortical system induce long-term neuronal plasticity, Neuron 75 (6) (2012) 1105–1113.
[116] G.B. Feld, J. Born, Sculpting memory during sleep: concurrent consolidation and forgetting, Current Opinion in Neurobiology 44 (2017) 20–27.
[117] G.H. Diering, R.S. Nirujogi, R.H. Roth, P.F. Worley, A. Pandey, R.L. Huganir, Homer1a drives homeostatic scaling-down of excitatory synapses during sleep, Science 355 (6324) (2017) 511–515.

[118] L. De Vivo, M. Bellesi, W. Marshall, E.A. Bushong, M.H. Ellisman, G. Tononi, et al., Ultrastructural evidence for synaptic scaling across the wake/sleep cycle, Science 355 (6324) (2017) 507–510.
[119] F. Lanté, J.C. Toledo-Salas, T. Ondrejcak, M.J. Rowan, D. Ulrich, Removal of synaptic Ca2+-permeable AMPA receptors during sleep, The Journal of Neuroscience 31 (11) (2011) 3953–3961.
[120] B.C. Clawson, J. Durkin, A.K. Suresh, E.J. Pickup, C.G. Broussard, S.J. Aton, Sleep promotes, and sleep loss inhibits, selective changes in firing rate, response properties and functional connectivity of primary visual cortex neurons, Frontiers in Systems Neuroscience 12 (2018), https://doi.org/10.3389/fnsys.2018.00040.
[121] W. Li, L. Ma, G. Yang, W.B. Gan, REM sleep selectively prunes and maintains new synapses in development and learning, Nature Neuroscience 20 (3) (2017) 427.
[122] G. Yang, C.S.W. Lai, J. Cichon, L. Ma, W. Li, W.B. Gan, Sleep promotes branch-specific formation of dendritic spines after learning, Science 344 (6188) (2014) 1173–1178.
[123] J. Durkin, S.J. Aton, Sleep-dependent potentiation in the visual system is at odds with the synaptic homeostasis hypothesis, Sleep 39 (1) (2016) 155–159.
[124] I.S. Stein, K. Zito, Dendritic spine elimination: molecular mechanisms and implications, The Neuroscientist 25 (1) (2019) 27–47.
[125] R. Evans, K. Blackwell, Calcium: amplitude, duration, or location?, Biological Bulletin 228 (1) (2015) 75–83.
[126] H. Park, Poo Mm, Neurotrophin regulation of neural circuit development and function, Nature Reviews. Neuroscience 14 (1) (2013) 7–23.
[127] E.J. Wamsley, Memory consolidation during waking rest, Trends in Cognitive Sciences 23 (2019) 171–173.
[128] N.P. Franks, General anaesthesia: from molecular targets to neuronal pathways of sleep and arousal, Nature Reviews. Neuroscience 9 (5) (2008) 370.
[129] H.C. Hemmings Jr., P.M. Riegelhaupt, M.B. Kelz, K. Solt, R.G. Eckenhoff, B.A. Orser, et al., Towards a comprehensive understanding of anesthetic mechanisms of action: a decade of discovery, Trends in Pharmacological Sciences 40 (7) (2019) 464–481.
[130] C.G. Abdallah, G. Sanacora, R.S. Duman, J.H. Krystal, The neurobiology of depression, ketamine and rapid-acting antidepressants: is it glutamate inhibition or activation?, Pharmacology & Therapeutics (2018) 148–158.
[131] T. Suzuki, K. Ueta, M. Sugimoto, I. Uchida, T. Mashimo, Nitrous oxide and xenon inhibit the human $(\alpha_7)_5$ 5 nicotinic acetylcholine receptor expressed in xenopus oocyte, Anesthesia and Analgesia 96 (2) (2003) 443–448.
[132] J. Westermann, T. Lange, J. Textor, J. Born, System consolidation during sleep–a common principle underlying psychological and immunological memory formation, Trends in Neurosciences 38 (10) (2015) 585–597.
[133] B.I. Somarajan, M.A. Khanday, B.N. Mallick, Rapid eye movement sleep deprivation induces neuronal apoptosis by noradrenaline acting on Alpha1 adrenoceptor and by triggering mitochondrial intrinsic pathway, Frontiers in Neurology 7 (2016) 25.
[134] A.C. Keene, E.R. Duboue, The origins and evolution of sleep, Journal of Experimental Biology 221 (11) (2018) jeb159533.
[135] C. Ma, P. Zhong, D. Liu, Z.K. Barger, L. Zhou, W.C. Chang, et al., Sleep regulation by neurotensinergic neurons in a thalamo-amygdala circuit, Neuron 17103 (2) (2019) 323–334.
[136] Y. Cherasse, Y. Urade, Dietary zinc acts as a sleep modulator, International Journal of Molecular Sciences 18 (11) (2017) 2334.

Index

H

I

K

L

M